"Drenda posted 'I a
Drenda, it was a ve
strong and courageous' was the beginning of a journey
Drenda's fight against cancer. It's a tale of terror, courage, friendship, support, love, faith, and family. 'I am strong and courageous' is proof that words mean something."

—Andi Pedersen Jordan, Friend and Former Co-worker

"At some point, one in eight women hears the terrible news: 'You have breast cancer.' Such news is never good, but it must be shared. Drenda's strength and courage have inspired everyone who knows her. I trust her story will inspire you, too."

—Honorable Lynn Peterson, Chair of Clackamas County Board of Commissioners

"Drenda Howatt has written a compelling story of what it's like to face a life-threatening illness. Her courage, her tenacity, and her strength are a testimony to all women who are breast cancer survivors. We can all learn from her example. This is a book all women need to share with their daughters and their friends."

—Honorable Martha Schrader, Oregon State Senator, District 20

"Drenda Howatt hasn't written 'just another book on cancer.' Instead, she lights the dark unknown path for anyone thrust into their own dreaded journey with this hated disease. Supported by her faith in God, a loving family, loyal friends, and the determination to be courageous, Howatt journals how living a 'normal life' one moment went to 'life with cancer' the next. Her honesty and courage answers the questions, 'What is it like?,' 'How can I get through this?' and 'Will life ever be normal again?' I highly recommend this to anyone facing cancer."

—Laura Wrede, National Women's Ministry Writer, Examiner.com

"Drenda Howatt has transparently combined personal notes from emails and social media to create a new kind of journal; one that allows family and friends to comment on your inner-most 'posts.' What emerges is a fascinating journey of hope through one of today's biggest battles. The love and encouragement of family and friends reaches beyond the page. Howatt's faith grows before the reader's eyes and transforms us with her brutal honesty and resolve."

—Kim Seeds de Blecourt, Author of A Willing Hostage

"As a cancer survivor myself, it has helped me tremendously reading Drenda's journey with breast cancer. Her strength, courage and ability to comprehend this disease is an inspiration to everyone."

—Mary Raethke, Friend and Co-worker

"Before the violent storms of life you must know that God is '100% for you.' He desires a personal relationship with you. The truth is... He cares, He never loses control, He is absolute goodness, and everything He does is motivated by His deep love for you. This is what sustained me through my own breast cancer, my sister's bone cancer, and my grand-daughter's leukemia. Don't get life and God mixed up. His precious presence in the 'eye of each storm' was His great gift to me. Nor will He ever leave you or forsake you, and He will go with you through every storm of life. We don't always know the 'why' of our storms but He does and that is enough!"

—Prof. Bonnie Kopp, Professor, Educational Ministries, Multnomah University

Strong & Courageous

A Survivor's Facebook Journey Through Breast Cancer

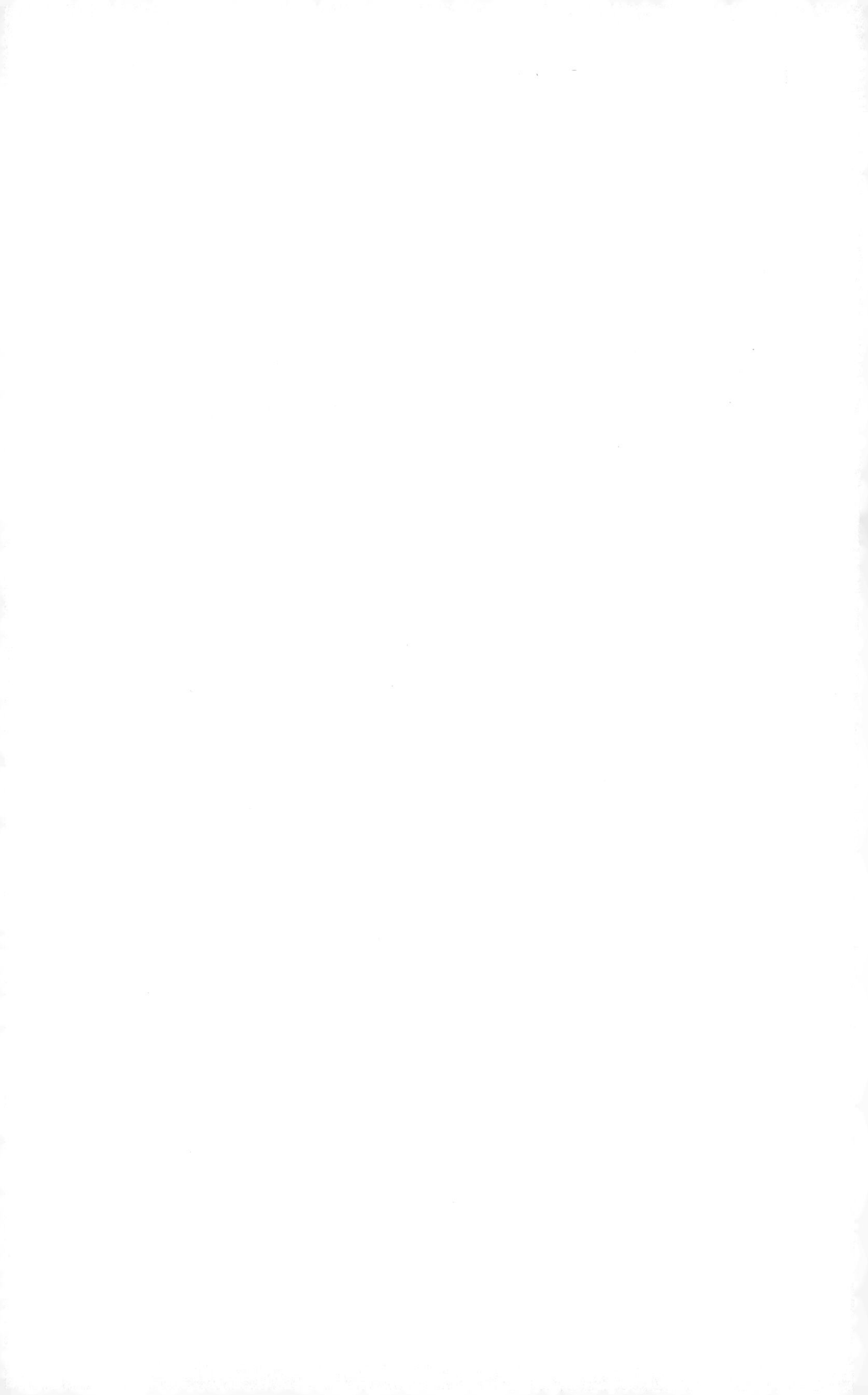

Strong & Courageous

A Survivor's Facebook Journey Through Breast Cancer

Drenda Lane Howatt

To Mary -
Thank you is not enough -
I appreciate your care +
support so much!
Drenda

Strong & Courageous: A Survivor's Facebook Journey Through Breast Cancer

Back cover photo by Kenneth Ulappa, Ponytail Photography, ponytailphotography.com

Front cover photo by Amber Lynn Montgomery Lane

Cover design by Faith Lichtenberg, LogoWorks.net

A portion of the proceeds from the sale of this book will be donated to Breast Friends. You can learn more about this organization online at www.breastfriends.com

To Don. Thank you for asking me
to be your wife. It is my honor.

To My Daughters. Anna, Rachel, and Ellie,
I am proud to be your Momma. Our experience
with breast cancer has made you even stronger
young women. Always remember where that strength
comes from. It does not come from cancer.
I love you.

Acknowledgments

How can I possibly thank each person who traveled alongside me through the fire of cancer? I know it is dangerous to start naming names – but I will do my best to have a comprehensive list.

First, my parents. Mom was not alive to be with me on this journey, but, with Dad, gave me lots of the 'ilities' that I used to keep moving forward. It is my hope that I have made them proud to be my parents.

My siblings and their families were a tremendous encouragement to me. Their constant care and love helped me keep afloat. They spurred me on to continued strength and courage.

Janette, Laurie, and Jory for taking the 'bad news' and meeting with Dad. I couldn't tell him. Thank you for loving us both enough to do the hard stuff.

Gilbert, Sally, Becky, Janis, Dad, Verta, Les, Nina, Dick, Cindy, and everyone who came to the hospital for my first surgery. Thank you for caring enough about my family to be with them through scary times.

Sally, Laurie, Scott, Becky, Linda, Janette, Wendy, Claire, Marilla, Sophie, and Ellie for planning, and prepping, the dinners that filled our freezer.

Becky, for the care packages and the chemo book. That book is a treasure that I will always cherish.

Sophie for the finger-knit scarf. I still wear it!

Claire, Sophie, Ellie and Zander. For the art in the 'chemo book'. It made me cry, but those were tears of joy over how I was loved.

Janette and Linda. You make me strong. To even consider going bald on my behalf is beyond my comprehension. To actually do it for me was amazing. You will never know how deeply your sacrifice touched me.

Thomas and Patrick. Thank you for shaving your heads…and for being present while my head was 'sheared'. You helped me laugh, and that kept me from sobbing.

Janis. Your immediate responsiveness to Don's call 'we think Drenda has cancer' meant so much. Your straightforward answers to our questions sharpened our focus and made us feel safer. Your willingness to look at all the medical paperwork gave much needed reassurance. "Thank you" is inadequate.

Les and Nina. You came home because we needed you.

Dad and Verta. You were among the first to encourage me to publish this chronicle. Thank you for your faith in me.

Dave and Cindy. Oh my goodness. How many times did you jump in your car just to come be with us? Your presence gave us moments of 'normal' and helped keep my panic away. Dave, thank you for being there for Don.

Shannon. Your ability to make me laugh, even in the midst of tears, speaks to our kindred spirits.

Kris and Abbi. The quilt, and the meals. Thank you.

Kate. The slippers. You are so sweet.

Karen. The tea. It helped to hold the cup of hot water and just smell the aroma. Thank you.

Ann Croze. Even in your own difficulties, you find time to send me a card and Papa Murphy's gift certificates. That was a huge gift. Thank you.

Tamara Anderson and Becky Coulson. Thank you for looking out for Ellie at PC. You have made a difference.

Cindy, Pam, and Shannon. You know I am always looking for a good excuse to go to Disneyland...

Kim and Kathy. Your emails and cards, and the incredible gift, helped me to keep going. Your friendship is precious.

Christina. You cared. You realized that Ellie was home alone with just her Momma and Daddy, and without her big sisters. You made her feel special and cared for. Thank you.

Evy and Maureen. Your experience with breast cancer, and survival, gave me hope. Your words of encouragement were heard – even through my sobbing.

Amber Lynn, Andi, Chelsea, Kristi, Caitlin, Barb, Danielle, Kathlin, Robin, Faith, Sherri, Amy, Abigale, Sally, Amanda, Susan, Denise, Erik, Laurie, Bethann, Zachary, Lori, Nancy, Karen, Lynn, Hollace, Elizabeth, Emily, Lindsay, Becky, Janette, Linda, Jessica, Abbi, Kris, Gail, Amy, Milt, Bobbi, Deanna, Cindy, Susan, Jennifer, Sandi, Kim, Shannon, Kortney, and everyone else who posted comments on my notes and wall. You were my facebook cheering squad. I don't think you could have known how much I drew from your comments. Oh, how I needed you!

Our Eastgate Church Family. Thank you for the cards, calls, meals and prayers. Knowing that I was being lifted up in prayer to our heavenly Father was the only thing that got me through some of the tough times.

Kaleb and Selah. Your sweet questions to me about how I was doing and your assurance that you were praying for me touched my heart.

My County work friends. Thank you for continuing to bolster me by telling me of my strength and courage. And your practical gift to me was a tremendous help and encouragement.

The Palm Spring Girl Friends. I have yet to meet even one of you…but your gift to me was more than the items in the huge basket. Thank you for reaching out to your UPS man and touching his family.

To all those who made a crane. 1001 beautiful testaments to the care and concern that others had for me. I don't know many of you, but your involvement in folding paper cheers me still. Thank you.

David Sanford. Thank you for sharing your expertise and encouraging me to finish this project.

Kelly and Kim. Thank you for using your 'eagle eyes' to read through this book.

Faith. Your willingness to lend your design expertise to Team Strong and Courageous was so kind. And then to design this book cover. You are amazing!

Erika Fitzpatrick. Thank you for your work preparing the manuscript for publication. Your attention to detail was a tremendous help!

Jerry. If I had it to do all over again, I would choose you for my doctor. You are amazing and I trust you and I feel safe knowing you're looking out for me.

My babies. Anna, Rachel, and Ellie. It was for you I kept on. What is a Mom going to do? She is going to take care of her babies, that's what. I am sad that I could not spare you the pain and terror, but you were oh so strong. My prayer for you is that, because of breast cancer, you know our Savior even more intimately and that you will rely on Him for all. I love you.

Don. Oh, Don. Words cannot express what you mean to me, or how I love you. Thank you for holding me up and pushing me forward. Thank you for loving me. I am a better person because I am your wife.

God the Almighty. Thank you for allowing me to have the experience of breast cancer so that I can claim the blessings that result. Thank you for speaking to me through Your Word. Thank you for the cross. Thank you for the empty tomb.

Preface

What follows is a journey. A journey that is relayed to you through my e-mails and Facebook postings. It is a normal life, interspersed with breast cancer. After I learned I had cancer, I used Facebook notes to update my family and friends on the status of my treatment. But before long, my notes changed from merely updates to more commentary on the things happening to me, and the people surrounding me. As hundreds of my friends can attest, it is an emotional 'read.' Believe me, it was an emotional 'write.'

I used the words "strong and courageous" in my Facebook status update on November 11, 2008 as I awaited my diagnosis. Not that I was 'strong and courageous' by any measurement. It was that I would be. I would be 'strong and courageous'...willing those traits to be present amid the terror.

Those words have taken on a life of their own. You'll read about where they came from (Joshua 1:9). Those dear family and friends that came alongside to support me used those same words to encourage me when I could not get up and go another moment. Team Strong and Courageous was 43 members strong at Walk for the Cure on September 20, 2009.

Strong and Courageous.

"Have I not commanded you? Be strong and courageous. Do not be terrified. Do not be discouraged. For the Lord your God is with you wherever you go." Joshua 1:9

Life is Normal

Drenda Lane Howatt is enjoying the scent of ham baking in the oven...and thinking about Christmas shopping.
November 2, 2008 at 3:55pm

Drenda Lane Howatt is glad to be staying home on this wet, dark night.
November 3, 2008 at 5:57pm

Drenda Lane Howatt is, once again, waiting for the man in brown to arrive to take her on the weekly date!
November 6, 2008 at 5:41pm

Drenda Lane Howatt is happy, so very very very happy, to have Miss Rachel home for the weekend.
November 7, 2008 at 9:16pm

Drenda Lane Howatt is trying to find the energy and courage to go to Costco.
November 8, 2008 at 2:07pm

Drenda Lane Howatt is getting ready to go to a dessert party with friends.
November 8, 2008 at 6:18pm

Terror

Saturday, November 8th. *After the dessert party, at home, in bed, I felt a burning, throbbing discomfort in my breast. I thought "that's weird..." and felt...a LUMP. Immediate terror. I had Don feel the lump. "Yes, it's a lump." He told me to stay calm, that it was probably nothing. I couldn't sleep. I got up and went into the bathroom to try and stifle my tears. I was so scared. And I KNEW.*

Sunday, November 9th. *Still terrified. Not much sleep the night before. We went to church, and it was hard to concentrate. I have never believed that God "gave" verses from Scripture to people...I believed that He gave the BIBLE. But that Sunday morning, God gave ME a verse. It was for me. Our church service always has a verse from Scripture to reflect on at our Communion Service. The verse is usually related to Christ's sacrifice on the cross. The verse this day was John 14:1.* ***"Do not let your heart be troubled. Trust in God. Trust also in Me."*** *I cried. I sat in the pew and cried. That verse was for me.*

Calm – Short-lived

Drenda Lane Howatt is calm again.
November 10, 2008 at 7:15pm

Monday, November 10th. After finally getting in to see the nurse practitioner, I was reassured by her calm assurance that the lump was most likely a fluid-filled cyst. But to be sure, a diagnostic mammogram and ultrasound scheduled for first thing the next morning.

> Andi Pedersen Jordan at 7:40pm November 10, 2008
> Implies that you weren't calm . . . and quick aren't I? ;-)
>
> Sally Park at 7:54pm November 10, 2008
> Me too...are our moons in the same orbit?

Concern

***N**ovember 11th. Veterans' Day. Diagnostic mammogram and ultrasound day. Radiologist "very concerned" after looking at the mammogram results. "Need to do a core biopsy". No words of reassurance. None. In fact, when the ultrasound tech saw my tears, she left the machine and came around to rub my shoulders in comfort. My thoughts amid my tears? "Oh shit."*

Strength
Courage

Drenda Lane Howatt is strong and courageous.
November 11, 2008 at 5:50pm

Strong and Courageous. These words just came to me that day. They are from Joshua 1:9. I remembered them from my study of the book of Joshua a few years ago. Strong and Courageous. Strong and Courageous. When I went back to read the passage again, I was struck with the other words. "Have I not commanded you? Be strong and courageous. DO NOT BE TERRIFIED. DO NOT BE DISCOURAGED. FOR THE LORD YOUR GOD IS WITH YOU WHEREVER YOU GO." Another verse for me. God was at work in my heart. I clung to this verse. I still do.

> Tom Turnbull at 5:56pm November 11, 2008
> You come from a good family!
>
> Drenda Lane Howatt at 5:56pm November 11, 2008
> Yes, even if I do say so myself! But strength can sometimes be hard to find.
>
> Sally Park at 6:51pm November 11, 2008
> We come from strong pioneers ~ no fluff. I believe strength is but a word for perseverance. I love you!

Waiting Waiting

Wednesday, November 12th…tried to work. Couldn't focus. Waiting, waiting, waiting for the test results. I left work early. Called the nurse practitioner in the early evening. She had no results, just a preliminary report. She said the radiologist was very concerned. "Drenda, make an appointment to see me late tomorrow afternoon; I should have the results by then. Oh – and, Drenda, bring your husband with you…"

Don made one phone call…to his sister, Janis. She is a physician and came over right away. Ellie had gone to bed unusually early that night. Janis was calm and reassuring. No false hope, but calm, matter-of-fact talking me through. "What have you told Ellie?" she asked. "Just that I found a lump in my breast, and that the doctor thought it was nothing…" "You have to tell her what is going on. You have to. Tell her that the doctor is concerned about the lump, and that you're going to go back tomorrow afternoon for the test results."

Life Turned Upside Down
The Long Long Day of November 13, 2008

November 13th...Don stayed home from work today. I told Ellie this morning that I needed to see the doctor in the afternoon to get the test results. She would go home from school with our friend Cindy, and Cindy would get Ellie to youth group.

My appointment was at 4:50...long day. We ran errands, and drove by Cindy's work to ask her if she could take Ellie in the afternoon. She knew about the mammogram earlier in the week, but not the lump. So I had to tell her...but not in her office surrounded by people. I asked her if we could go somewhere for a minute. We went into the teachers' lounge. I told her the reason I had the mammogram, and tried not to cry. She, of course, was wonderful. She already had plans, but would change them and would take Ellie. Such a true friend.

Drenda Lane Howatt is puttering around the house trying to stay busy. Shouldn't be hard, but it is!
November 13, 2008 at 9:41am

> Andi Pedersen Jordan at 10:37am November 13, 2008
> Shouldn't you be at work? :-)

"It IS cancer, Drenda."

Such awful words.

So many tears.

Terror so real and overwhelming that it cannot be described. I don't even remember what we did immediately after the doctor appointment. Came home? I just remember sitting in my bed crying. "Don! How did this happen?" "What am I going to do?" "We have to tell the girls." Don said he'd call Anna and Rachel, both away at college. "NO. I should call them. They have to hear from me."

I made three phone calls that night. I don't even remember if I called Anna or Rachel first. I had to ask them if they could go somewhere alone to talk to me…I didn't want them surrounded by people when they heard my words. They thought I was calling about Christmas lists. Those were the hardest phone calls I have ever had to make. I realized that I was about to shatter their worlds. Moms are not supposed to shatter worlds…they are supposed to hold worlds together.

Then I called my sister, Janette. Again, a terrible call to make. I asked her, too, if she could go somewhere away from her family to take my call. She thought it was a Christmas question. But, no, not Christmas. cancer. I don't remember my words to her...just my plea that she call the rest of my family. Especially Dad. I knew I could not talk to my Dad. I just could not tell him.

Then Don had to make a few calls. He called his parents who were out of town. His Mom wanted to talk to me, but I could not talk anymore. Too many tears. He asked them to come home early.

And then he called our friends, Dave and Cindy. Cindy came right over. More tears. And a few laughs.

From my sister, Sally:

On Nov 13, 2008, at 8:20 PM
Drenda and Don,
Lonnie and I will be in Tacoma on Saturday and if Rachel would like to come home we would be more that happy to swing up and bring her back with us. It would be close to 5 ish, after Calvin's game.
I can imagine this is a very stressful time for you, but I know that it's going to be okay. Just a bump in the road.
I know you aren't up to chatting, so just let me know via email, that's fine.
Love you very much.
Sally

Date: November 13, 2008 9:09:25 PM PST
Sally,

Thank you so much. Rachel does want to come home, but I want to wait until I know more about when the surgery will be. We are hoping to be able to get in to see the surgeon tomorrow, and I am really hoping I can have surgery next week. This waiting stuff is HARD. Yesterday I was so upset -- Janis prescribed tranquilizers for me, and as a result I was able to sleep. My understanding is that surgery first, and then chemo and/or radiation. I never thought this would be me. Lots of crying around here, I can tell you. I think we're in shock.

Don is on his way to pick up Ellie from youth group, and when she gets home, we'll tell her. I called Rachel and Anna tonight after we had the pathology report. Hardest phone calls a mom has to make, I think. Rachel is very upset and was sobbing.

Anna is taking it in slower, I think.

Can we let you know tomorrow evening about bringing Rachel home?

Thank you,
Drenda

Ellie came home from youth group. She came into our bedroom and sat on the bed. "Did you get the test results?" "Yes, Ellie", I said. "The doctor told me that the lump in my breast is a form of breast cancer. I'll have surgery next week to take it out." I don't remember the rest of the conversation, except for the last part. Don asked "Ellie, do you know what cancer is?" "Yes. It's the virus that kills people." "Oh, Sweetie! Cancer can kill people, but the doctor believes that mine has been discovered early and can be taken out with the surgery. If that changes, we will tell you. But it was found early, and that is a very good thing." I thought my heart would break at that moment. My baby, only 12 years old, and her world is crashing.

From my sister, Janette:
On Nov 13, 2008, at 9:53 PM:
Drenda and Don,

Between Laurie and I we have called the siblings. Tomorrow a.m. Laurie and I will go out and tell Dad.

Of course everyone wants to know what they can do. There are offers to go get Rachel if she would like to come home this weekend. Truly whatever you need we can cover.

Does Ellie need a place to hang out this weekend? And get extra hugs? I will try to call you tomorrow but don't want to bother you. We love you all very much.
Janette

Drenda Lane Howatt is going to try and sleep.
November 13, 2008 at 10:27pm

Drenda Lane Howatt is tired of the "what ifs" and wants to focus on the "I knows"...I know God is in control. I know He cares for me. I know He is at work in my life.
November 13, 2008 at 10:51pm

> Anna Howatt at 11:17pm November 13, 2008
> It'll be just fine...
>
> Sally Park at 5:23am November 14, 2008
> Atta girl!

Time to let my two dear, life-long friends know of the latest news:

To: "Kim Burns"
Cc: "Kathy Hopman"
Sent: Thursday, November 13, 2008 11:08 PM
Subject: my week

Dear Kim and Kathy,

I write with shocking news...I can't bring myself to make phone calls, so I must share the latest in my life via email. Please forgive me, but do understand that emotion is high at our house right now.

This week has been one of incredibly difficult and trying times for me. I was diagnosed with breast cancer today and will be facing surgery in the next week or so.

I am struggling to follow the scripture in John 14:1 where Jesus says, "Do not let your heart be troubled. Trust in God and trust also in Me." But, my heart is troubled. I would appreciate your prayers -- prayers for peace of heart, prayers for the peace of my family, prayers for healing, and prayers that I will be a true and faithful witness to God's unfailing love and grace.

Please pray especially for Don, Anna, Rachel, and Ellie that they will not be overcome with fear. We are all still reeling from the news, but knowing the outcome of the testing is better than the waiting wondering.

I am hoping to be able to see the surgeon tomorrow and will know more once I have met with him. My understanding is that surgery will be followed by chemo and/or radiation. As far as I know, only my right breast is involved. We do not know the extent of the cancer, and most probably will not until surgery. The initial reports indicate that it has not mestastized and that it looks like it is still contained in the breast. We are of course hopeful that the cancer has not spread into the lymph nodes. I will let you know when I know more.

Thank you for your friendship and prayers.
Drenda

Cancer Day 2

From my friend Shannon:

On Nov 14, 2008, at 1:02 AM, Swope wrote:
Hello friend,

Well, I'm up and about after having tossed and turned…thinking of you and just saw your note.

I am so sorry dear friend that you have been diagnosed with breast cancer! Wow, and it will be a long haul...my prayer has been that you and Don will remain strong in your walk through this, that God will be proud of you both and that somehow it will reflect greatly of His glory.

My heart is saddened by all that you face...I truly wish that you didn't have to go through any of it at all but I also know without a doubt that God did allow this to happen in your life because He does know the bigger picture and He obviously knows you're up to the task.

I'm sorry my dear friend that you will have some really lousy times ahead...some good times too of course...I want you to know WHATEVER you may need help with just let me know. Of course your thoughts are on your sweet girls and Don. I have been praying for them...just a 'normal' day turned all topsy-turvy….one never knows. I've shed many a tear the past couple of days….all on your behalf but I also have such faith in our Lord and Jesus Christ and aim to be His faithful servant. I have much hope too and will be one of your strongest encouragers and advocates along the way….So, my dear here we go on another adventure....this one's not so funny.....but I'm glad to be by your side.

I wish I could come and lay my eyes on you and give you a good hug...but...having the 'camp board' retreat this weekend...so, alas I can't. I've made all the food up ahead and AR actually has to get it out to them on Saturday because I have a clinical all day....I'll fumble through starting IV's, foley catheters, chest tubes etc. etc. all the usual 'nursey' hands on stuff.... sounds like so much fun huh?....Ok, I'm rambling....just wanted to talk with you a bit....

I'm not sure what your next week looks like but my ONLY plans are studying and I can do that anywhere. So, if you end up having surgery and Don would like to work some of the days....I'd be happy to hang out with you during the day...pick up Ellie.... or whatever....just say the word

Later,

S

From: drenda-howatt@comcast.net
Date: November 14, 2008 9:35:27 AM PST
To: Shannon Swope

Thank you. I do ok as long as I am on the sedatives Janis gave me. When the medicine wears off, the panic rises, literally, from my toes to my throat.

Telling the girls last night was the hardest thing I've ever done. Don offered, but I thought it was important they hear my voice. Rachel is taking it VERY hard. Ellie had questions that we answered. I even had her feel the lump. She slept in our bedroom last night, sweet girl. She said, "don't people die from cancer?" "Yes, but most people do not."

Don called his parents, and has asked his Mom to come home early. I need a Mom right now.

I just found out that I won't be able to see the surgeon until Wednesday - with a slight possibility of Monday opening up. That is a disappointment as I was hopeful of getting in today. Unfortunately, he is in surgery all day today. Perhaps I could just go to Providence and wait outside the surgery area and catch him there? Janis has been wonderful and offered to go with us to the surgeon if we wanted.

After I had called the surgeon's office, my nurse practitioner called. She, too, had called the surgeon's office and was told I'd already called. She spent 30 minutes on the phone with me trying to calm my tears. "Drenda, it's only a few days. You have to wait your turn…it will be ok."

What? A few days? Only? Are you kidding. I wanted the cancer out…NOW. Second opinion? I DON"T CARE. Take it out!

Drenda Lane Howatt thinks the surgeon should have saved time to see her today.
November 14, 2008 at 9:49am

> Andi Pedersen Jordan at 10:57am November 14, 2008
> ??? Everything a-ok?

Date: November 14, 2008 12:56:49 PM PST
To: My Family (siblings)
Hi all,
Just a quick note to thank you for all of your notes and concern. I am doing ok...but with the help of sedatives. When the medicine wears off, the panic tide rises. I know you all probably want to call, but right now, I'd prefer to have fewer phone conversations. Thank you for understanding.

We just returned from seeing the surgeon. The fact that we got in today was in itself a little miracle. He had nothing open until next Wednesday, but in between his surgeries, his office told him about me (and my upset) and he came back to the office in between surgeries to see me. I am scheduled for an MRI on Monday (to check my left breast again just to be sure), and surgery at Providence Portland on Tuesday at 2 p.m. If all goes well, I'll be home Tuesday night.

The current plan is to do a lumpectomy and take a few lymph nodes to check for the presence of the cancer. If circumstances warrant, a full mastectomy of the right breast will be performed. My cancer is infiltrating ductal carcinoma (invasive -- it has breached the wall of the ducts) and also in situ ductal carcinoma (not yet breached the walls). A little bit confusing, I must say.

Don's parents are coming home early from Maui and are scheduled to arrive around midnight on Monday night.

At this point, I don't know what we need, or if we need anything. I feel fine everywhere except my heart! Rachel is not yet sure if she wants to come home for the surgery or stay in Seattle. At this point, I think Ellie has decided to be at the hospital for the surgery -- we've left the choice to her and told her either way is fine. She thinks it odd that I might have my breast "amputated". She has had questions ("don't people die from cancer?" "Yes, sometimes, but it looks like they found my cancer early and can take it out in surgery", etc.) Anna was not scheduled to come home for Thanksgiving, but I am thinking we'll throw lots of $$ at the airline and get her home anyway. Good to be all together for a few days.

Janette, if you'd make sure Dad is up to date, I would really appreciate it. It is still very difficult to talk about what is happening, and I am getting quite tired of crying all the time.

I am so very relieved to have the surgery scheduled and to know that there is a plan in place to take care of the cancer. Of course, this will be a loooong haul, and follow-up treatments will ensue, but at least we're on the way to eradication and recovery. Thank you all for your kind notes and thoughts. Keep praying!

Drenda

The surgeon asked me if, during surgery it was determined that I needed a mastectomy, what did I want done? "Some women want to know what they are going to wake up to…and then have a second surgery to remove the breast." Me? Take it off. I want the cancer out. Do what you need to do, Dr.

When he told me that I may end up later having my ovaries removed (depending on the type of cancer), I asked him if he could just take the ovaries out while I was on the operating table for the tumor. "Uh, Mrs. Howatt, uh, NO. That wouldn't be a good idea." "Well, I was just thinking, no sense having another surgery if you could take care of it all at once…" Silly me.

From: Laurie Lane
Subject: Re:
Date: November 14, 2008 1:05:05 PM PST
To: Drenda
Cc: The siblings

Drenda,
Thank you for keeping all of us up to date on what's happening. I trust that you will continue to be direct and let us know what you need and don't need. You are one awesome person!

I love you and am thinking of you!!

Oh, Janette offered to shave her head if I told Dad this morning.... I told Dad so she needs to follow through on her end of the bargain....

Laurie

Drenda Lane Howatt is thankful for change of events that allowed her to see the surgeon this morning!
November 14, 2008 at 12:57pm

> Amber Lynn Montgomery Lane at 1:13pm November 14, 2008
> Wonderful. We're waiting to hear details, and of course prayers are constant.
>
> Rachel Howatt at 1:22pm November 14, 2008
> Psalms 103:1-3
> Praise the LORD, O my soul; all my inmost being, praise his holy name. Praise the LORD, O my soul, and forget not all his benefits — who forgives all your sins and heals all your diseases

On Nov 14, 2008, at 10:44 AM, David Sanford wrote:
Dear Drenda,
Please keep me posted so I can keep you in my prayers during the days ahead. Thankfully, we live at a time when recovery from breast cancer is so high. Still, the prospects of facing surgery and then chemo and/or radiation are not pleasant. The past few months Renée and I have been walking through this with a dear family friend at SMBC who is about your age and has three children. May I share this with Renée so she can join me in praying for you? In John 14:1, we might understand Jesus saying, in effect, "Do not let your heart *continue to* be troubled. Trust in God and trust also in me." Trouble has come, but God will never leave you or forsake you. Knowing He is with us every moment is so important. We love you, Drenda, and earnestly pray that "the God of all comfort" (2 Cor. 1:3) will be your comfort, solace, encouragement, joy, strength, and peace. With your permission, I'd like to ask everyone at SMBC to join us in praying for you. Would that be okay?

David

From: Drenda Howatt
Subject: Re: Praying for you...
Date: November 14, 2008 1:10:04 PM PST
To: David Sanford, Arden Trautman, Gilbert Gleason

Thank you for your encouragements and prayers. We have chosen, consciously, to not be secretive about my condition or diagnosis, so please feel free to share with your prayer partners.

I did experience a miracle this morning. The surgeon had no openings to see me until Wednesday, and he is in surgery all day today. In between surgeries, he called his office, who informed him about me (and my upset about not being able to get in to see him), and he came back to the office in between surgeries just for me! I was so very happy! Don's sister, Janis (a physician) accompanied us to see the surgeon, which was a great help. Long story short, I will have an MRI on Monday to check the unaffected breast to be sure it is clear, and then surgery at 2 p.m. on Tuesday at Providence Portland. The plan is for a lumpectomy and removal of a few lymph nodes to check for the presence of cancer. If circumstances warrant, a full mastectomy may be done. If it is just the lumpectomy/lymph-nodes, I'll probably be back at home Tuesday night. I am so thankful to have a plan in place.

The cancer is infiltrating ductal carcinoma, meaning it has breached the walls of the ducts, and also in situ ductal carcinoma, which hasn't yet breached the walls. Hopefully, the breaches are minor and close.

We all take our lives, and our schedules for granted. Since finding the lump on Saturday, everything about my world has been shaken and turned upside down...but I am focusing on what I KNOW to be true about our God.

Drenda

Drenda Lane Howatt can't wait for Tuesday at 2 p.m. God Bless surgeons.
November 14, 2008 at 1:43pm

Andi Pedersen Jordan at 3:04pm November 14, 2008
All will be well!!

Abigale Mary Lane at 5:30pm November 14, 2008
Brian and I are thinking of you! Forester too!

Rachel had just begun her freshman year at Seattle Pacific University.

Rachel's Note:
Request for Prayer

Friday, November 14, 2008 at 11:45pm

Hey guys -
I didn't know how to let everyone of you know about the situation my family is currently in. I've seriously started typing mass emails, but it's just too overwhelming. So I'm telling you via Facebook note, because it's quick, simple, and easy access. If you've heard the story before from me through Facebook messages or chat, then sorry... I am guilty of cutting and pasting on this one.

Last night my mom called me with some scary news. She wanted me to go somewhere private so she could tell me what it was.

On Saturday night she found a lump in her breast...
Monday she went in for a mammogram and last night, Thursday, she got the results back.

It's cancer, you guys. My mom has breast cancer. Please, please, please. Pray.

I am really really scared right now. I'm not mad at God, this isn't causing me to doubt Him. I trust Him, but I am still worried about what His plans are and how they may differ from mine and what I want His plans for my family to be.

My mom has to get surgery to get the lump out and to make sure that's all there is, so it's part exploratory. After that she'll most likely go through chemo/radiation just as a precaution. The doctors are confident because they've caught it at an early stage. But, cancer is cancer, and cancer is bad.

Her surgery is scheduled for this Tuesday at 2 P.M. I'm going to head home to Portland on Monday morning, after my USEM and after I take a Spanish quiz, and then come back to Seattle sometime on Wednesday. We're going to try and get me scheduled for a mammogram too - just to make sure everything is ok with me.

Please be praying. This isn't to be kept under wraps, obviously, I'm writing a Facebook note, aren't I? As far as I'm concerned, the more people that know = the more people who are praying.

I have been so encouraged and felt so blessed. I have been showered in prayer. I can't tell you how much love I feel for myself and for my family right now. Tonight a ton of girls packed into my room while I told them what was going on (we organized a "floor meeting" because I wanted people praying and I hated telling people individually over and over and over). They prayed and cried with me. Hugged and comforted me. God is so good.

Feel free to talk to me about this you guys. Tell me what you're feeling - it's ok. I would much rather you get in touch with me - ask me questions, give me advice, if you have something you think would be encouraging - say it! Talking about it is my therapy.

And remember to pray. I think we've forgotten how powerful our God is - how powerful praying in His name can be. Brad was healed from scoliosis last week at a prayer meeting. They put their hands on his back, prayed over him, and they *felt* his spine realign. HELLO. Prayer is powerful. God is capable of doing IMMEASURABLY more than all we ask or imagine. Pray in faith - believing that God will come to the rescue. That's what I'm striving to do right now.

And we know that all things work together for the good of

those who love Him, who have been called according to His purpose.
Romans 8:28

We'll be talking, then.
Love you guys.

Cancer Day 3

Drenda Lane Howatt is going to attempt to have a normal day. IKEA anyone?
November 15, 2008 at 7:52am

> Cindy McElmurry at 8:39am November 15, 2008
> I was thinking of going myself. Would you like company?

Drenda Lane Howatt forgot how exhausting it is to shop at IKEA. oh my goodness.
November 15, 2008 at 3:43pm

> Karen Buehrig at 4:33pm November 15, 2008
> IKEA has some sort of energy vacumn installed. I never cease to be amazed at the expereince of that store. Even when I go in knowing what I am looking for, it takes at leaset an hour and I end up getting lost in the maze. Did you buy anything interesting?
>
> Drenda Lane Howatt at 8:48pm November 15, 2008
> Just candles for my fireplace and a few Christmas items...

Drenda Lane Howatt is going to try and get some deep, restful sleep. Please.
November 15, 2008 at 9:07pm

> Sally Park at 9:28pm November 15, 2008
> Sweet dreams

Drenda Lane Howatt is, to use Miss Rachel's words, scared but not worried. Make sense? No? Message me and I'll explain!
November 16, 2008 at 3:58pm

Breast Cancer...

Sunday, November 16, 2008 at 4:32pm

...is the pits. I found a lump in my right breast last week and after waiting an agonizing 4 days, received the diagnosis of cancer on Thursday evening. I am scheduled for an MRI tomorrow to make sure the cancer is really only in my right breast, and then surgery on Tuesday afternoon. It seems the cancer was found early, as the tumor is estimated to be 1.5 cm. We'll know more about the extent and stage of the cancer after surgery. So, yes, I am scared. I am tired of crying. I am tired. But, I am not worried anymore. I am not worried because I know God is in control, and I rest in His hands. I know He is able to heal me, and I know that He is able to take care of my family. "blessed be the God and Father of our Lord Jesus Christ, the Father of mercies and God of all comfort, who comforts us in all our affliction..." He comforts me.

Janelle Flanagan: Drenda, I will keep you and your family in my prayers. I am sorry to hear that you have had such difficult news, however, your words are encouraging and very true...God is able...
November 16, 2008 at 6:08pm

Rachel Howatt: Praise Jesus!
November 17, 2008 at 1:54am

Amy Hickman: Drenda, I am so very sorry to hear this...I know you have some dark days ahead of you, but I praise the Lord that you are finding comfort and peace in Him. I will pray that God's peace, comfort and hope will surround you and your family during this time. I will surely be praying for you. Would you mind if I passed on this prayer request to the body at

Westside? Keep us posted...

God is our refuge and strength,
a very present help in trouble.
Therefore we will not fear though the earth gives way,
though the mountains be moved into the heart of the sea...
...be still and know that I am God.

Psalm 46:1,2,10
November 17, 2008 at 10:12am

Elizabeth Lundquist Calhoun: Dear Drenda - I am so very sorry to hear your news. You can count on me and my family for our prayers. Please keep us all posted as things progress. He is more than able!
November 17, 2008 at 4:52pm

The Treatment Odyssey Begins

Drenda Lane Howatt is leaving to go have an MRI. And, she will NOT be claustrophobic.
November 17, 2008 at 10:38am

> Amber Lynn Montgomery Lane at 10:50am November 17, 2008
> My best wishes for you. If there's something to find, I hope they find it thoroughly. But of course, the best hope is a clean bill on this one. Love you!
>
> Isaac Lane Koval at 10:54am November 17, 2008
> You're in my thoughts Drenda. I'm sending love your way!

Drenda Lane Howatt had her MRI and all in all, it was a pleasant experience.
November 17, 2008 at 3:44pm

> Andi Pedersen Jordan at 3:54pm November 17, 2008
> Whew!
>
> Robin Reilly at 5:25pm November 17, 2008
> Cool!

Drenda Lane Howatt is going to relax and watch Dancing with the Stars. Oh yeah.
November 17, 2008 at 8:01pm

Breast cancer, Part II

Tuesday, November 18, 2008 at 8:06pm

I am home from the hospital!

Yesterday's MRI apparently showed my left breast is a.o.k. whew. This morning, a phone call from the hospital to come earlier than planned so that they could do more stuff to me. So I got through the insertion of two "guide" wires into my breast - not fun, but hey, who cares. The wires were to help guide the surgeon, one wire at the front of the cancer, one wire at the back. The wires were about 7 inches long sticking out of my breast. Blue dye inserted into the cancer to stain the tissue. Radioactive something injected to find the sentinel lymph-node. a bit early to surgery (amazing -- and a wonderful thing). Making the anesthesiologist stop in the hallway as he wheeled me to surgery..."I didn't get to say goodbye to Ellie, just Rachel. Get Ellie". So the Dr. left me in the hall, went back to the waiting room -- "she wants to see Ellie". Ellie came to the hall, and I can't remember what I said! Hopefully, I told her I loved her.

In the recovery room after surgery, I was ECSTATIC to hear that two pathologists and the surgeon believe the entire cancer was removed, and the lymphnode was negative for cancer. PRAISE GOD. That is the prelim report, final pathology report due on Friday. If they do find more cancer cells (not uncommon), I will probably have a mastectomy at that point (if I understand correctly what Don told me). And let me add just a quick note about my most wonderful husband. Don has been a rock for me. He has been my helpmate and my best friend. I love you, Donald Kent Howatt!

The outcome of the surgery is the best possible, as far as we know without the final pathology report. I am so thankful. So thankful.

Thank you, each one of you, who have offered such tremendous encouragement and support over these last few days. Just a few days, but also a lifetime. The journey is not over, but I do believe a major step is behind me.

Hug your family tonight and tell each one how much you love them.
Drenda

Andi Pedersen Jordan: YIPEEEE!!!! Been thinking about you all day . . . and boy did the day drag!
I finally sent Anna a note to ask if she had any news. Thanks, Anna!
November 18, 2008 at 8:27pm

Zachary Lane Koval: =D
So wonderful to hear!!!!!
November 18, 2008 at 8:43pm

Amber Lynn Montgomery Lane: BIG sigh, and halleluia! So glad to hear things went so well. May the future continue to be so full of rich blessings.
November 18, 2008 at 9:15pm

Marilla Park: =) I am really happy everything went smoothly!!
November 18, 2008 at 9:22pm

Sally Park: Oh my goodness! As Don relayed the news from the surgeon I blurted out "that's fabulous!" Felt kinda oinky cause...I just did.
But I was ecstatic and excited and relieved and the best of the best was reality!
Do you realize the fabulous family you have gathered about you?

Your husband and daughters are treasures!
November 18, 2008 at 9:31pm

Amy Hickman: Praise to our gracious God that things went as well as could be hoped! Thank you for the update. Your comment about Ellie was so sweet it made me tear up. =)
I will keep praying for you, Drenda, and will anticipate any more news you will have. God is faithful!
November 18, 2008 at 10:02pm

Rachel Howatt: I love you, Mom!
November 18, 2008 at 10:07pm

Anna Howatt: This was so good to hear!
November 19, 2008 at 12:10am

Kristi Smith: Drenda, that's great that they think they removed all the cancer and that it hadn't metastasized into the lymph system! I'm praying that the pathology reports confirm the optimism of the Drs.
November 19, 2008 at 3:31am

Karen Buehrig: Drenda~
Of course words cannot explain how relieved we are. I was thinking of you yesterday during the AOC conference. The conference was a good experience and you definately should go next year.

As you said, the journey is not over. Hopefully you will be able to rest and recover, taking your time to heal. We have got things totally covered here at the office. Lynn and I came up with a good plan for staff assistant coverage while you are healing and for the wild and crazy transition that will happen next year.

Today is a good day to snuggle up in bed and rest rest rest!

Karen

November 19, 2008 at 8:08am

Kris Howatt: I was glad to hear how well things went. Anything you need, let me know
November 19, 2008 at 2:08pm

Drenda Lane Howatt is happy happy to have surgery behind her and healing in front of her.
November 19, 2008 at 6:44am

Note from Rachel:

Breast Cancer: Post Surgery

Wednesday, November 19, 2008 at 10:25am

Surgery is over and mom is doing well. We are blessed.

It was a scary thing, this surgery. Waiting in the main lobby of Providence for 3+ hours was frustrating - but I enjoy hospitals. They're fascinating. People, we're broken - all of us. We're brrrrrroken, so, naturally, hospitals are fascinating. Broken people getting fixed is a wonderful thing.

We went and saw my mom before she went in. I was crying when she was being wheeled away for surgery - it's an unnerving thing to see your mother lying on a gurney.

Then we waited.

And waited.

Yeah, still waiting.

I played musical chairs, sitting with people from my church, with Aunt Becky and Aunt Sally, with Dad.

Finally, Dad was paged and he, Aunt Janis, and I went to meet the surgeon. Long story short, the lump is out. The cancer was localized - it had not spread to her lymphatic system (which is what we were worried about). They believe that the perimeter of breast tissue surrounding the lump is cancer free. However, that is only based on what their eyes can see and their hands can feel, so they will not know for sure if the tissue is cancer free until they look at it under a microscope. We'll get the results on Friday, hopefully, and then know for sure if the tissue is cancer free.

If the tissue *does* have cancer, mom will have to go in and get her entire breast removed. Apparently, they already took out a good amount of breast tissue - any more and it would be a sad day in booby town. So anymore taken out means all of it will be taken out. Pray it doesn't come to that.

You guys, the surgery is over! Praise God! My mom made it out beautifully.

Let me just stand on a soapbox for a minute. My mom wasn't *lucky*, she wasn't taken care of by the cosmos, no amount of passing on good energy or whatever else caused the wonderful good news we received. It was the God of Abraham that blessed us. The Christ who lived, died, and rose again to pay the ultimate price for His creation. The power of prayer is impossible to stand against. Faith is only as strong as the object is placed in. Jesus is the author and perfecter of mine and my family's. We are firm believers in the redeeming power of Christ and that He takes care of us. It was all Him you guys - with all my heart I believe that.

Praise Jesus!

A Little Bit of Normal Life?

Drenda Lane Howatt is bored
November 20, 2008 at 8:37am

Andi Pedersen Jordan at 8:47am November 20, 2008
Welcome to my world!

Karen Buehrig at 8:51am November 20, 2008 via Facebook Mobile
Drenda- I wish you were around so we could yak it up about staff asst stuff. I'm out at my leadership class

Drenda Lane Howatt at 8:52am November 20, 2008
Let's talk tomorrow

Drenda Lane Howatt is going to take a nap
November 20, 2008 at 11:32am

Drenda Lane Howatt is shopping on-line. Let Christmas be delivered!
November 20, 2008 at 7:22pm

Caitlin Lopez at 3:21pm November 21, 2008
So wise.

Caitlin Lopez at 3:21pm November 21, 2008
I wish I could afford all the shipping. I hate running all over town!

Drenda Lane Howatt at 4:51pm November 21, 2008

No, my dear. You get free shipping. Sometimes, just asking for free shipping gets you free shipping. Try it!

Caitlin Lopez at 5:01pm November 22, 2008
Seriously? That's so cool.

Tremendous Relief!

Drenda Lane Howatt received good news...tissue margins all negative for cancer. Praise God.
November 21, 2008 at 5:55pm

> Karen Buehrig at 6:00pm November 21, 2008 via Facebook Mobile
> Yeehaa! I am so glad that you got such good news! - am wacthing Kate at her swim lessons now.
>
> Amy Hickman at 6:01pm November 21, 2008
> Praising God with you, Drenda!!
>
> Amber Lynn Montgomery Lane at 6:18pm November 21, 2008
> WAHOOOO!!! Does this mean you're all done other than preventative measures for the future, or will you still have to go through some drug treatments? No mastectomy, right?
>
> Andi Pedersen Jordan at 6:24pm November 21, 2008
> Hip Hip Hooray!!!!! ;-)
>
> Drenda Lane Howatt at 6:33pm November 21, 2008
> I THINK it means no mastectomy. I am assuming I'll still have follow-up treatments, but not sure exactly what those will consist of.
>
> Amber Lynn Montgomery Lane at 6:35pm November 21, 2008
> In any case, it sounds like this is the best we could hope for. You are a blessed woman, Drenda.

Kristi Smith at 4:06am November 22, 2008
Hooray! Thanks for sharing the good news. :-)

Caitlin Lopez at 5:00pm November 22, 2008
Wooo hooo!!!!!

Robin Reilly at 8:01pm November 22, 2008
YES!! PTL!

I don't think there are words to describe my euphoria upon receiving the surgeon's phone call and the news that the tissue margins were clear. I was, literally I think, on cloud nine. I was so very thankful and happy and ecstatic. Then reality set in. "Still a long road ahead..."

Drenda Lane Howatt is going to convince Donald to go to Starbucks on the way to church...
November 23, 2008 at 8:58am

Drenda Lane Howatt is going to try and work for a few hours tomorrow. Watch out Clackamas County! Here I come!
November 23, 2008 at 5:25pm

Drenda Lane Howatt is trying to recover from working yesterday...
November 25, 2008 at 11:28am

> Andi Pedersen Jordan at 12:16pm November 25, 2008 via Facebook Mobile
> Thumbs up or thumbs down?

Drenda Lane Howatt is working on getting ready for Christmas! Trying to use time wisely.
November 28, 2008 at 12:08pm

Cancer Update

Saturday, November 29, 2008 at 9:00am

I still can't seem to get my head to accept that I have cancer. Life goes along, and then, all of a sudden, "I HAVE cANCER" hits me over the head. So very odd -- this is not what I had planned. I don't have time to have cancer! But, alas, I will find time to beat cancer.

I saw my surgeon last week. He believes that I'll have radiation and chemotherapy. ugh. Probably radiation first (every day for 5-6 weeks), then the chemo. The pathology report did confirm that the tissue margins and the lymph node were negative for cancer cells. It did show, though, that the cancer was on its way to the lymphatic system. My cancer is considered stage 1 (best possible) and grade 3 (worst possible -- most aggressive on a scale of 1-3). Good news and also scary news.

When my panic rises, Don reminds me of the surgeon's words: "the cancer is OUT of your body" and the treatment is to make sure it doesn't come back. That helps. When I can't sleep at night (every night), I try to remember Jesus Christ's words "Do not let your heart be troubled. Trust in God, trust also in Me." The Psalms are also so helpful.

I have been so worried about my girls through this. I don't want them to have to experience the pain of Mom having breast cancer. But then I realized, if I had my desire, they would be robbed of seeing what God has for all of us in this -- the joys as well as the pain. They would be robbed of the strength they will gain by walking through this fire. I think one of the hardest things in life is trusting God with the lives of my children. He is able, and does, care for them more than I could ever.

I have appointments on Wednesday with two oncologists -- one a radiation oncologist and the other a regular (?) oncologist. That day will be overwhelming, I am sure. So if you think about me on Wednesday, please pray that I'll have a calm heart and clear mind so that I can hear and process the information I receive from the doctors, and that my questions get asked and answered.

So now I am thinking I should have joined the "Biggest Loser" contest at work -- the contestant who loses the most weight wins! I would be ahead, I'm sure. Stress is a great weight loss inducer.

I'd rather stay fat.

Andi Pedersen Jordan: Tell it to go away . . .
November 29, 2008 at 9:02am

Cindy McElmurry: Drenda,
I know it's scary. My prayer for you is that you can REST in the arms of your Savior. That when you wake up at night that you will feel His peace. That when this is over and you are able to look back and see how He carried you through. I love you my friend. C
November 29, 2008 at 10:10am

Amy Hickman: Your words are so true...it's when we go thru the fire and the valley that we see God and His comfort, compassion and grace so much more clearly. While I wouldn't ASK to go thru hard times, I am truly grateful for those times because I have grown so much more intimate in my relationship with the Savior.
November 29, 2008 at 2:03pm

Don Howatt: The Doc said he took it out~
I Love You
November 29, 2008 at 2:44pm

Tara L Koch: The best book I ever read was 'Crazy Sexy Cancer Tips' by KRIS CARR. There is a DVD as well. It is much different than the title might indicate. Bless you Drenda.
November 29, 2008 at 2:57pm

Tayler Younge: We at the Younge's will most definitely be praying for you and I'm so glad they got it out of your body!!!
November 29, 2008 at 6:58pm

Lynn Peterson: Whatever you need to help you beat it! Your Clackamas County buds are there for you!
December 1, 2008 at 8:17am

More Normal

Drenda Lane Howatt is going to stop at SBUX (again) on the way to church!
November 30, 2008 at 9:17am

Drenda Lane Howatt is going to eat lunch and then take the obligatory Sunday nap.
November 30, 2008 at 12:49pm

Drenda Lane Howatt is getting ready to re-enter the real world...going to work in the morning!
November 30, 2008 at 5:45pm

Drenda Lane Howatt is enjoying the pancakes Ellie made for breakfast. Thanks, Miss Eleanor!
December 1, 2008 at 6:48am

Drenda Lane Howatt successfully completed two full days of work. woo hoo. Tomorrow, two oncologists. Busy Day.
December 2, 2008 at 5:08pm

> Andi Pedersen Jordan at 8:13pm December 2, 2008
> How did it go?

Another Cancer Update If You're Interested

Wednesday, December 3, 2008 at 4:28pm

Ok, so two oncologists and one entire day --Radiation Oncologist seen first -- radiation will be AFTER chemo. great Medical Oncologist, Dr. Segal, seen next - 2 1/2 hour appointment, 1 1/2 hours of which is with the oncologist. Too much information.

My cancer is stage 1 grade 3. Hormone receptor strongly positive for estrogen and progesterone. The pre-surgical MRI of my breasts showed a benign very little something in one lymph node (new news) on the right side. HER2-neu positive (new info). Her2-neu positive is the most aggressive type of breast cancer. This type of cancer apparently can travel to the brain. The Dr. doesn't think my cancer has gone there, but I will have an MRI of my brain to be certain.

I will have a port inserted surgically (probably next week) for the administration of the chemotherapy. On Friday (12-5) I have the brain MRI, a CT scan of my body, and an echocardiogram of my heart. I see Dr. Segal again on Wednesday 12-17 and anticipate the chemo beginning the next day.

The first round of chemo consists of two different drugs administered every 2 weeks for a total of 4 treatments. The side effects of this first regiment are total hair loss and vomiting/nausea. Then, I'll have Taxol administered every week for 12 weeks. Along with this, I'll have herceptin which is a drug specfically to target the HER 2-neu issue. Dr. Segal has asked me to consider being part of a trial to try a new drug Tykerb either instead of or in conjunction with Herceptin. The possible advantage to Tykerb is that it does pass the blood/brain barrier and would attack any cancer cells in the brain. Herceptin does not go into the brain. Herceptin would be injected regularly (weekly? can't remember what he said) for one year. So I have a decision to make -- and soon. There is a 24-page consent form that I have to sign if I agree to the trial.

After the chemo regiment, I'll have 33 radiation treatments -- every day M-F for 6.5 weeks. The first 28 radiation treatments are to the entire breast area, and the last five are a "boost" to the tumor bed. Either in conjunction with the radiation or after it is concluded, I'll begin taking Tamoxifen for hormone therapy (suppression). That will continue for 2-3 years, and then I'll switch to a different drug for more years.

Too much information.

Oh, and Dr. Segal thought I was quite intelligent because I used the word "cumulative" in a sentence..."I've NEVER had a patient who has used that word!" My response: "that concerns me..."

Andi Pedersen Jordan: First, of course we are interested!

I agree . . . too much information. I know I feel overwhelmed by it, so I can't imagine how you are absorbing all of this.

Here if you need me.
December 3, 2008 at 5:28pm

Kathlin Gabaldon: Praying for you Drenda! Thanks for the update! keep 'em coming!
December 3, 2008 at 6:13pm

Kris Howatt: Thank you for sharing the info - it is alot to deal with. Let me know what your transportation needs are - I am available to help get you to/from many of these treatments (and of course any meals you or your family need). Kris
December 4, 2008 at 11:00am

Kristi Smith: So sorry to hear about the lymph node and her2neu news. I'm praying for your strength and healing and for wisdom in decision-making.

Thanks for sharing the "cumulative" anecdote. Made me chuckle even after reading the sobering news about the further diagnosis and treatment plan.
December 5, 2008 at 1:37am

Drenda Lane Howatt doesn't want to have cancer.
December 3, 2008 at 4:30pm

Karen Buehrig at 6:08pm December 3, 2008
I don't want you to have cancer either! :(

Laurie Lane at 6:18pm December 3, 2008
Drenda,
Thanks for letting all know what's going on. How are you doing with all of this "cumulative" information???
(Tell the doctor that smarts run in your family... however spelling errors are in my 1/9 of the family...!)
I love you!
Laurie

Drenda Lane Howatt is, hmmm, still not wanting to have cancer.
December 4, 2008 at 5:51am

Andi Pedersen Jordan at 7:08am December 4, 2008
Strong and courageous . . . let's go back to Drenda is strong and courageous.

Drenda Lane Howatt at 5:39pm December 4, 2008
Ok. Strong and courageous. Drenda WILL be strong and courageous.
"Have I not commanded you? Be strong and courageous. Do not be terrified or discouraged. The Lord your God is with you wherever you go".

Andi Pedersen Jordan at 5:51pm December 4, 2008
:-)

Karen Buehrig Hey Drenda- Thanks for sharing the different things you are experiencing. - know you must get tired of talking about it.
December 5, 2008 at 5:51pm

Drenda Lane Howatt is upset that insurance doesn't want to pay for tests the doctor says are a must...
December 5, 2008 at 4:42pm

> Laurie Lane at 4:56pm December 5, 2008
> Is the doctor going to fight it for you?
>
> Drenda Lane Howatt at 5:03pm December 5, 2008
> Yes, he is trying. I also called the insurance company and launched an official appeal. Now we wait. I don't know if this delay in the testing will delay the start of treatment. Frustrating!
>
> Kris Howatt at 5:46pm December 5, 2008
> My experience with most insurance is that they deny first and make you appeal - whether it is medical or dental or car. Very frustrating, and I deal with it every time.

Drenda Lane Howatt is trying to decide about participating in clinical trials.
December 6, 2008 at 1:28pm

Drenda Lane Howatt is still working on strong and courageous. Strong and courageous. Strong and courageous. YES I AM.
December 6, 2008 at 8:48pm

> Kristi Smith at 8:56pm December 6, 2008
> Don't be afraid, for I have redeemed you. I have called you by name; you are mine! When you pass through the waters I will be with you. And when you pass through the rivers they will not sweep over you. When you walk though the fire you will not be burned, the flames will not set you ablaze. For I am the Yahweh, the Lord your God, the Holy One of Israel, your Savior. Isaiah 43:1-3

Kristi Smith at 8:56pm December 6, 2008
Praying for you, Drenda.

Drenda Lane Howatt had a normal day at work, and gets to go back tomorrow. I love my job!
December 8, 2008 at 6:14pm

Drenda Lane Howatt at 6:15pm December 8, 2008
I really, truly, love my job! Clackamas County is a great place to be.

Drenda Lane Howatt is chatting with her sister about being bald. Woo hoo!
December 8, 2008 at 8:14pm

Becky Annus at 8:44pm December 8, 2008
You'll be BEAUTIFUL and bald!

Rachel Howatt at 12:11am December 9, 2008
I'll crochet you as many hats as you want

Becky Annus at 5:41am December 9, 2008
Maybe Rachel could crochet matching hats for all of us?!

Rachel Howatt at 9:16am December 9, 2008
Sure!

Becky Annus at 12:08pm December 10, 2008
Please!

Drenda Lane Howatt had another normal day at work. Gotta love normal, she thinks!
December 9, 2008 at 8:05pm

Another Cancer Note

Tuesday, December 9, 2008 at 8:37pm

Insurance update: Appeal denied. Doctor upset. Doctor dictating letter to insurance company. Drenda distressed that MRI of brain seems so very important. Doctor not so upset that CT scan denied -- good news is that all blood tests came back normal, so CT scan not so imperative.

More good news(?) is that delay of testing does not cause delay in treatment. Chemo slated to begin next week -- Thursday.

So here is my schedule, as it stands at this moment, for the next few days:
Wednesday (tomorrow) -- appointment with the surgeon to check incision sites; echo-cardiogram to check heart health
Friday, Dec. 12 -- surgery to insert port
Saturday -- cut that hair off!
Sunday - Tuesday: normal days (hopefully!)
Wednesday, Dec. 17: appointment with oncologist for blood work and ?
Thursday, Dec. 18: first administration chemo -- 4-5 hours
Christmas Day: remainder of hair should be falling out. Could be worse. It is only hair, and a "renewable resource" as my husband so lovingly reminded me! Sustainable, in other words :-) That is us -- we're all about being sustainable around here~

It is good to have a plan. I am anxious to start treatment so I can be done with treatment. Then I realize, I will never be done with this cancer thing. That is difficult. I find myself dividing my life into "before cancer" and "after cancer". Life was so simple and, in retrospect, care-free "before cancer". But the interesting thing is that I thought I had problems then. If only.

So, if you think about me in the next few weeks, please pray that God will give me peace of heart, especially in the evenings and nights, that I'd be able to get through the chemotherapy with the least possible physical hinderances (aka vomiting), and that the treatment would be COMPLETELY successful and that I will be declared cancer-free. Pray, too, for Don, Anna, Rachel and Ellie. This is so difficult for them as well.

Laurie Lane: It's nice to have your doctor dealing with the insurance company! AND great news about your blood test results!!! For getting such a scary diagnosis, everything else is going your way.
December 9, 2008 at 9:06pm

Andi Pedersen Jordan: Happy for the good news.

As always, thank you for keeping us updated. . . . you are at the forefront of all of my thoughts.

I'm sending "PEACE" your way.
December 9, 2008 at 9:49pm

Drenda Lane Howatt visited the surgeon, did Christmas shopping downtown, had an echo-cardiogram, made banana bread AND worked from home. Busy day!
December 10, 2008 at 5:05pm

Drenda Lane Howatt is nervous about snow, surgery, and shopping. But not in that order.
December 11, 2008 at 5:23pm

Drenda Lane Howatt is happy, oh so happy, to have all three of her girls home for Christmas!
December 13, 2008 at 8:47am

One More Surgery Down

Saturday, December 13, 2008 at 8:45am

Yesterday, I dutifully reported to Providence Portland Medical Center at 6 a.m. for my 9 a.m. surgery to insert the port into my chest. Three hours is a long time...
Due to complications in the surgery prior to mine, my surgery was delayed until about 10:30. Long time waiting. Valium helps tremendously, I've learned.

General anesthetic again. Surgery was successful, and after waking up in the recovery room, I waited an hour and a half for "transport" to take me back to the post-op area of day surgery. Fine for me, but I was worried about Don, worried that he'd be worried. hmmm. too much worrying, perhaps. But then I'd doze off again.

Long story short, I was home by about 2:30 and went back to bed. Nice to be groggy and get to sleep. The pain from this surgery was significantly more than from the lumpectomy, but still not so bad. I am sore in my arm and shoulder muscles, and the surgery site is tender. Advil is all I am taking now.

The big news is that I am getting my hair cut today. And I mean CUT. Not bald, but shorter than I have ever had it in recent and not so recent memory. According to the calendar, I should be going bald on Christmas day or the day after, so I am taking the first step this afternoon. I may allow Miss Rachel to document the day, so stay tuned for the first photos!

Thank you, all, for your notes and words of encouragement. They help me weather this storm. I am trying to take one day at a time and not think or worry about "tomorrow". That is difficult, Very difficult. I go back to God's instruction to Joshua "Have I not commanded you? Be strong and courageous. DO NOT BE TERRIFIED. DO NOT BE DISCOURAGED. For the Lord your God is with you wherever you go."

Terrified is often a good word to describe my state of mind. But I know God and I know God's Son. Knowing them is different than knowing about them. I know I will be carried through this. I know God is at work in my life. I trust Him.

Andi Pedersen Jordan: I am so happy that you are willing to share all of this with us. I care, and I know so many others care about you.

I think you should find a very hilarious movie to watch today. Laughter has great medicinal qualities!
December 13, 2008 at 8:55am

Sally Park: Drenda we are waiting for pictures. =)
Love you.
December 13, 2008 at 6:43pm

Drenda Lane Howatt has the shortest hair she's EVER had...except for when she was a newborn baby.
December 13, 2008 at 6:12pm

> Amy Hickman at 8:22pm December 13, 2008
> Drenda, it seriously looks super cute!
>
> Danielle Becker at 8:44pm December 13, 2008
> I love it! It is VERY stylish! :-)
>
> Andi Pedersen Jordan at 11:40pm December 13, 2008
> You look great . . . can't believe that you've never had short hair!

My sisters Linda and Janette accompanied me to get my hair cut, and they had theirs cut just as short. They decided to go 'bald' with me. Upon first hearing this, I thought they were crazy. But, as time progressed, it was a great comfort to me to know I was not alone in my baldness.

Linda, Drenda, and Janette before getting haircuts.
(December 13, 2008)
Photo by Rachel Howatt

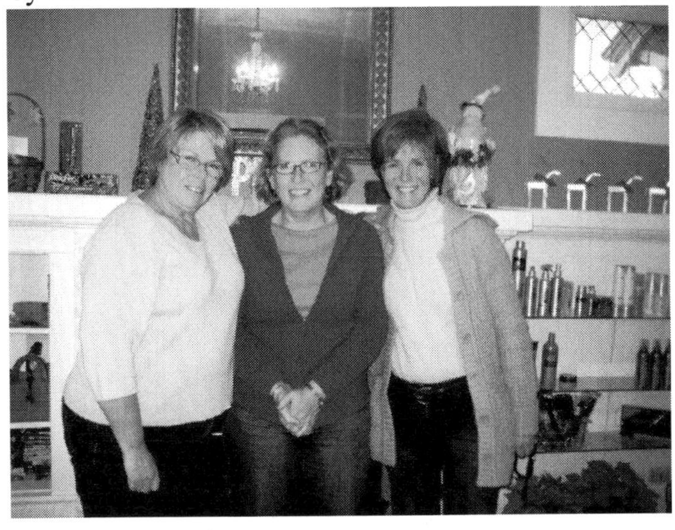

Drenda getting her hair cut short. (December 13, 2008)
Photo by Rachel Howatt

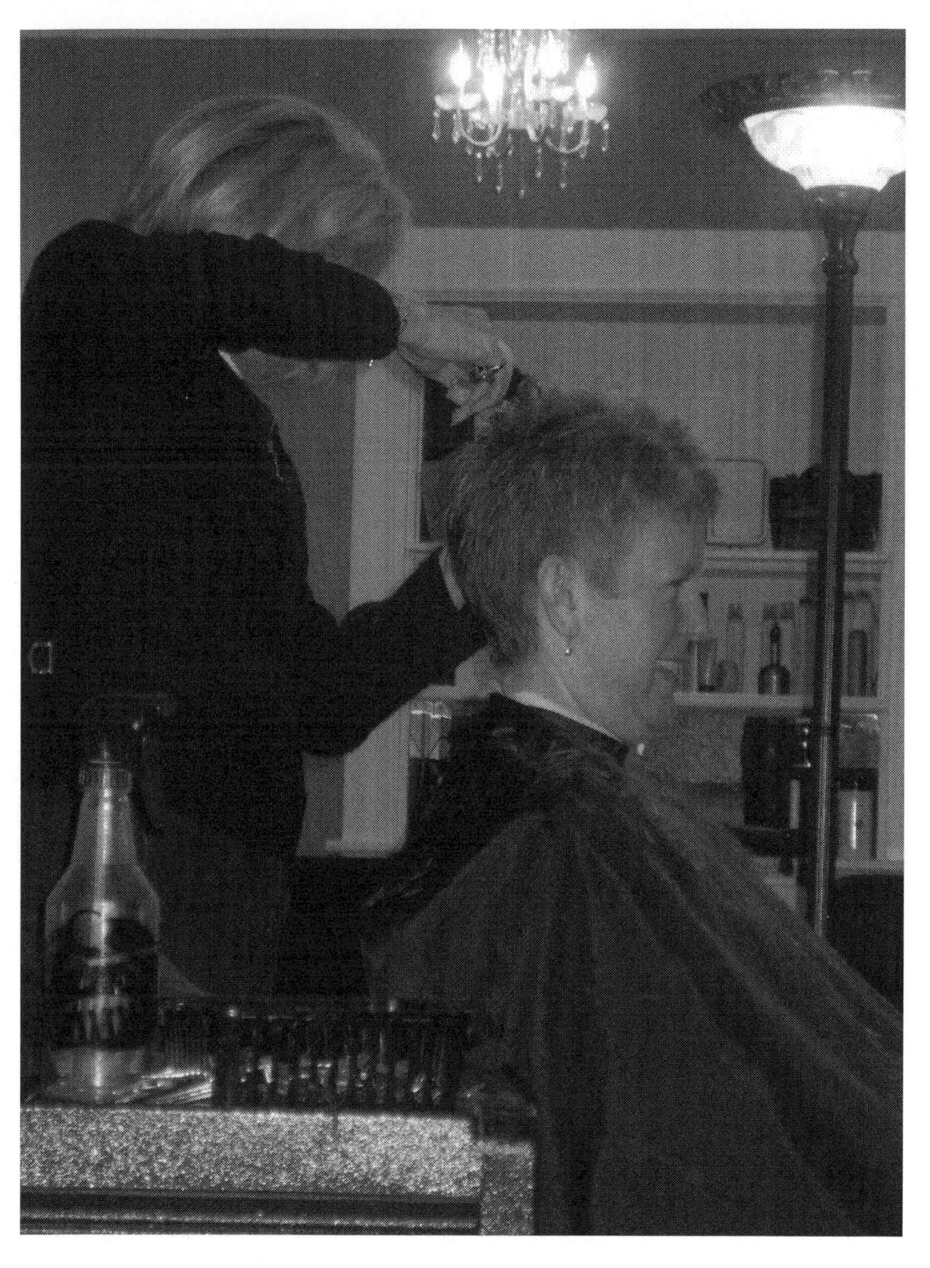

Sister Janette's turn! (December 13, 2008)
Photo by Rachel Howatt

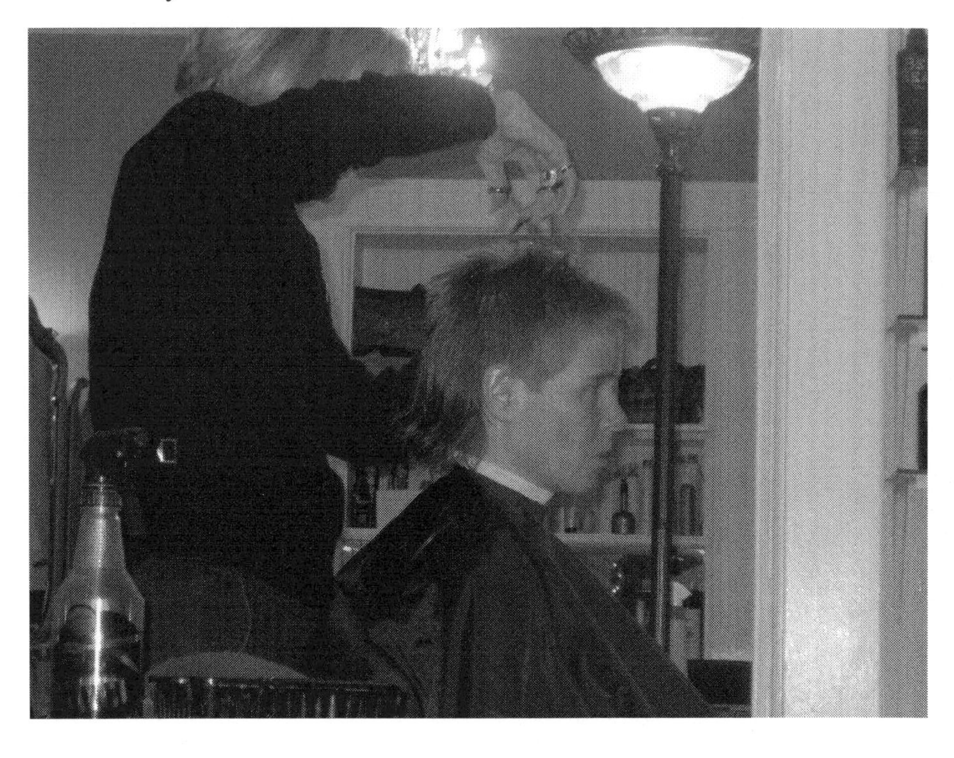

Rachel came to lend moral support, and to document the day with photos. (December 13, 2008)

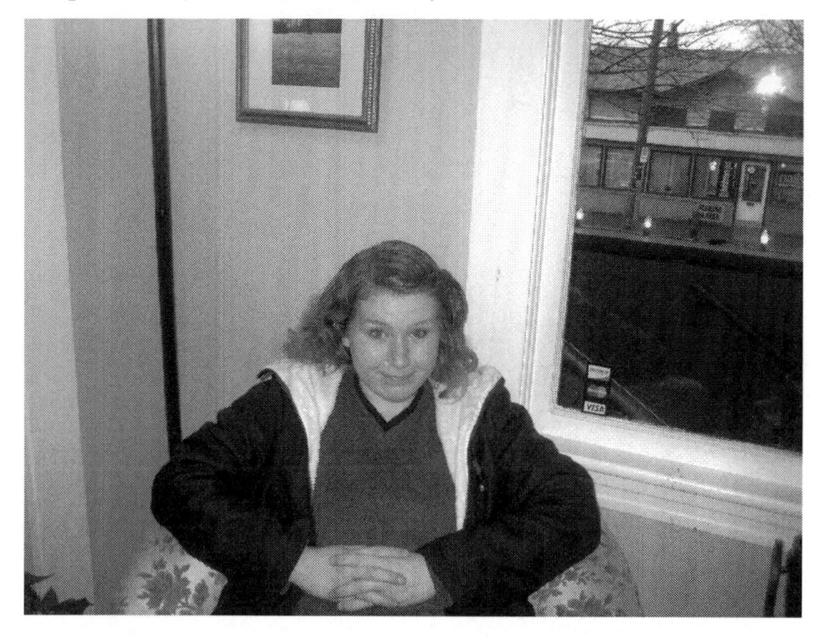

Linda waits her turn. (December 13, 2008)
Photo by Rachel Howatt

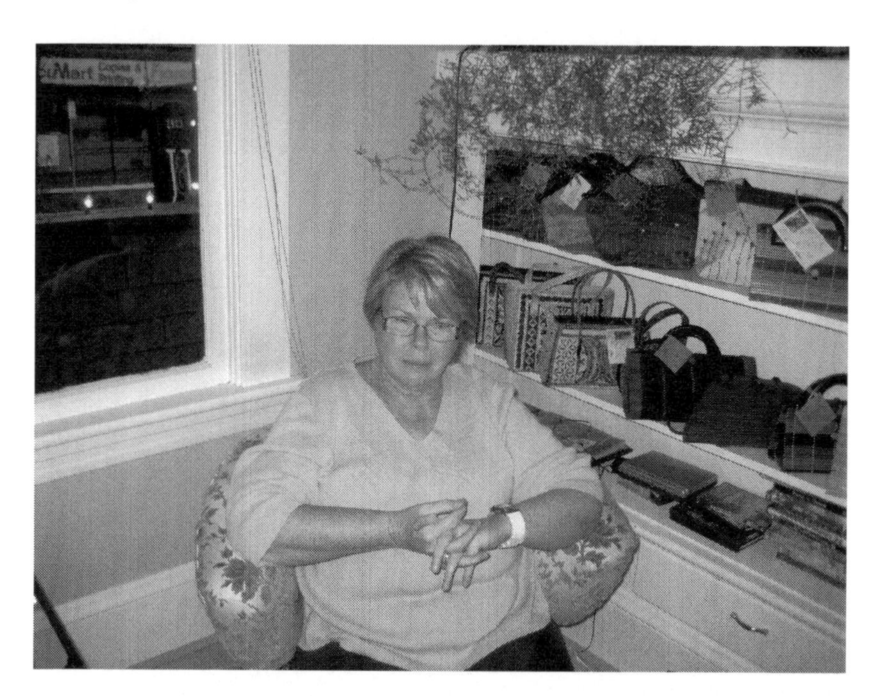

Linda's haircut begins. We found many things to laugh about in the midst of the solemn situation. (December 13, 2008)
Photo by Rachel Howatt

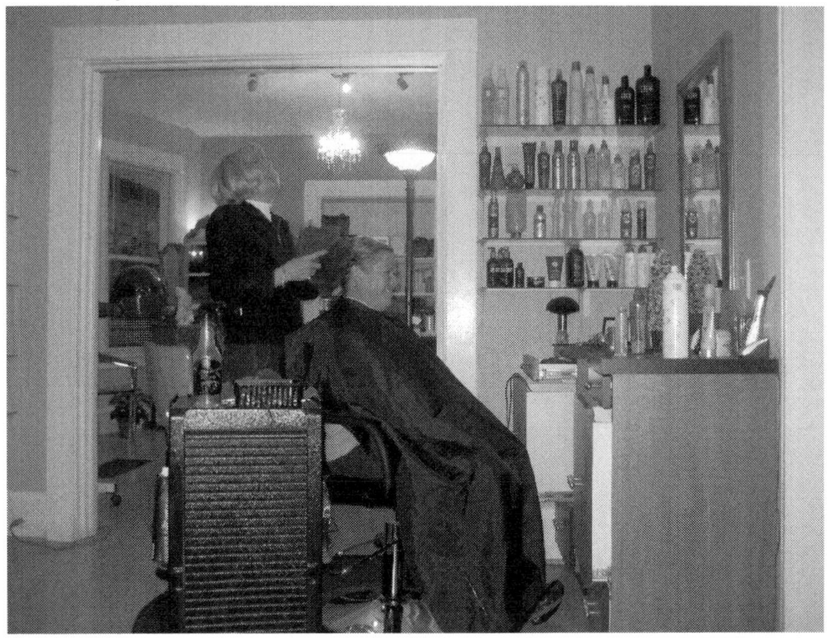

Drenda models her short hairstyle! (December 13, 2008)
Photo by Rachel Howatt

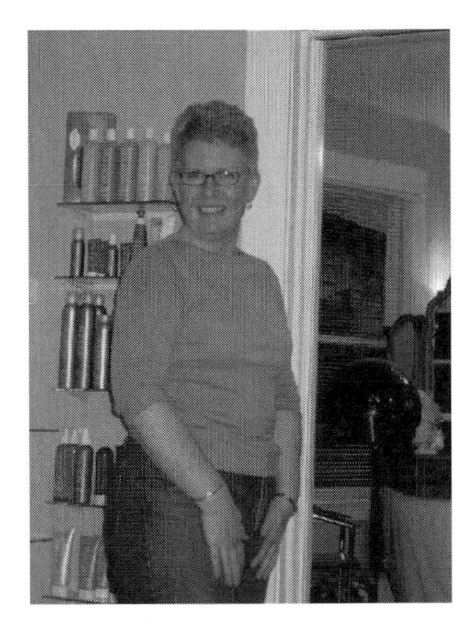

All done! Short hair…first step to baldness. (December 13, 2008) Photo by Rachel Howatt

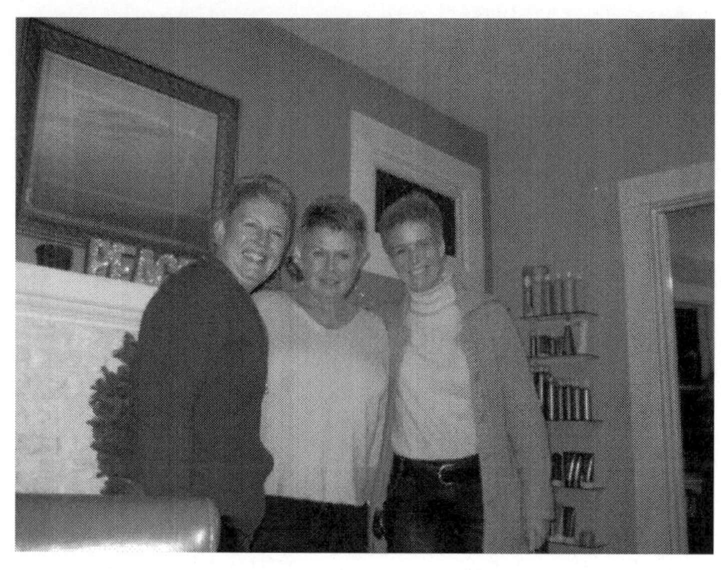

Drenda and Rachel pose for the camera. (December 13, 2008)

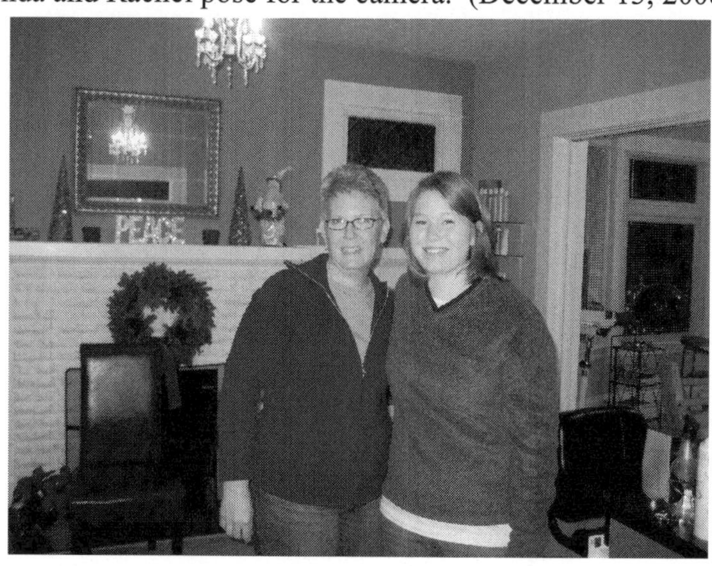

Drenda Lane Howatt has a cold head. brrr
December 14, 2008 at 8:35am

Abbi Howatt at 12:30pm December 14, 2008
I empathize completely.

Encouragement

Sunday, December 14, 2008 at 11:57am

I received a card in the mail yesterday from Joyce McElmurry. It contained such encouragement for me, I wanted to share it with all of you.

"Do not look forward to what may happen tomorrow; the same everlasting Father who takes care of you today will take care of you tomorrow and every day. Either He will shield you from suffering, or He will give you unfailing strength to bear it. Be at peace, then, put aside all anxious thoughts and imaginations, and say continually: "The Lord is my strength and my shield; my heart has trusted in Him and I am helped. He is not only with me but in me and I in Him." St. Francis de Sales

---

Drenda Lane Howatt is amazed how little shampoo is needed when one has an almost shaved head...
December 15, 2008 at 8:26am

> Janette Wilkinson at 8:31am December 15, 2008
> I am going to go take a shower right now and see how much time is shaved off my morning by having this haircut...I will let you all know!
>
> Brian Torres at 8:59am December 15, 2008
> Are you done yet?
>
> Becky Annus at 7:37pm December 15, 2008
> What about now? Done yet?
>
> Janette Wilkinson at 9:08pm December 15, 2008
> You will be happy to know that from pajamas on, undress, shower, to dressed, hair done, face on and teeth brushed was 17min. Almost 15 minutes off my old time! Woo Hoo! There is no time for drying. By the time I am dressed my hair is too dry for the hair dryer! Now what to do with all my free time...hmmmmmm

Drenda Lane Howatt is trying to finish Christmas...oh my goodness.
December 17, 2008 at 4:01pm

Oncologist Visit #2 (Not That I'm Counting, or Anything...)

Wednesday, December 17, 2008 at 3:50pm

Saw Dr. Segal this morning. Original appointment scheduled for 2:30 -- moved earlier due to the weather. Problem was that Don was working until noon, and then planning to come home and take me to the Dr. visit. Ended up that I slowly drove to the appointment by myself, and Don met me there when it was almost done.

First, blood work. Even though I now have the handy-dandy port, I declined to allow the lab tech to draw blood from it -- incision still very tender. So, bring out the heating pad, and heat up those arm veins! The lab tech (probably has a professional label, but I don't know what it is...) brought out a "port" to show me what is inside my chest. Very interesting. Metal backing so that the needle can't go too far in. Nice safety feature.

I was reassured when I saw Dr. Segal in the hall -- he addressed me by name and asked if I'd received the official insurance denial of the brain MRI. He knows me! smile. I am not just a number.

Dr. Segal spent considerable time, again, explaining things to me. First, reassurance about the brain/cancer link. No reason to believe I have any cancer in my brain (no jokes, please), but he thinks a baseline test is imperative for comparative purposes. He will follow-up with the insurance company. He also explained the process should cancer ever be found in my brain, and while the situation would be very serious, it would not be a death sentence. whew. Treatable with surgery and drugs, and brain radiation if needed.

Chemo treatment will begin tomorrow at 9 a.m., if weather permits. If not, and the office is closed, I have an appointment for Friday at 9 a.m. One thing I learned today is that, because I am having "dose-dense" treatment with treatments every two weeks instead of every three weeks, I have to go back the day after each chemo for an injection of "neulasta" (sp?). This is the drug that allows for the two week treatment schedule. That means if I have chemo on Friday, I'll have to go to Providence hospital on Saturday to get the injection of neulasta. Dr. Segal also is calling in prescriptions for me for two or three anti-nausea drugs, plus a numbing cream I can put over the port area to help facilitate inserting the needle for chemo. Along with the chemo, they will administer a new anti-nausea drug that is supposed to last for three days. I will also see the Dr. 7 days after each chemo treatment to check my blood counts, etc. We're going to be great friends!

I had lots of questions -- "should I come to chemo with an empty stomach?" "No, eat a light breakfast". "If I do get sick, when would it hit?" "Probably that evening or the next day". "should I call you if I get sick?" "YES! We have a doctor on call 24 hours a day, and if you're having trouble, we'll take care of you -- get you on iv's, or whatever is needed. We will be aggressive and pro-active in combating nausea". whew.

Dr. Segal asked me again about the drug trial. Still not decided. Dr. Segal said there is no rush, I have 2-3 weeks before a decision is needed. We did talk about the trial more, and he is so convinced the new drug is of great benefit based on the research so far, and even his own patients' response to it. I am leaning toward participating.

Then, Dr. Segal took us upstairs to see the treatment room. Filled with leather recliners, and quite busy! It was as comfortable and welcoming looking as probably possible. But no wireless access. That means you all will be spared the detailed account of what is happening as it is happening.

So, I am almost ready to start the next step in this journey called breast cancer. Thank you for traveling alongside me, and propping me up when I collapse. I am feeling very loved and supported by my family and friends. A number of you have told me how strong you think I am. But, alas, I am not. It is the strength of my God upon which I am forced to rely. I am putting aside anxious thoughts and imaginations, and saying continually "the Lord is my strength and my shield; my heart has trusted in Him and I am helped. He is not only with me but in me and I in Him."

Drenda

Laurie Lane: Drenda,
Thanks for taking us on the journey with you. You will be in my thoughts all day tomorrow (and/or Friday). Sounds like you have a great doctor! I love you!
Laurie
December 17, 2008 at 6:48pm

Becky Annus: That was a positive Dr. appointment. Good information!
December 17, 2008 at 8:17pm

Linda Waggoner: Drenda,
I always forget to check Facebook -- maybe it's a sign of my age! Good luck today and tomorrow! Oh, did you find out when we need to cut our hair shorter?
I love you!

Linda
December 18, 2008 at 10:03am

Drenda Lane Howatt: I'll keep you updated on the "fall-out"...
December 18, 2008 at 8:02pm

Linda Waggoner: OK!
December 19, 2008 at 10:33am

Chemo #1

Drenda Lane Howatt is preparing for war. Cancer cells WILL be killed today.
December 18, 2008 at 7:01am

> Jennifer Stady at 8:07am December 18, 2008
> Yes they will!!!
>
> Andi Pedersen Jordan at 8:34am December 18, 2008
> We've got your back. You go girl!
>
> Laurie Lane at 9:14am December 18, 2008
> Although I'm generally a pacifist, this is a war I totally support! Be aggressive, kill those cells!

Chemo Therapy #1 December 18, 2008

Friday, December 19, 2008 at 8:35am

Yesterday was the first chemo treatment. Don and I were on our way to the appointment just before 9, when Don's phone rang. It was Ellie saying that school was closing, and we needed to pick her up! So, Don dropped me off at the Dr. office and turned around to get Ellie and take her home. Then he came back to be with me. By the time he arrived, everything was under way.

First stop is vitals -- weight (even lost a bit since the day before -- cancer is an odd way, and awful way, to lose that unwanted weight). Blood pressure and temp next - BE CAREFUL, Miss Vitals Taker -- no blood pressure to be taken on the right side where the lymph node was removed. (I have to remind every time).

Then upstairs to the "Infusion Suite". I chose recliners near a window so that I could watch the beautiful snow, turned on the hot pad (supposed to use for warming arm veins for IVs, but in my case, I used it as a wonderful neck and upper back warming and relaxation pad). Wonderful! I asked for a hot blanket, and then I was set. I had my "Chemo Bag" with me. My sister Becky brought me the tote bag filled with goodies. A notebook that is titled "Drenda is Strong and Courageous" and filled with encouraging notes from family and friends, as well as lots of Christmas memories that my family wrote to each other a few years ago. I had magazines and suduko puzzles in the bag, too.

So, for the actual treatment. The nurse numbed the area over the port with "freezing spray" that was very very cold. Numb. Then for the needle into the port. Not bad, except she had to press really hard to make sure it was all the way in because of the amount of swelling I have over the incision. That wasn't the most fun.

Saline injected to clear the line, and then the meds and IV fluids start. First was one of the two anti-nausea drugs. I don't remember the order of the others, except that when it was time for the adriamyican, the nurse had to sit with me and push it in slowly. Three large vials. RED. I am receiving very close to the maximum life-time allowed dose of this drug. I can NEVER have it again. It harms the heart. I also received cytoxan, another cancer killer, and then another anit-nausea drug. All this along with fluids to make sure I stay hydrated and that the poisons don't stay in my body any longer than necessary.

Beginning to end, my visit lasted about 4 hours. Less than I had been told to anticipate.
I have been taking two more anti-nausea drugs regularly upon arriving home in hopes that the bad reactions can be held off. The weird part was that yesterday afternoon, I could literally feel each organ being attacked as the medicine/poison moved its way through my body.

After treatment, we raced to Costco and made a huge purchase of food to stock up freezer and pantry, and even managed to get a few Christmas presents checked off the list.

Don's sister Janis brought dinner for us. That was so sweet of her -- and a surprise for us, and it tasted very good. I risked eating because I was SO hungry... So far, so good.

Ok, there you have it - the blow-blow account of my first Chemotherapy. I return today to receive more IV fluids and an injection of neulasta. Neulasta is the drug that spurs the bone marrow to produce more white blood cells so that the chemo can be administered every two weeks instead of every three weeks.

On another note, if you're missing these updates and want to receive them, I think you can subscribe -- but I am not sure how to do that. You are all probably much more Facebook savvy than I....

Amber Lynn Montgomery Lane: Thank you so much for sharing Drenda. I really had no idea what chemo treatment is really like. You ARE strong and courageous.
December 19, 2008 at 9:31am

Janette Wilkinson: Strong and Courageous! Strong and Courageous! Strong and Courageous is
Drenda AND her family!
December 19, 2008 at 9:49am

Abigale Mary Lane: Wow! And then you went shopping! :) I love you!
December 19, 2008 at 10:58am

Zachary Lane Koval: Love and healing thoughts are being sent your way!!!!
December 19, 2008 at 11:26am

Andi Pedersen Jordan: Thank you . . . I had no idea what this is like so, and I agree that you are filling the informative role in our lives as well as the strong and courageous one!
Sending lots of warm holiday hugs your way.
Be strong and courageous . . . and nausea free!
December 19, 2008 at 11:37am

Tom Turnbull: Our thoughts are with you Drenda! You are fortunate to have such a strong group of supporters around you!
December 19, 2008 at 1:25pm

Denise Lane: Drenda, thank you for keeping us updated on this. You are in my prayers!
December 19, 2008 at 1:37pm

Lynn Peterson: I echo the comments from above...not only are you stong and courageous but a good story-teller. Thank you for sharing it with us!
December 19, 2008 at 3:12pm

Linda Waggoner: Drenda,
You are a wonderful advocate for yourself! I really admire you for telling the medical professionals what you want and need from them. You are, as always in my prayers!!!

I love you!
Linda
December 19, 2008 at 4:56pm

Karen Buehrig: Kate and I are thinking of you as well. Karen
December 19, 2008 at 7:28pm

Amy Hickman: You are in my prayers, Drenda. I admire you and know the Lord is with you.
December 19, 2008 at 9:34pm

Bobbi Gurney: Drenda,
What an amazing story. Your journey is sure to help others as so many who love you are connected through this community. I am endeared to you, by the spirit your writing brings. I know we met a long time ago, and you may not remember me…but know that my thoughts and prayers are with you. Warm Wishes~ Bobbi
December 20, 2008 at 3:16am

Sally Park: Ditto ~ Ditto ~ Ditto!! Love ya dear sister
December 20, 2008 at 8:57am

Drenda Lane Howatt knows the battle has begun -- and is hoping that she doesn't suffer too many casualties of healthy cells.
December 18, 2008 at 3:10pm

Abigale Mary Lane at 3:42pm December 18, 2008
Oh! How many treatments to go?

Andi Pedersen Jordan at 6:27pm December 18, 2008
Yeah!! You did it . . . one down . . .

Drenda Lane Howatt at 7:49pm December 18, 2008
Abi, dearie, I have 3 more war treatments; one every two weeks. Then I have 12 re-inforce the troops treatments; one every week. Next comes 33 daily radiation treatments. Then, 52 weekly treatments. Somewhere in this timeline, I'll begin taking oral medication to suppress my hormones. In between all those chemo treatments, I have numerous dr. and blood checks. My new part time job: CANCER ERADICATION

Sally Park at 7:25am December 19, 2008
How are you feeling this morning?

Drenda Lane Howatt at 7:52am December 19, 2008
Nauseated...but not terrible terrible. I keep taking the anti-vomiting medicine and praying that it works...

Sandy Hagstrand at 8:03pm December 19, 2008
You go girl! You've got the biggest comfort measure down - you took the pill!!! I'm so glad to hear that this hasn't been too bumpy for you. You're words educate and encourage others. Thank you for being vulnerable!

Snuggle down, watch the snow and enjoy being surrounded by your girls and of course Don.

You are in my prayers...

Sandy Hagstrand

Drenda Lane Howatt is going to bed. Good Night.
December 18, 2008 at 7:51pm

Drenda Lane Howatt is going back to bed with hopes of keeping the chemo vomiting at bay.
December 20, 2008 at 9:58am

Drenda Lane Howatt is enjoying the blizzard.
December 20, 2008 at 3:47pm

Sally Park at 3:51pm December 20, 2008
How are you feeling?

Drenda Lane Howatt at 4:41pm December 20, 2008
Blaaah. Terrible. Need to eat and drink but am afraid to

Kathleen Hopman Damon at 6:29pm December 20, 2008
Yes this is almost a blizzard to me; we may give Walla Walla a run. We officially canceled the anniversary party for tomorrow. Since we will be celebrating just the six of us tomorrow, we baked a small three tier cake today in case we lose power. I have assembled candles and flashlights. Girls playing outside in the dark.

Thinking of you constantly.

Drenda Lane Howatt risked retribution and ate dinner anyway. a small bit of dinner.
December 20, 2008 at 6:40pm

Sally Park at 8:21am December 21, 2008
Did it stay in place?

Drenda Lane Howatt at 8:23am December 21, 2008
Yes, thankfully

Drenda Lane Howatt still has hair. Note to Janette & Linda.
December 21, 2008 at 7:39am

Janette Wilkinson at 8:19am December 21, 2008
That is good because it is pretty cold out to be bald!

Drenda Lane Howatt at 8:20am December 21, 2008
Yep.

Janette Wilkinson at 8:20am December 21, 2008
Remember that you have to give us a heads up on the baldness so we can all go bald together. Ladies, sharpen those razors!

Drenda Lane Howatt at 8:21am December 21, 2008
That is why you had the special note today. When the clumps start falling, I'll tell you to shave!

Another update from Rachel:
In November my mom was diagnosed with breast cancer. I found out over worst phone call of my life. That night I worked out with my friends because I didn't want to just sit around and do nothing. I pushed myself harder than I ever have. I went faster, pounded harder, worked more... and I didn't feel any of it. I remember thinking that if I pushed hard enough, I could make the cancer go away. If I felt pain, no one else would. I didn't feel anything. I wish that numbness would have lasted. But at the same time I know that the joy of Christ would be harder to grasp without this hurt.

Drenda Lane Howatt just finished cooking a Sunday dinner her Mom would have been proud of. And, even better, Drenda was able to eat some of it!
December 21, 2008 at 1:55pm

Sally Park at 3:54pm December 21, 2008
Fried chicken? It is a cooking kind of day

Kris Howatt at 4:22pm December 21, 2008
Yeah! Especially the getting to eat part of it!

Drenda Lane Howatt at 4:26pm December 21, 2008
No, porkloin roast with garlic, onion, and rosemary (frozen rosemary!) and baked potatoes...salad, and viola, Sunday dinner. With a bit of leftovers

Janette Wilkinson at 5:51pm December 21, 2008
You must be feeling better?

Don Howatt at 5:57pm December 21, 2008
eh excuse me-who went out in the deep snow to fetch the rosemary....Hmmmmmmmm.....

Janette Wilkinson at 6:10pm December 21, 2008
That is such a long walk to the rosemary bush! Drenda is lucky to have a husband that will make that long trek for rosemary!

Sally Park at 6:14pm December 21, 2008
Yummmmm. We had broiled costco chicken dogs with french fries and salad. Goooood eating.

Drenda Lane Howatt is amazed it is snowing again. Beautiful!

Wondering if Clackamas County Administrator thinks the same thing?
December 21, 2008 at 4:32pm

> Andi Pedersen Jordan at 5:17pm December 21, 2008
> Why don't you get him on FB. . . and we could all find out! :-) lol
> Oh, wait . . . I don't have to worry about that . . . I'll worry for you!
>
> Jennifer Stady at 6:46pm December 21, 2008
> Hope so...it's probably worse WAY out there...

Don, Drenda, Ellie, Rachel, and Anna posing for family Christmas photo. (December 2008)

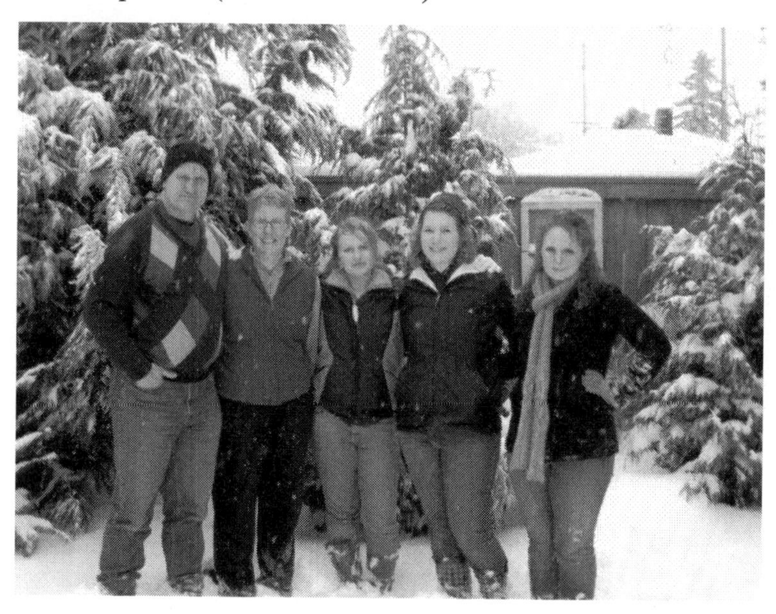

Don and Drenda in the snow. (December 2008)

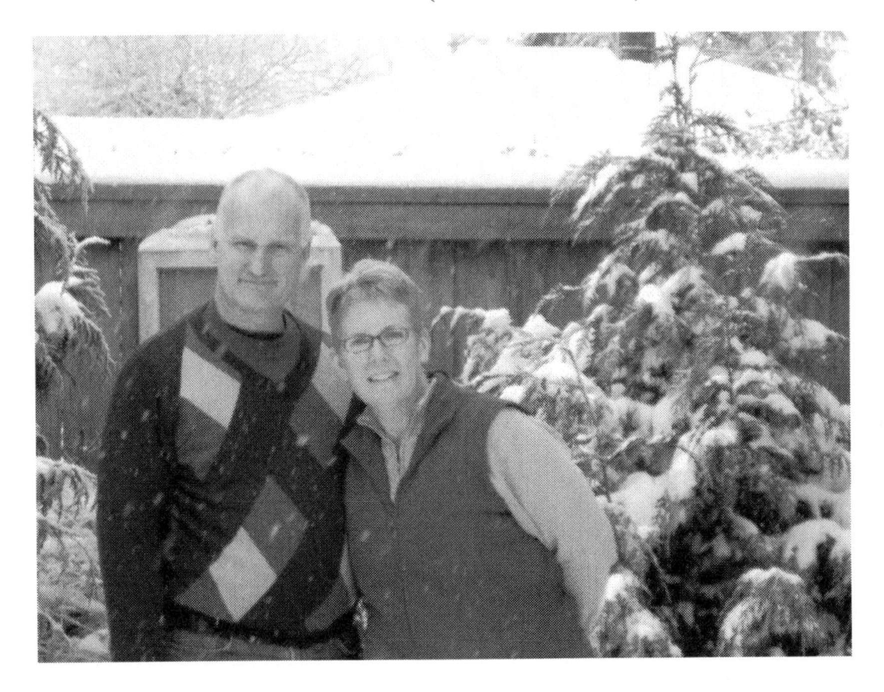

3 Days After Chemo…

Monday, December 22, 2008 at 6:48am

…and I am still nauseated...but not complaining! I made it through without throwing up, and for that I am extremely thankful. The medicine the Dr. gave me really worked -- didn't stop the nausea, but made it bearable. If you were to look at me, you might think I am dehydrated...my lips are dry and cracked and peeling, but I have been doing my best to drink fluids. I don't know if the "cumulative" effect of the chemo will cause the side effects to worsen with each treatment, but I will continue to be hopeful that I have experienced the worst, and know that I only have three more of the "bad" treatments to go. That means I am already 25% done! with the first part...

The Dr. tells me that, after these first four treatments, the next twelve weekly treatments are much more easily "tolerated". And that the following 33 radiation treatments are also "tolerated" with only fatigue and leathery radiation-burned skin. Not awful when you consider the benefits derived from the treatments -- killing cancer is a good thing.

I am still trying to decide about participating in the new drug trial. I want God to give me a scroll from heaven that says "Drenda, do this: ____________". BUT, I want the blanks filled in! If it were only so easy. I know God has said "Drenda, trust ME", and "Drenda, I will CARE FOR YOU". He is the God of the universe, creator of heaven and earth, and He cares for ME. I WILL trust Him, and will use the brain he has given me to make the best decision I can.

I go back to the Dr. on Friday to have my blood counts checked.

Then, back again on New Year's Eve for chemo #2.

Amber Lynn Montgomery Lane: Do you want my Sea Bands? I know they have helped me with nausea from car sickness and pregnancy.
December 22, 2008 at 11:45am

Drenda Lane Howatt: what are sea bands?
December 22, 2008 at 11:46am

Amber Lynn Montgomery Lane: They're little wrist bands than keep pressure on a pressure point that affect nausea somehow. No pain, possible gains...
December 22, 2008 at 11:48am

Drenda Lane Howatt: sure, I'll try them...any possible gain is worth an attempt
December 22, 2008 at 11:50am

Andi Pedersen Jordan: Hey, Drenda...I used those as well, but ginger worked just as well. Ginger tea, gingersnaps...anything ginger.
December 22, 2008 at 1:32pm

Laurie Lane: So, these first 4 treatments are every two weeks but after that the treatment is weekly... is that right? I think you should have a paper chain that you remove a link every time you have one of your treatments, just like we do to count down to a special occasion!
December 22, 2008 at 1:35pm

Robin Reilly: I agree with Andi, ginger always works for me. I just take the capsules.
December 22, 2008 at 10:23pm

Andi Pedersen Jordan: you can try tea . . . though or just smelling it . . .
Thinking of you . . .
December 22, 2008 at 11:14pm

Gail Stempel Hilderbrand: I understand what you are going through. I have been doing chemo for 1 1/2 years now, once every three months. I go again Jan 9. Because it was so spaced out, my hair thinned a lot but I didn't lose all of it. Because of my MS, when I have it I am bed ridden for 4-5 days. The nausea is nothing I have ever experienced. I take zofram for it, and it does stop the throwing up, but I am still very sick. It is so hard to just drink water, although they say to drink as much as you can to flush it through. I just mentally picture the chemo killing the bad cells in my body. It is a scary thing, and the only thing getting me through is clinging close to my family and God. Where are you having your chemo? I go to Providence cancer center. I am praying for you Drenda. Praying that God will cradle you in his arms and keep you safe.
December 23, 2008 at 10:56am

Drenda Lane Howatt is loading up on potassium -- her booklet "Chemo and You" suggests bananas and oranges. Cuties it is!
December 22, 2008 at 7:43am

> Kris Howatt at 5:07pm December 22, 2008
> I ate so many bananas when I was pregnant, it was the only thing that helped with the 9-month-morning-noon-and-night sickness

Drenda Lane Howatt is nauseated. yuck
December 22, 2008 at 8:45pm

Drenda Lane Howatt is waiting for her wonderful father-in-law to deliver Costco shopping. Thanks, Les!
December 23, 2008 at 3:06pm

I was surprised to learn that losing one's hair due to chemo hurts. A lot. It felt like each hair strand was a needle in my scalp. Each one. And they were sharp. Who would think hair could cause such pain?

Drenda Lane Howatt is still nauseated, and her scalp hurts. Sign of impending hair loss. Oh my goodness.
December 23, 2008 at 5:57am

> Cindy Knight at 8:19am December 23, 2008
> I am so sorry that you are having to go through this. I will be praying for you.
>
> Jennifer Stady at 9:56am December 23, 2008
> I'm sorry too...I'm hoping that it will hurt less soon.
>
> Andi Pedersen Jordan at 10:37am December 23, 2008
> Strong and courageous.
>
> Faith Jossi Lichtenberg at 6:29pm December 23, 2008
> We love you Drenda...I hope you will feel better for Christmas.

Drenda Lane Howatt can't believe it is Christmas Eve!
December 24, 2008 at 7:05am

> Becky Annus at 8:00am December 24, 2008
> I hope Corbett's Man in Brown makes it down my street...
>
> Sally Park at 8:21am December 24, 2008
> How are you feeling Ms Drenda?
>
> Drenda Lane Howatt at 8:24am December 24, 2008
> Still nauseated, but the medicine is helping some.

Drenda Lane Howatt is well cared for. Thank you Janette!
December 24, 2008 at 1:59pm

Becky Annus at 3:07pm December 24, 2008
Tell us more!

Drenda Lane Howatt at 4:06pm December 24, 2008
Scalloped potatoes delivered to my kitchen...and a visit with both Jim and Janette! Wonderful, wonderful

Becky Annus at 6:06pm December 24, 2008
Is the ham for tonight or Christmas Day?

Drenda Lane Howatt at 7:01pm December 24, 2008
Tonight and the morning breakfast

Drenda Lane Howatt is upset with fedex...pay for 2nd day air, and where is the package? gonna get a refund, she is.
December 24, 2008 at 4:10pm

Laurie Lane at 5:02pm December 24, 2008
Let me know how successful you are. I too paid top dollar to get packages here before Christmas and they haven't arrived yet.

Becky Annus at 6:05pm December 24, 2008
hmmmmm I wonder if I too might request a refund of the shipping....along with the rest of the USA

Janette Wilkinson at 6:52pm December 24, 2008
Oh dear! Who is going to be sad on Christmas morning with not a present to open?

Drenda Lane Howatt at 7:00pm December 24, 2008
Miss Ellie and Grandma Nina at our house...

Amanda Ouellette at 7:23pm December 24, 2008
Drenda, FedEx???

Drenda Lane Howatt at 7:25pm December 24, 2008
I know...but sometimes one has no choice in the matter...

Laurie Lane at 8:46pm December 24, 2008
One of the packages I paid top dollar for was Isaac and he won't make it---so I guess it will be me that is sad on Christmas morning. But he is healthy and happy and for that I am thankful!

Don Howatt at 9:05pm December 24, 2008
What do you expect form Fed Ex...Oops I just said the F word

Laurie Lane at 11:01pm December 24, 2008
Some of my packages were sent UPS... I saw a Budget truck delivering packages yesterday and was hopeful, but all for naught, they stopped next door but had with nothing for me. Don, where were you and your truck when I needed you????

Drenda Lane Howatt is going to bed and hoping Santa comes tonight...
December 24, 2008 at 9:54pm

Becky Annus at 12:59pm December 25, 2008
Did Santa make it to your house?

Drenda Lane Howatt is happy that the nausea is gone (yeah! -- only lasted 7 days), and anxious about going to see her oncologist today.
December 26, 2008 at 7:25am

Drenda Lane Howatt is back from the doctor. Low white blood counts. No fresh veggies or fruit until after the weekend. That means no lemon with the ice water, remember.
December 26, 2008 at 3:29pm

> Andi Pedersen Jordan at 3:34pm December 26, 2008
> Huh? So why no fresh fruits or vegies?
>
> Drenda Lane Howatt at 4:32pm December 26, 2008
> Bacteria...make me sick. Hopefully my white blood count will recover enough by early next week so that the next chemo treatment can occur as scheduled on Wednesday.
>
> Gail Hilderbrand at 6:35pm December 26, 2008
> Don't worry this happens. Just listen to your doc, the wbc's will be back!

Drenda Lane Howatt is doing laundry and trying to keep warm.
December 27, 2008 at 1:20pm

Drenda Lane Howatt is going to take her Sunday nap.
December 28, 2008 at 1:15pm

Drenda Lane Howatt is going bowling. Whee! She means "wii".
December 28, 2008 at 3:40pm

> Becky Annus at 4:16pm December 28, 2008
> Sophie is a champ at wii bowling!

Drenda Lane Howatt has 17 high school and college age "young people" at her house -- 13 of whom have not yet gone to sleep!
December 29, 2008 at 6:50am

Janette Wilkinson at 8:47am December 29, 2008
I had three "dead" boys in my car on the way home. Henry couldn't even tell me about his night he said, "Mom! I just need to sleep right now!"

Becky Annus at 9:18am December 29, 2008
Zander had no energy for any details...he crashed on the couch. check out the pix...

Becky Annus at 3:19pm December 29, 2008
It's 315pm and he's still sleeping

Gail Hilderbrand at 6:16pm December 29, 2008
I bet Don had a great time since he seems to be a bit of a kid himself!

Drenda Lane Howatt at 7:03pm December 29, 2008
Don slept through the entire party...until it was time to get up and go back to work.

Gail Hilderbrand at 7:18pm December 29, 2008
Wow...I wish I could do that. It must be a gift:)

Drenda Lane Howatt is home from work and trying to figure out how to get a flat tire fixed AND get back to work in the morning.
December 29, 2008 at 7:04pm

Drenda Lane Howatt is preparing emotionally for chemo #2 tomorrow.
December 30, 2008 at 8:22pm

Andi Pedersen Jordan at 8:30pm December 30, 2008
Strong and courageous

Amy Hickman at 8:32pm December 30, 2008
I will pray for you, Drenda!

Amber Lynn Montgomery Lane at 8:33pm December 30, 2008
Deep breath.

Drenda Lane Howatt is going to get hooked up...to an IV
December 31, 2008 at 9:46am

Gail Hilderbrand at 11:39am December 31, 2008
Stay focused. Chemo is your friend even though it doesn't feel like it. Hold onto Jesus, he is holding onto you.

Cancer War, Chemo #2 Battle

Wednesday, December 31, 2008 at 6:55pm

After seeing my doctor, I had the second chemo treatment today. Apparently, the doctor I saw last week (must have been a newbie, me thinks) over-reacted about the white blood count level. Mine was 2400, and I was told to not eat anything that had not been cooked. No fresh fruits or veggies. hmm. Today, my doctor said a "low" count that would be worrisome would be 900. 2400 was quite good considering the treatment.

I had been doing very well at controlling the panic - I was quite panic free for almost two weeks. But then, I stupidly read an obituary...of a young mom with breast cancer that traveled to her brain. Panic returned. Dr. Segal called in a refill of my sedatives, so should I need them I'll have them.

I am not sure if the panic is a fear of dying, or a fear of the process of dying. Breast cancer is testing my faith -- I SAY I believe that absent from the body is present with the Lord, and I THINK I believe that absent from the body is present with the Lord, but I admit that I have to go back to God's word to reassure me. I am coming to the conclusion that my fear is of the process of dying, not death itself, and it is fear for my family. Again, a test of my faith. As tremendously difficult it was for me when my Mom died, I am OK. I am OK. And my family can be OK, too. Surely, the Lord of the universe, the creator of heaven and of earth and of me, and of Don, Anna, Rachel and Eleanor, is capable of caring for His creation. And they all have accepted the gift Christ offers all by his death on the cross and resurrection. They too have eternal life with God in heaven. So what worries me? Still figuring it all out I guess. Please don't think I am expecting death from this round of cancer. But it is possible that I will always struggle with breast cancer. I am just being honest about my panic and fears and thoughts.

I did mention to Dr. Segal that I have had headaches (I have -- no lie!) since the last treatment. So he ordered another brain MRI, and this one was approved! Brain MRI scheduled for Monday, January 5th. Dr. Segal also gave me samples of a different anti-nausea medicine to try after the iv meds wear off in three days. We're hoping that will shorten the number of sick days.

Don had to work today, so Linda, Ron, and Janette worked together to make sure I was not alone for the appointments. THANK YOU. Even though I've done this once before, it is still scary and upsetting. It helps so very much to have someone with me. I enjoyed reading my "Chemo Notebook" that my family has prepared for me with photos and notes of encouragements. The additions for chemo #2 included precious art work and notes from my sweet Ellie and some of my younger nieces and nephews. One niece signed her art "your favorite niece Claire" and the other signed "from your dear Sophie". They are all so dear to me! I admit I cry easily (as in very) these days, but my chemo notebook had me teary again. I know I am so completely loved and supported by my family. Thank you Thank you Thank you.

Things seemed to go faster today, and we were done with everything in under four hours. Ron dropped us off, and drove in to pick us up as we literally stepped out of the office. Perfect timing!

I came home and ate lunch, had some raisnets, liquids, then took a short rest. I return for the neulasta injection on Friday afternoon. That isn't too bad, but it does make my bones and joints ache and ache and ache. But, hey, what's an ache or two, or five, when you're in the business of killing cancer cells?

Laurie Lane: Drenda,
You are a great writer! Again, thanks for taking us along on your journey. I thought of you often today and sent my caring thoughts your way. I hope to see you tomorrow if you are able to join us.
Love you!
Laurie
December 31, 2008 at 11:28pm

Gail Stempel Hilderbrand: I agree you are a fantastic writer. You mention the headaches, I wonder if you should rethink the zophram. It does cause headaches. I end up taking advil to get rid of the headaches caused by the zophram. Just a thought.
January 1 at 12:09pm

Drenda Lane Howatt has a New Year's Resolution: Cancer Free in 2009!
December 31, 2008 at 7:32pm

Andi Pedersen Jordan at 8:06pm December 31, 2008
Happy New Year! I'm with ya on that one!!

Laurie Lane at 11:31pm December 31, 2008
Yes!

Drenda Lane Howatt had a nice time at the barn with her family, then came home and slept for almost 4 hours. Fun party, great nap!
January 1, 2009 at 9:08pm

Becky Annus at 9:22pm January 1, 2009
Love naps!

Drenda Lane Howatt knows her days with hair are winding down....
January 2, 2009 at 7:32am

Don Howatt at 10:34pm January 2, 2009
Once you try bald you'll never go back...it's the breve' of head fashion

Emily Chandler Lawler: Hi Drenda,
I was praying for you yesterday when this passage came to mind, and I have been praying it for you...
"Yet this I call to mind
and therefore I have hope:
Because of the LORD's great love we are not consumed,
for his compassions never fail.
They are new every morning;
great is your faithfulness.
I say to myself, "The LORD is my portion;

therefore I will wait for him."
The LORD is good to those whose hope is in him,
to the one who seeks him;
it is good to wait quietly
for the salvation of the LORD...
Though he brings grief, he will show compassion, so great is his unfailing love."
Lamentations 3:21-26, 32

Drenda Lane Howatt is having a rough day.
January 3, 2009 at 12:27pm

Andi Pedersen Jordan at 1:19pm January 3, 2009
I'm sorry...wish I could make it go away!

Drenda Lane Howatt at 3:17pm January 3, 2009
I wish you could, too

Abigale Mary Lane at 3:37pm January 3, 2009
Drenda, are you working right now too?

Drenda Lane Howatt at 5:55pm January 3, 2009
I am working as much as I am able.

Abigale Mary Lane at 7:20pm January 4, 2009
Gosh, that must be something to juggle.

Drenda Lane Howatt is going bald at 3:30 this afternoon.
January 4, 2009 at 12:50pm

> Andi Pedersen Jordan at 1:19pm January 4, 2009
> Strong and courageous!
>
> Amber Lynn Montgomery Lane at 1:34pm January 4, 2009
> At least you have one of those good-looking Lane heads. Hang in there!
>
> Cindy McElmurry at 2:54pm January 4, 2009
> You are an amazing Lady. See you at dinner! Chicken Soup and cheese rolls!

So, the afternoon of January 4th held a shaving party in my living room. My sister Janette, her sons Patrick and Thomas, Don and I all went from 'hair' to 'no hair'. My sister Linda was fighting a cold, so she stayed home and had her husband shave her head at the same time as we were shaving. It was an emotional party. But we had some great laughs.

Drenda sits waiting for the head shaving to begin. (January 4, 2009)

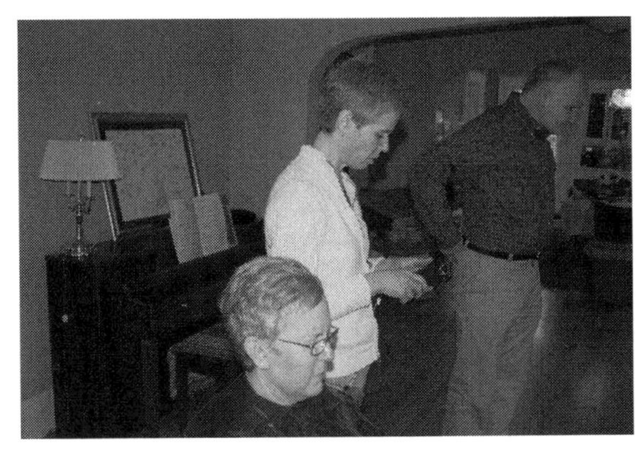

Beginning the shaving. It was very painful, physically and emotionally. (January 4, 2009)

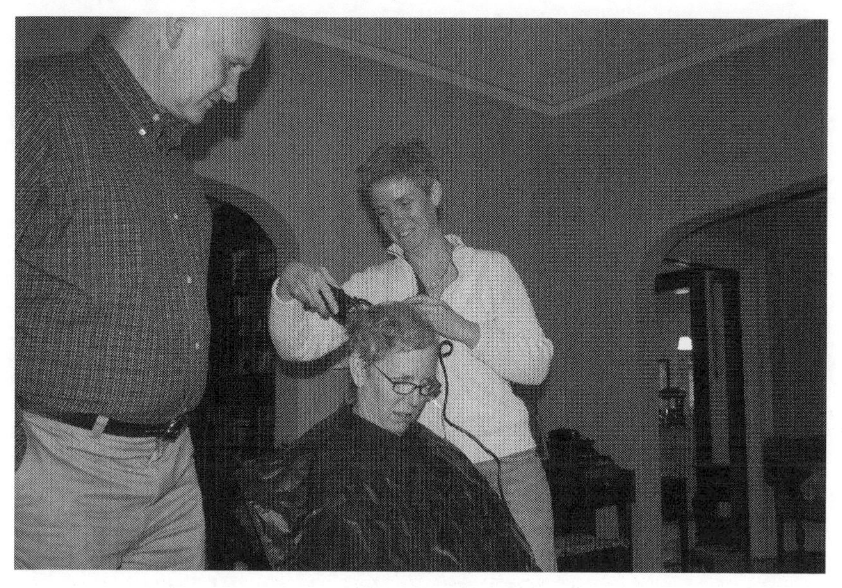

Anna and Ellie watching their Mom get her head shaved. (January 4, 2009)

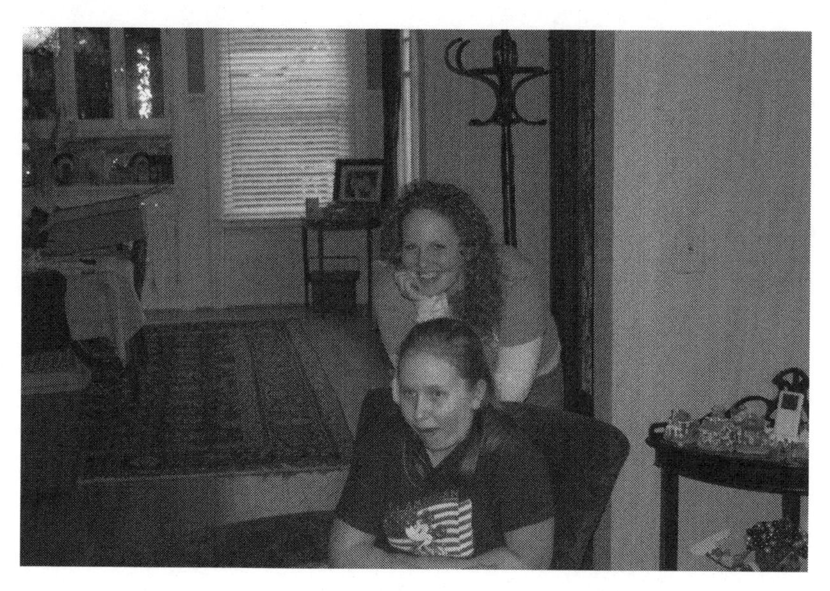

Janette shearing Drenda
The hair is coming off…(and out!) (January 4, 2009)

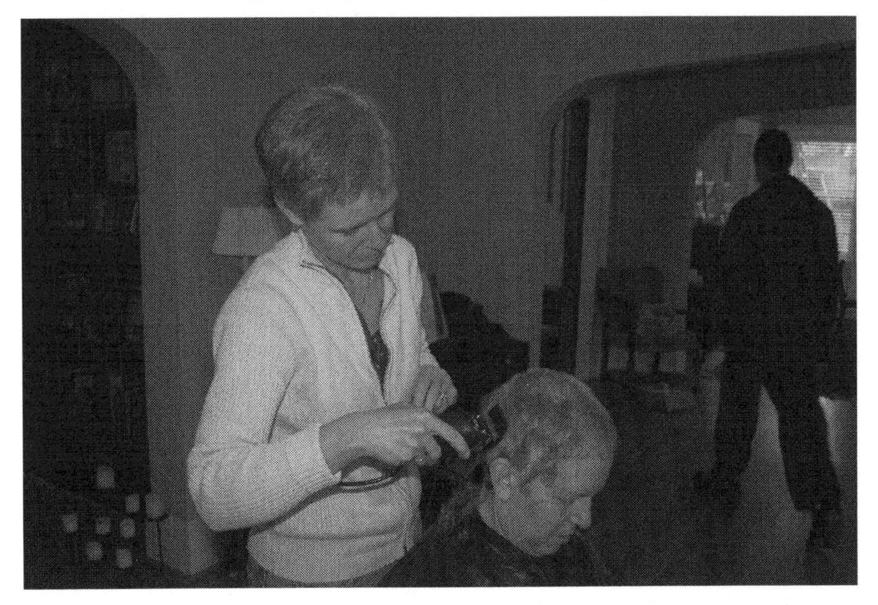

Don watching Drenda as she gets her head shaved. Cancer is hard on Don. (January 4, 2009)

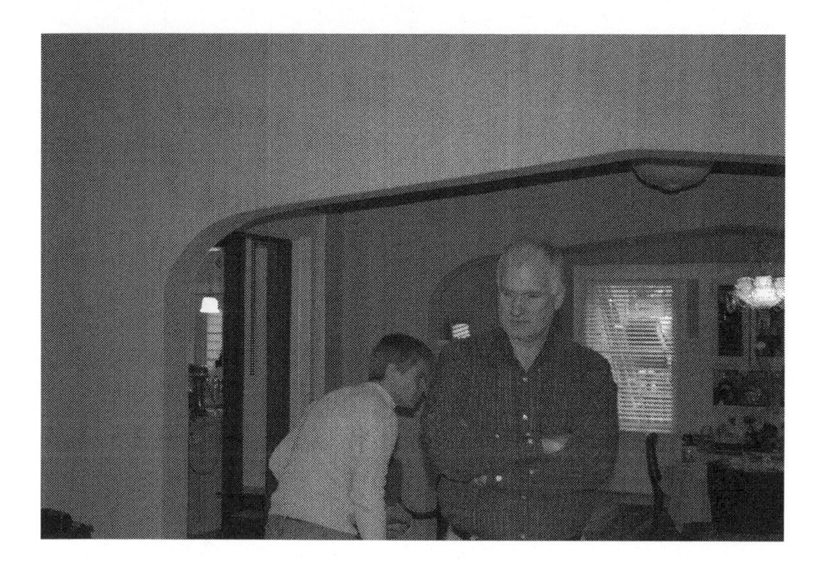

Drenda Lane Howatt did it! Along with Don, Janette, Linda, Patrick, and Thomas, Drenda now has a shaved head. Woo hoo! January 4, 2009 at 3:31pm

> Gail Hilderbrand at 4:26pm January 4, 2009
> SEXY!
>
> Drenda Lane Howatt at 4:27pm January 4, 2009
> Hmmm. Not sure about that! But I do realize how much I look like my brothers!
>
> Janette Wilkinson at 4:34pm January 4, 2009
> Oh my goodness! There seemed to be two Jory look-a-likes at Drenda's this afternoon!
>
> Jennifer Stady at 7:10pm January 4, 2009
> Who needs hair? You all look fantastic!
>
> Abigale Mary Lane at 7:17pm January 4, 2009
> You look great...is it open participation in the bald head event?
>
> Drenda Lane Howatt at 8:10pm January 4, 2009
> Open indeed! The Bald Support Corp is open to all who would like to make a bold/bald statement in support of me!

All done…and bald~
(January 4, 2009)

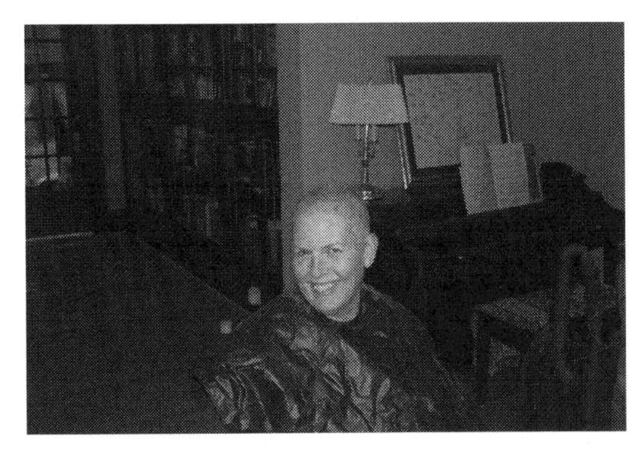

Janette is next! (January 4, 2009)

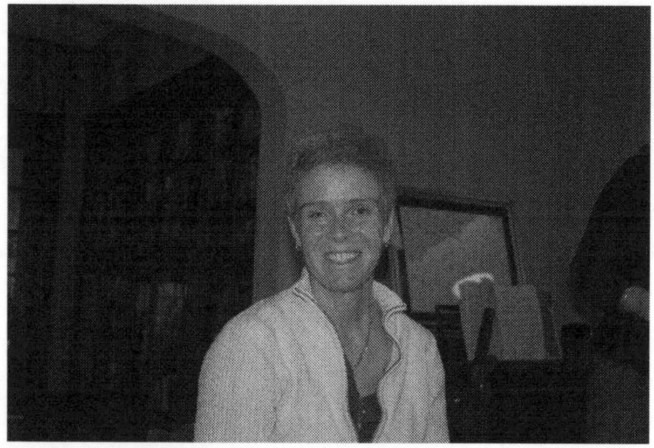

Janette's shave
in progress. (January 4, 2009)

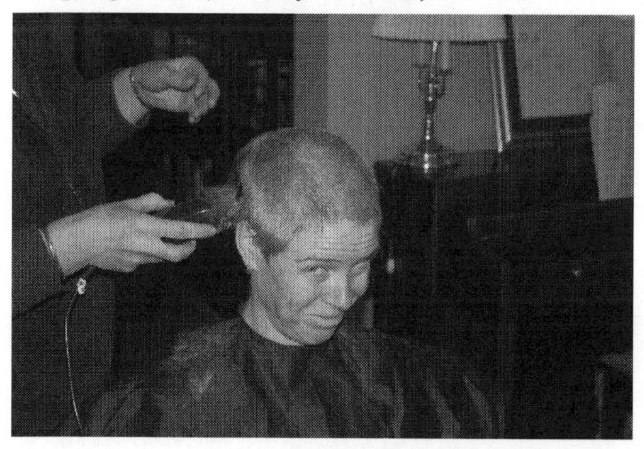

Janette is done! (January 4, 2009)

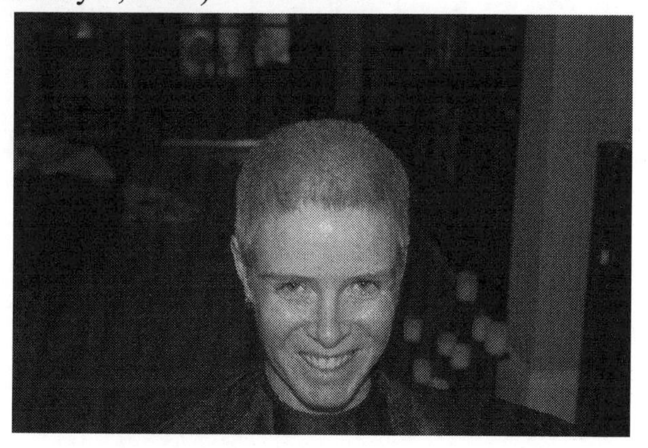

Don's turn to have his head shaved. (January 4, 2009)

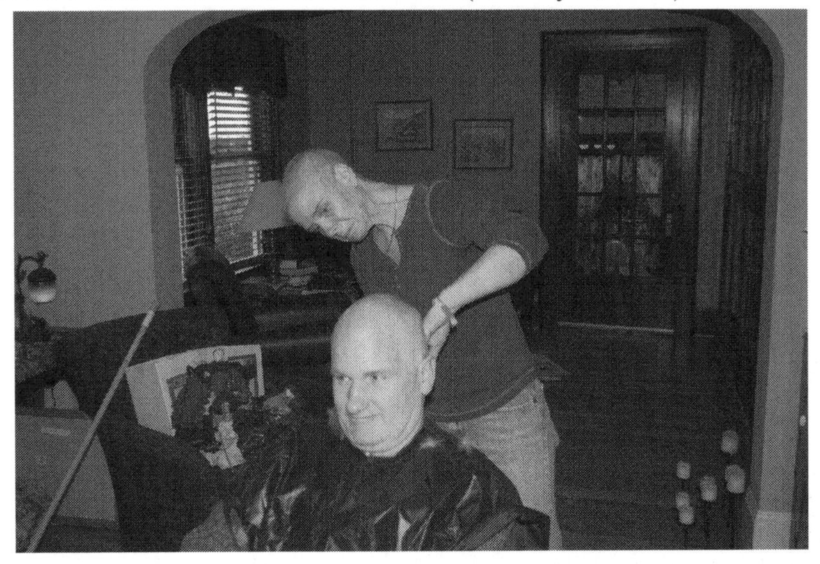

Drenda's nephew Thomas gets his head shaved. (January 4, 2009)

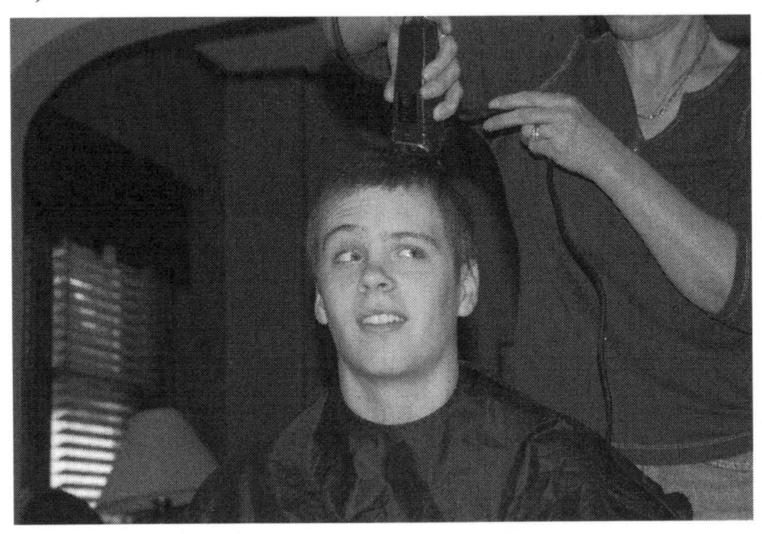

A little fun with Patrick's head shave…(January 4, 2009)

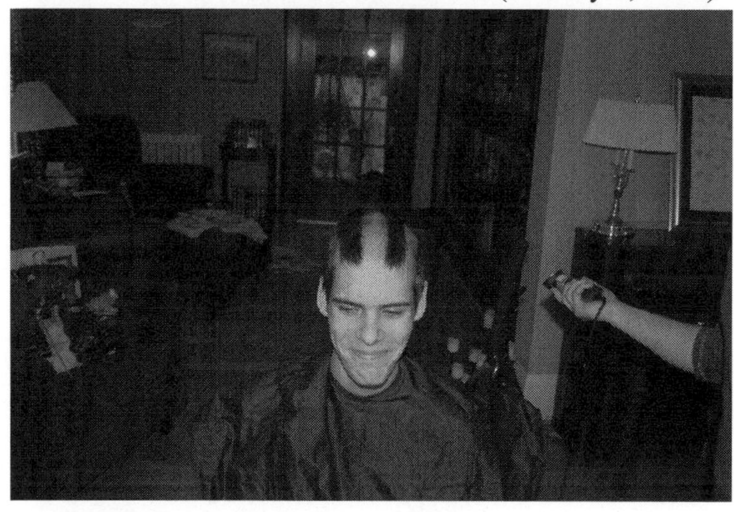

Shaving all done. (January 4, 2009)

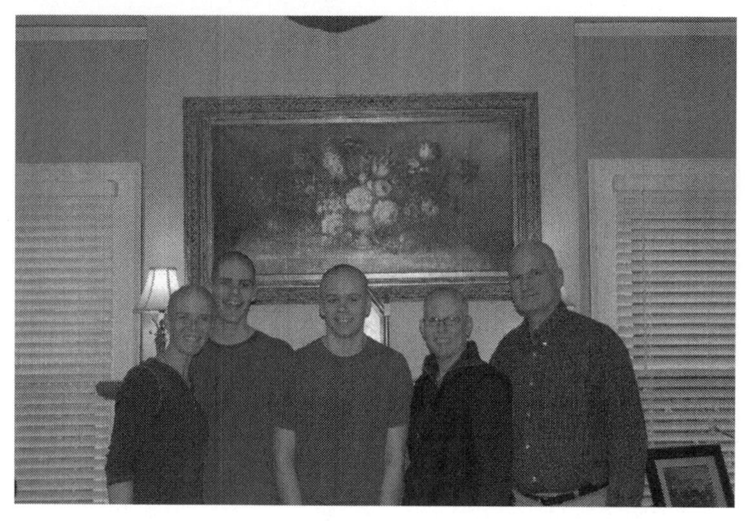

Linda shaved her head the same day as Drenda and Janette. Linda was fighting a sore throat and head cold, so she stayed away from the 'shaving party' and shaved at home. (January 4, 2009)

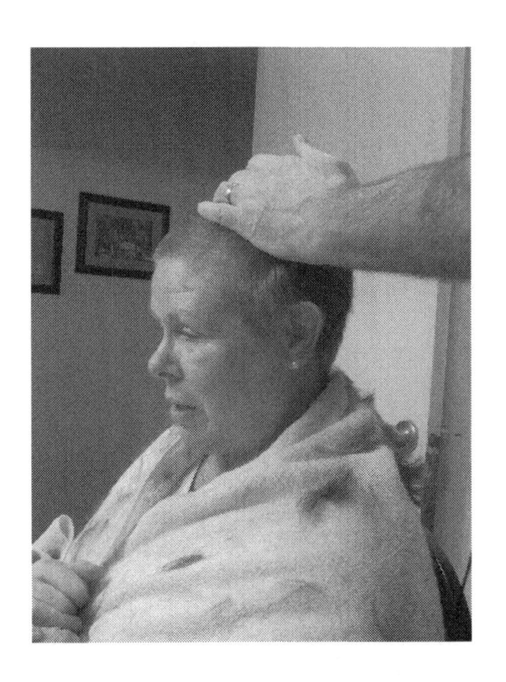

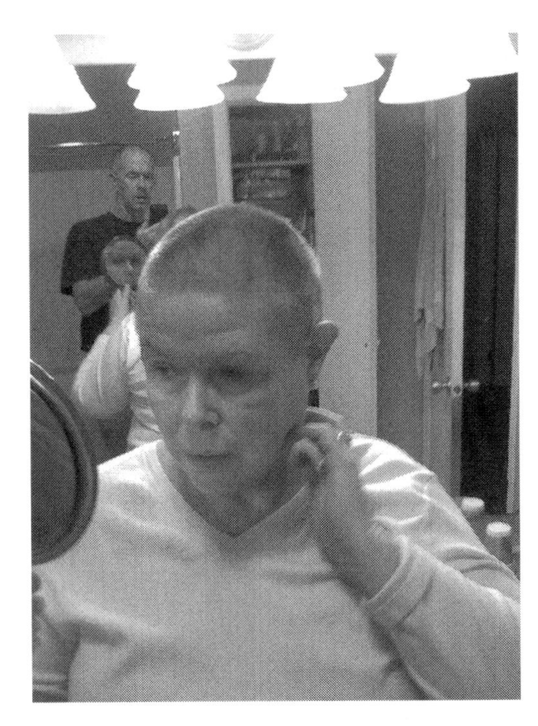

Linda taking her first look in the mirror. (January 4, 2009)

Drenda Lane Howatt is on her way to have a brain scan. No iodine, please.
January 5, 2009 at 8:14am

Becky Annus at 9:19am January 5, 2009
We're thinking about you...

Gail Hilderbrand at 1:20pm January 5, 2009
I hope you get an A on that test!

Claustrophobia...Worse Than I Thought

Tuesday, January 6, 2009 at 7:01pm

Brain MRI on Monday. In anticipation, I did take a sedative...but it did not sedate nearly enough. My Mother-in-law graciously gave up her morning to drive me to the appointment, and after filling out more paperwork, I was sent right in for the test. I learned from a friend at work that if you wear clothes without any metal, you don't have to change for the MRI. Good information!

This MRI exam was worse than the one I had of my chest because this time I was on my back (with back and hip pain, it is no fun to have to lie flat on your back for 40 minutes). The "tube" that they put me in for the MRI is so narrow that my arms cannot be at my sides...they have to be on my stomach. Because this test was of my brain, they had a contraption over my head that only made the "tube" seem more shallow and narrow. On top of the head gear, they attached a mirror so that I could see out of the enclosure. But looking in the mirror only confirmed how small the space was, so I did my best to keep my eyes closed. I did have ear plugs, but the noise is so loud that the plugs don't give much relief. But I came to appreciate the loud noises..."count the clunks, Drenda" "Breathe, Drenda, breathe. don't move. don't move". Every time I opened my eyes, the panic of claustrophobia started to set in. "Keep your eyes closed, Drenda, breathe." I did have a "panic" button that, if squeezed, would stop the test and rescue me. But then, I would just have to start over. So I REFUSED to squeeze, even though I desperately wanted to.

After 25 minutes, I was brought out, and the contrast was

injected into my hand. The injection was very slow, almost 5 minutes, during which time I was instructed to lay perfectly still...can't move my head. Problem is that when one can't move one's head, somehow, one's nose starts to itch tremendously. I managed to lay still, and then I was taken back inside the "enclosure" for more images...15 more minutes of silently talking to myself, calming my itches and my panic. yikes. Brain MRI is not something I'd be too excited about doing again, I must say.

The MRI tech told me that they were able to get some great images. Cool. I go to the doctor tomorrow for blood count checks, so I am hoping to hear about the results then.

Sally Park: Sounds like a rough procedure. You are a tough cookie!!
January 6, 2009 at 7:06pm

Drenda Lane Howatt: I didn't feel too "tough"...I felt weak and puny. Trouble getting through a little procedure in a little tube? What's the problem?!
January 6, 2009 at 7:07pm

Gail Stempel Hilderbrand: Good job, I couldn't have described that experience better. The nose itch part made me laugh, because that happens to me everytime!
January 6, 2009 at 8:34pm

Laurie Lane: I am so glad you are writing down your experiences. It helps me and will help you, if not now, later. AND you are a GREAT writer!
Sounds like you did an awesome job at keeping yourself calm and that's not easy.
January 6, 2009 at 8:36pm

Amber Smart: Drenda - I'm so proud of you! I've always been afraid of MRIs. I get claustrophobic with the covers over my head! You are continually in our prayers!
January 6, 2009 at 9:22pm

Tracy Cram: I know its been what seems like a million years since I've actually seen you, (I'm guessing its actually closer to 18 years rather than a million, although 18 still is a lot of years!) but I wanted you to know that you have been in my prayers since finding you here on FB.
January 6, 2009 at 11:43pm

Andi Pedersen Jordan: so Drenda, I haven't seen any pictures of your "new" look on here . . . someone must have gotten a picture Monday night . . .
January 7, 2009 at 8:49am

Pamela Zarek: Only the LORD can give you strength and the peace you need. HE is with you each step and each MRI you take. And believe or not your faith is growing with each test you take and have to trust in HIM for the results...I am praying for you dear sister...Hang in there. You are NOT alone. We, your sisters and brothers of the Faith are there with you!!!
January 7, 2009 at 11:03am

Kris Howatt: I know about the MRI claustrophobia - even with the sedative the only thing that kept me from pressing the panic button was not wanting to repeat the test.
January 8, 2009 at 3:47pm

Drenda Lane Howatt has, apparently, a brain that is "entirely normal", and "amazing bone marrow". According to Dr. Segal, oncologist extraordinaire.
January 7, 2009 at 4:42pm

Sally Park at 4:55pm January 7, 2009
Whoop Whoop!!!!! Celebrate tonight! Call out for dinner!!!!!!

Amber Lynn Montgomery Lane at 5:10pm January 7, 2009
That is good news! :)

Andi Pedersen Jordan at 5:13pm January 7, 2009
As if we didn't know . . . :-)

Janette Wilkinson at 5:21pm January 7, 2009
I knew your brain was "normal" as soon as we saw the shape of your head and it was without "dents". We now can assume that Linda and my brain must be entirely normal or even perhaps extraordinary! Now if we could just find out... "why do you talk like that?" Perhaps Dr. Segal could consult? Would it be a "cumulative" effect?

Drenda Lane Howatt at 5:25pm January 7, 2009
Yep. Entirely normal. I was a bit perplexed why it was just "normal"...doesn't he remember my outstanding intellect?

Gail Hilderbrand at 5:57pm January 7, 2009
I never doubted it for a minute! Celebrate!

Caitlin Lopez at 9:25am January 9, 2009
Yay! That's great!

Fall Out

Drenda Lane Howatt now knows that losing one's hair is a messy ordeal -- no matter how closely one's head is shaved...
January 8, 2009 at 6:26pm

Drenda Lane Howatt felt GOOD today, and tried to accomplish too much. Now her bones ache and ache. Oh my goodness.
January 9, 2009 at 7:01pm

> Drenda Lane Howatt at 7:14pm January 9, 2009
> I tried to do too much because I only have 5 good days left until my next treatment. Feeling well 6 days out of 14 doesn't give nearly enough time to do all a wife, mom, policy coordinator, and manager needs to get done. yikes! But the "good" news is that I only have two more of these treatments to go. I have been assured that after those two treatments, the next twelve are much easier. Here's to hope!
>
> Cindy Knight at 7:58pm January 9, 2009
> I have nothing to complain about. When I read this, it sure makes me thankful for my health. I am so sorry that you are having to deal with this but I will be praying for you. I love that you post updates on your status. Thanks and have a good weekend.

Drenda Lane Howatt is having another good day and is determined to get the house de-cluttered and CLEAN. dang nab it.
January 10, 2009 at 10:10am

Drenda Lane Howatt is happy to be home from work and trying to not think about cancer and treatment. Oh my. Thursday is coming fast.
January 12, 2009 at 4:55pm

Benefits of Total (Almost) Baldness... Let Me Count the Ways!

Tuesday, January 13, 2009 at 6:07pm

So, first let me explain. I am not (yet) totally bald. The sad thing is that all of my hair that had any discernable color is out. What is left is white. As in completely. Now, who knew I had so much hair without the red? (Ok, be quiet. Not a real question I wanted an answer to. You could not have known. No way.)

This means that I have approximately 1/3 of my hair still on my head. Stubby and white, and worst of all, patchy. But I am not complaining, because:

Not having hair has its advantages!

1. Shampoo? A little dab ‘ll do ya
2. Conditioner? what? who needs it?
3. Drying time? done! the ultimate in towel dry.
4. Brushing through tangles? ha ha
5. Hair in your food? not a chance (not now that most of it has fallen out!)
6. Bad Hair Day? no such thing
7. Pre-Menopausal Hot Flashes? a cold bald head helps the cooling process immensely!
8. I can take a deep, hot, bubble bath without worrying about my hair getting wet and soggy. aaaahhh. that’s nice.
9. Saving $$ on hair cuts/colors
10. shower time cut way down - in and swish and out and you’re done

At this point, I still have my eyelashes and eyebrows...maybe they'll defy the poison and stay. I am hopeful.

On another topic, I got the information on the bill for the brain MRI today. Just under $2000. Makes me thankful we waited for the insurance to pre-authorize (the second MRI order -- they're still denying the first). We had considered going ahead with the MRI and paying for it ourselves, but that is ALOT of money.

My next treatment is Thursday morning. If you think about me on Thursday or the next 8 days after that, please pray for me -- pray that I'll be able to get through with the least amount of nausea and cramping. Pray that I'll remain encouraged and hopeful about the outcome of these treatments, and most of all, please pray that the treatment is successful and I will be declared cancer free at the end of chemo and radiation (end of June/early July).

Drenda

Laurie Lane: Drenda,
With your attitude the cancer doesn't have a chance!
I will be thinking of you over the next several days, whoa, what am I saying.... You are in my thoughts every day. Every day I send positive thoughts your way and every day I am impressed by your attitude, courage, and your willingness to share your struggles, both your bad ones and your funny ones. I love you!
January 13, 2009 at 6:58pm

Drenda Lane Howatt: Thank you. I have been appreciative that this week I've actually had a few hours at a time on different days where I almost forgot I had cancer! Those times are a true gift.
January 13, 2009 at 7:05pm

Andi Pedersen Jordan: Hi, there... I've been away but haven't

stopped thinking about you. . . and that lunch that we get before I have lunch with anyone else in “your” office gets. :-)
January 13, 2009 at 10:55pm

Lindsay Chandler Mandjek: Other advantages to hairlessness?

1. Ride in a convertible or on a speedboat without getting the “wind-blown” tangles
2. Don’t have to take your hair out of the drain
3. You can actually feel a head massage!
January 14, 2009 at 2:32am

Drenda Lane Howatt: Lindsay, excellent additions! Thank you.
January 14, 2009 at 5:17pm

Drenda Lane Howatt is wondering if she ordered too many Girl Scout cookies...but she has a great Brownie to purchase from!
January 13, 2009 at 7:38pm

> Janette Wilkinson at 7:57pm January 13, 2009
> how many did you order?

Drenda Lane Howatt is going to take a hot bath and then go to bed...all in preparation for Chemo #3. Gotta be emotionally ready and rested.
January 14, 2009 at 7:20pm

> Andi Pedersen Jordan at 7:33pm January 14, 2009
> Strong and courageous . . . go, Drenda!
>
> Maureen Gatens Thompson at 7:35pm January 14, 2009
> Just remember what I told you...I celebrated being 24 years breast cancer free on November 20th. I will be sending healing thoughts your way tomorrow. Maureen
>
> Drenda Lane Howatt at 7:38pm January 14, 2009
> I do remember, Maureen...every day! It helps. I think the stats say about 85% of women with the type/stage cancer I have are cancer free in 10 years. I am hoping to be in the majority this time...
>
> Maureen Gatens Thompson at 7:44pm January 14, 2009
> Just remember...my prognosis was very, very dismal because I was only 30 years old and age works against you in breast cancer. The chemo levels they gave me were too toxic to give now. So getting old is grand and increases your odds. Another reason to be thankful for each day we have and to celebrate. Hugs!

Becky Annus at 7:45pm January 14, 2009
Your family loves you...

Drenda Lane Howatt at 7:47pm January 14, 2009
Becky - I so know it! Thank you for all your care of and for me and Don, Anna, Rachel, and Ellie.

Janette Wilkinson at 9:07pm January 14, 2009
Drenda, STRONG and COURAGEOUS are we! You will be fore front in my thoughts tomorrow. I love you!

Drenda Lane Howatt is going back to war today...killing cancer cells.
January 15, 2009 at 8:11am

Shannon Swope at 11:25am January 15, 2009
Hey friend, thinking of you and praying for you today. Let me know if you'd like some company...

Gail Hilderbrand at 1:16pm January 15, 2009
You are incredible how you snap back after chemo. You inspire me!

Caitlin Lopez at 4:15pm January 16, 2009
Kick some butt lady!

Drenda Lane Howatt hates the recovery from cancer war...ugh.
January 17, 2009 at 8:50am

Andi Pedersen Jordan at 1:50pm January 17, 2009
I'm sorry.

Drenda Lane Howatt is quite nauseated and thus totally unmotivated.
January 19, 2009at 8:23am

Kris Howatt at 1:47pm January 19, 2009
It was hard to get motivated yesterday and today with no electricity - everything I wanted to do required a power source.

Sally Park at 4:37pm January 19, 2009
I am sorry you are feeling so icky. I think about you all the time.
Looking forward to Saturday, hopefully you will feel up to making it.

Drenda Lane Howatt tried to work today, but was overcome by nausea. Oh, this is getting old.
January 20, 2009 at 5:05pm

Andi Pedersen Jordan at 5:21pm January 20, 2009
Bummer...hope it's only temporary!

Drenda Lane Howatt at 5:28pm January 20, 2009
My hope as well...but I do think 6 days is much too long. Of course, what I think does not, apparently, matter.

Jennifer Stady at 5:46pm January 20, 2009
I'm so sorry Drenda. Is the nausea supposed to subside soon? Does anything work in making you feel better once it sets in?

Drenda Lane Howatt at 5:48pm January 20, 2009
Nope. I am thankful for the five meds I have that supposedly make it better...can't imagine what it would be like without them. Last time, the nausea was gone by end of day 8...that's only two more days.

Andi Pedersen Jordan at 5:53pm January 20, 2009
Wish I could help make it go away.

Jennifer Stady at 7:15pm January 20, 2009
Well, I will be sending you lots of strength and love for the next two days!

Gail Hilderbrand at 7:29pm January 20, 2009
"Come to Me, all who are weary and heavy-laden, and I will give you rest" (Matthew 11:28)

Drenda Lane Howatt is only a "tad bit" nauseated...woo hoo! It was a GREAT day. And thanks to Miss B for coming to clean my kitchen (including the frig!). Great day.
January 22, 2009 at 5:17pm

Maureen Gatens Thompson at 5:34pm January 22, 2009
You've crossed another bridge, rounded a corner, beat the monster & lived another 24 hours. The nausea is lessening...YIPEE! You can only feel better from here on out. I remember after I finished chemo, I went back about 3 months later for a check-up and threw up as soon as I got inside the doctor's office. Fortunately, I made it to the bathroom ...

Drenda Lane Howatt at 5:36pm January 22, 2009
Yikes. That's a story to remember! I'll have chemo through April, but only one more that is so awful, supposedly. One more.

Sally Park at 6:58pm January 22, 2009
What a relief!!

Amanda Ouellette at 9:38pm January 22, 2009
WOOHOO!!! I'm glad that today was a good day. I'll pray that tomorrow is just as good!

No “Sorry Buts”...

Wednesday, January 21, 2009 at 2:39am

...allowed at our house. We’ve tried to teach our girls that an apology cannot come with a “but”. As in “I’m sorry I hurt you, BUT you made me mad”. True repentance and requesting of forgiveness cannot include rationalization for your wrong.

I was all set to apologize for complaining here on fb, but the apology was going to come with a “but”. So, following our house rule, I will not apologize, because I am not truly sorry. I am discouraged. Deeply discouraged.

I have completed three chemo treatments so far. And they are not fun. Almost not even tolerable. I am awake now with pretty severe stomach cramps. I know, I know, there are people much worse off than me. But it doesn’t feel that way. I have been sick for 6 days. SICK. However, given my experience with hyper-emesis (acute vomiting) and hospitalization with each of my pregnancies, I am doing my best to REFUSE my over-active gag reflex and avoid throwing-up. I know I would not be able to stop, and would probably end up in the hospital. But sometimes...

So many people have encouraged me. “You’re 75% done with the bad treatments!” “Only one more to go!” Yikes. I CAN’T do one more. I will do one more, but let me tell you, it is not easy to willingly walk into Northwest Cancer Specialists and submit to more poison. Hard to keep my eye on the “prize”, so to speak. These are the times that I recognize the enemy at work. But I am too weak to fight him. I rely on the prayers and support of family and friends.

So, we careen along this journey of breast cancer, with so many ups and even more downs. The difference between us? Some of you can choose to stop reading. I will continue to write, and live, this journey. And why, exactly, do I write? Many reasons. Probably therapy. Education. Notification.

But the real reasons?

My babies. Anna, Rachel, and Ellie. My sisters. Linda, Laurie, Sally, Becky, and Janette. My nieces. Audrey, Dustine, Jessica, Amanda, Denise, Abi, Marilla, Sophie, and Claire. All of whom must now answer the question "history of breast cancer in your family?" with "...yes..." I write so that they can know this journey, and not be as frightened as I have been. That we all can look back and learn from the struggles and joys we experience. That, through it all, God will be glorified and I will be a faithful and true witness to His goodness.

Now, for sleep.

Drenda

Drenda Lane Howatt: I knew this was a bad idea -- to name people. Chemo brain is a real condition you know. I forgot sweet niece Natalie. For her, too.
January 21, 2009 at 6:03am

Andi Pedersen Jordan: Happy anti-nausea thoughts your way. Go, away, cancer . . . you are not welcome here!

Strong and courageous, Drenda. Strong and courageous.
January 21, 2009 at 8:23am

Susan Rasmussen Lane: Don't worry about it. Natalie was not

offended, and neither was I. You're in our prayers.
January 21, 2009 at 8:39am

Amber Lynn Montgomery Lane: You are so brave to share how difficult this is. To be honest about it. To fight this fight in the first place! I always feel like typing encouraging words, and then think how trite they sound compared to what you're really going through. Good thoughts. Prayers. Faith. You'll make it.
January 21, 2009 at 10:57am

Sally Park: Sally Park at 5:08pm January 21
You are incredible! You are sharing and giving all of us a real tangible gift. I had no idea cancer treatment could be so hard, physically or emotionally. Give Rachel a big hug this weekend (from me)
January 21, 2009 at 5:11pm

Miles Purcell: I havent thought about this that way before with the sorry but thing thats very true I'll remember that
January 21, 2009 at 5:24pm

Andi Pedersen Jordan: And I whole-heartedly agree with Amber's thoughts. It's hard for me to figure out what to say . . . so let us mumble, jumble our way through figuring out a way to show you we care about you.
January 21, 2009 at 5:27pm

Drenda Lane Howatt: You are all so wonderful to me! I truly do not know how anyone could get through this cancer thing without such a tremendous support group such as I have. Your encouraging words are read over and over, trust me.
January 21, 2009 at 5:31pm

Laurie Lane: You are awesome! I love you!!!
January 21, 2009 at 5:46pm

Megan Kochendorfer: I'm praying for you to have restful, refreshing sleep...and that the nausea will recede.

January 21, 2009 at 6:15pm

Marilla Park: you are so strong Auntie Drenda =) you are always in my prayers
January 21, 2009 at 7:57pm

Tara L Koch: I taught my kids that if they say 'but', it erases everything they just said. So they have to say 'and'. I am sorry...and, I wanted to tell you... Anytime they wanted to say 'but'...they had to say 'and'. It changes the whole dialog!

It was nice to connect with you again Drenda...thank you!
Praying for His grace to cover you...
Blessings,
T
January 21, 2009 at 9:18pm

Jennifer Stady: Drenda, I'm so touched by your words and what you are going though. I think of you every day.
January 22, 2009 at 6:58pm

Drenda Lane Howatt is making room in her freezer...
January 23, 2009 at 6:50pm

Suzanne Lee Laisner at 7:14pm January 23, 2009
What are you making room for??? Don't be tempted to use it when the hot flashes come!

Drenda Lane Howatt at 7:37pm January 23, 2009
My sisters are filling my freezer with ready-to-cook meals!

Laurie Lane at 8:05pm January 23, 2009
Some brothers may be involved too!

Sally Park at 9:03pm January 23, 2009
I am so excited!!!

Sally Park at 12:43pm January 25, 2009
I hope you have room in your freezer. 14 casserole size dinners worth of room....

Drenda Lane Howatt is dreading tomorrow, but looking forward to a week from Friday! Keeping her eye on the end of nausea. It WILL come, she knows, and she is happy for that.
January 28, 2009 at 4:30pm

Kris Howatt at 6:41pm January 28, 2009
Last one - I hope it has gone quickly for you.

Gail Hilderbrand at 6:57pm January 28, 2009
Think happy, joyous thoughts...I will be

Becky Annus at 8:38am January 29, 2009
A week from Friday-end of nausea-will be cause for celebration!
Thinking of you today.
Becky

Chemo #4

Thursday, January 29, 2009 at 7:20pm

Today was the day for chemo battle #4 -- the last treatment of the nasty (but, hopefully, effective) adriamyiacin and cytoxan. These are the drugs I can never have again, as at least one of them would prove to be fatal. I was a bit emotional as I sat in the blue recliner waiting for the poisons...and then, as I worked through it and calmed myself, I came back to the "it is what it is, and this is what it takes to make it different".

Dr. Segal was not happy with me when he learned that I had informed the research people at the clinical trial that I would sign up for the trial but would not stay in it if I was assigned to receive just the new drug. Shouldn't have told them that because they will think Dr. Segal is in "collusion" with me. So far from the truth -- he thinks I should do the study no matter which part I am assigned. Oh well.

I have continued to impress Dr. Segal in so many ways (other than the one mentioned above...) I know big words, my bone marrow is amazing (repeated today), AND I have continued to work. "That is impressive. So impressive. Hardly anyone works through this treatment." Perhaps I should reconsider and stop working? NO! It helps me to take my mind off of cancer. Besides, there are still those pesky bills to pay, darn them.

I have an echocardiogram (again) on February 6th, and a chest xray the same day. This is in preparation for the next steps in the treatment. I start weekly chemo with Taxol on February 12th. Taxol can cause an allergic reaction...so pray that I will be immune from that. There is an alternative, chemically related drug, but from what I've heard of the alternative, it is harder to handle. Taxol rarely causes nausea (!), but can cause loss of finger and toe nails. Can also cause neuropathy (numbness?) in fingers and toes. In conjunction with the Taxol, I will start the her2-neu inhibitors. Depending on the clinical trial, those drugs could be started at the same time. If I am on herceptin, I'll have injections weekly for one year. So I am glad that it will start with the beginning of Taxol and not wait until Taxol is done. That saves me 12 weeks. I should know more about the trial next week.

I have been reading in the book of James from the Bible. In verse of 2 of the first chapter, James tells us to "consider it pure joy when you face trials of various kinds..." Pure joy? Yes, because trials test my faith, and testing produces endurance and lets me grow as a whole person, to develop spiritual maturity, and stability of character. It is through tackling what I don't want that I am forced to look to God. James does not promise that God will take away the problem, or make it any easier, only that, if I let Him, God will give me what I need to get through. The trial might test me to the limit, but I will be the better for it. Hard advice, but liberating. Accept the cancer, trust God, and grow. In the end, that will bring peace.

Philip Yancey wrote "Faith means trusting in advance what will only make sense in reverse".

My faith has already been strengthened by looking in reverse...finding the lump through pain ("early stage breast cancer is painless" --not mine, apparently!), the fast trip to surgery, oncology, etc. The complete removal of the cancerous tissue, the cancer-free lymphnode, the availability of excellent health insurance. The wonderful support of family and friends.

I am convinced that God is at work here -- even through my tremendous weakness, His strength is evident to me. I hope He is evident, at least through my cancer journey, to you as well. There are no coincidences with God. None. And there are no surprises to Him. None. He is not just my God. He is THE God, Creator of Heaven and Earth, of you and of me. You can bet I have asked Him lots of hard questions...most beginning with the word "why". But every day that I can read His word, He answers me. With Scripture that speaks directly to me. Like this morning's passage in James -- every trial pure joy? And, how exactly, Lord, do I do that? But then He tells me! Just ask Him for the strength and wisdom, and He will supply it.

I must trust and obey, for there's no other way, to be happy in Jesus, but to trust and obey. And with His help, I will be strong and courageous and make it through this battle of cancer. But it is His strength that strengthens me.

Accepting. Trusting. Growing.

Andi Pedersen Jordan: Yes, you are ever so strong and courageous.
So proud of you ... I just ached . . . and you still work! :-)
January 29, 2009 at 11:38pm

Lori Buckelew: I have been blessed to read your journey through this "trial" of cancer. Your strength through Christ is an encouragement and blessing to all. Having been one of the "impressive" ones to work through the same treatment, I understand the peace there is in keeping yourself busy and focused. It helps to not dwell on the situation but to focus on The God that is giving you the strength to have pure joy in the midst of it. I heard the saying that "Joy is not the absence of trials, but the presence of God in the midst of those trials". Thank you for living that everyday to those around you!
January 30, 2009 at 10:21am

Caitlin Lopez: I'm so proud to know you. And so privileged to be encouraged by watching your unfaltering faith in God.

I'm glad you're my landlady:)
January 30, 2009 at 3:45pm

x + 32 = 50

Friday, February 6, 2009 at 7:11am

What does "x" equal? The number of days out of the last 50 that I have felt functional, o.k., or close to "normal". As in not terribly nauseated and/or receiving treatment.

For those of you who may struggle with math, the answer is that "x" = 18. 18 out of the last 50 days. I was beginning to feel like a baby - always complaining and crying about how awful I felt. No matter how hard I tried to control them, the tears were (and are) so often present. But when I did the math, I felt better. Because 18 is not very many. Add in to the mix that within those 50 days, we had college girls come and go, prepared for and celebrated Christmas, got through big snow storms, I continued to work two jobs (semi), and lived normal life. In retrospect, I did pretty good, I think.

End of math lesson for today.

Dan D Davis: Drenda,

Math is good. Math is our friend. Math can make us feel better.

I pray God's best is yours today and in the coming weeks...
February 6, 2009 at 7:47am

Tara L Koch: You are so inspirational! I love the way you write...
February 6, 2009 at 9:07am

Rachel Howatt: my mom is strong and courageous!
February 6, 2009 at 12:56pm

Ginger Clausen: "Do not fear for I am with you. Do not

anxiously look about you for I am your God." Isaiah 41 is my favorite passage. You're doing a good job of letting His light shine through your cracks even if sometimes you feel more cracked than whole! I'll keep praying for you to pass this math test!
February 6, 2009 at 7:58pm

Sally Park: You are right! Mom always used to say that we are never given more in life than we are capable of handling. You have proved that to be true. One day at a time is my motto!
February 6, 2009 at 8:31pm

Sally Park: Love you! by the way
February 6, 2009 at 8:33pm

Drenda Lane Howatt: :-) thanks
February 6, 2009 at 8:35pm

Drenda Lane Howatt is back! Hosting 242 once again this week.
February 15, 2009 at 5:18pm

Janette Wilkinson at 5:52pm February 15, 2009
What is 242?

Drenda Lane Howatt is attending the Breast Cancer Issues Conference at the Convention Center on February 28th because she is a breast cancer survivor.
February 15, 2009 at 9:17pm

Becky Annus at 7:57am February 16, 2009
...a strong and courageous breast cancer survivor...

Drenda Lane Howatt hates going out at night for meetings. Especially in the cold. Hates it.
February 17, 2009 at 6:29pm

Abbi Howatt at 6:46pm February 17, 2009
:-(I'm sorry

Drenda Lane Howatt just got the call from Dr. Segal...treatment postponed yet again. That means another echo-cardiogram, more lab work, and a physical exam. oh my goodness.
February 18, 2009 at 5:00pm

Sally Park at 7:49pm February 18, 2009
That is disappointing…I am sure you want to get moving.

Drenda Lane Howatt at 9:16pm February 18, 2009
YES! These delays are throwing major problems into my plans...need to go L.A. in May for a certain someone's college graduation (still able to, with another little delay), and now no more family vacation in June. Drat.

These delays mean radiation treatment will last until at least July. ugh

Shannon Swope at 9:30am February 19, 2009
Hey friend...that's a bummer but ya just gotta go with it. Can you get dirty hands tomorrow? You know...."all in God's timing..." :) There's always the ENTIRE picure we don't get to see...you're in my thoughts and prayers-s-
What an absolutely gorgeous drive home yesterday!

Drenda Lane Howatt is back from the doctor visit. ekg normal (no change from the one two weeks ago). Echo-cardiogram tomorrow. This cancer thing sure takes a lot of time.
February 19, 2009 at 6:54pm

Andi Pedersen Jordan at 9:13pm February 19, 2009
Good news then! Tell that cancer thing to go away!

Kim Burns at 9:25am February 21, 2009
Ugh... how hard to spend so much time in doctor offices or medial clinics. Yes it does add so much time to your already full schedule.
Ok there must be a lot of sitting around. Can you catch up on some reading? Start some of those novels you have set aside for another time. I am so glad to hear the ekg was normal.

Drenda Lane Howatt is visiting Anna in two weeks!
February 20, 2009 at 3:43pm

Drenda Lane Howatt is preparing to go downtown with Ellie for the traditional 13th birthday overnight including ear piercing and make-over! All to mark the passage to teenager.
February 21, 2009 at 9:52am

Rachel Howatt at 10:28am February 21, 2009
Take lots of pictures!

Don Howatt at 11:44am February 21, 2009
Don't worry about me Rachel, I'll be fine!

Rachel Howatt at 12:39pm February 21, 2009
Aw Dad! You should have a batman marathon

Kim Burns at 3:52pm February 21, 2009
Can I come for a piercing and make over? Don and Rachel are making me smile. The kids never worry about poor old dad. He can take care of himself... right? Well maybe.... :)

Drenda Lane Howatt is home. Ellie's ears are sufficiently pierced...and we had a GREAT time downtown. Highly recommend The Nines hotel (at Macy's downtown).
February 22, 2009 at 2:35pm

Screaming

Sunday, February 22, 2009 at 4:53pm

I still have hair. Some. White. And it was long. 1/4 inch or so. But no more. As I progress through this "cancer thing", I find myself growing stronger, and even more courageous. For I am beginning to not care about convention. As in having hair, or having my bald-ish head covered in public. As a result, I just finished completely "buzzing" my head. Not shaved with a razor, but as close to that as possible. I was more self-conscious with 1/4 inch long hair than I think I will be with hair so short it cannot be measured.

I have pretty much stopped wearing my "hair" (as in wig). And, while having a bald-ish head is COLD, I am beginning to cut back on wearing hats as well. I need to be comfortable enough with my body to be able to take the hat off at any time -- especially during a hot flash. Because hot flashes are HOT. And sweaty. Hmmm. What would be worse, being a bald woman in public, or being a bald woman who has fainted in public?

Friday morning, I had the second echo-cardiogram. And I went without a hat. It was freeing. Even the second glances and stares from strangers -- while a bit difficult at first -- did not bother me enough to put my hat on. I still always travel with an emergency head-covering. Friday, I grew stronger.

Being bald in public is hard. Not the bald part. But the part that screams, without anyone saying a word, to passersby "I have CANCER". THAT is the hard part.

But I do have cancer.

And I am bald.

So, I'll just continue to live while my body screams.

My new normal.

Andi Pedersen Jordan: Yes, you are so very strong and courageous.
February 22, 2009 at 6:32pm

Annette Mattson: I think you should wear fabulous earrings and/or sensuous and or bright lipstick/lipgloss to show off and draw attention to the beauty of the strength you carry, inside and out.
February 22, 2009 at 10:30pm

Rachel Howatt: I love you mom!
February 22, 2009 at 11:27pm

Shannon Swope: NOW you're talkin'! :) Love you friend~
February 23, 2009 at 8:09am

Amanda Lane: You go girl! You're making bald the new hot... Such a fierce woman I get to call aunt (without lying). Sending you all my love.
February 23, 2009 at 8:35am

Zachary Lane Koval: You're amazing. :D
February 23, 2009 at 8:36am

Laurie Lane: I agree with Zachary!
February 23, 2009 at 6:50pm

Drenda Lane Howatt is loving the fact that she thought ahead enough to get a frozen dinner entree out this morning and set the oven timer to cook it for her while she was at work.
February 24, 2009 at 5:41pm

Drenda Lane Howatt worked on taxes and FAFSA...still more to do. ugh
February 24, 2009 at 9:21pm

> Carri McClure: Drenda, I am incredibly touched by your courage. I absolutely adore your entries and I think they can speak to so many women. Have you approached the Oregonian, Willamette Weekly with an idea for a column?
>
> I will touch base with my contacts at several magazines and the Oprah Winfrey show as well as the View. I have been so inspired by reading your entries.
>
> best, Carri

Perhaps More Waiting...

Wednesday, February 25, 2009 at 8:00pm

I heard late this afternoon that I am still not "randomized" (is that even a word?) in the clinical trial. FRUSTRATING! I have been assured that the randomization will be done tomorrow morning. That is important because I am scheduled to begin (after two delays) the second phase of chemotherapy tomorrow at noon.

As it stands currently, I have a 50% chance of being able to go ahead with treatment tomorrow. And a 50% chance of having to wait, yet again. If I have to wait, it would be for the trial drug to be delivered, and that takes two days. Waiting means that treatment would start on Monday or Tuesday, or so I've been assured.

I don't know if participating in the trial is the best thing, the right thing to do. It's a risk. A guess. A gamble, either way. And a lot of stress.

Waiting.

Wondering.

Questioning.

Sally Park: Keep us posted. You have alot to deal with. Through this you are a wave breaker and an exceptional role model for

the women in this family, young and old (er) =)
Thank you !
February 26, 2009 at 7:35am

Amber Lynn Montgomery Lane: I agree with Sally. You are so strong and courageous! It is a gamble. Related story: signing up for trial treatment for breast cancer prolonged my own Grandma's life 15 years longer than they had given her to live. Unfortunately I never knew her in person, but she DID leave me an amazing legacy of strength and courage.
February 26, 2009 at 7:58am

Drenda Lane Howatt: thank you for your kind words! I don't "feel" strong, but I know I am getting STRONGER every day. It is what it is, and I am what I am...I am slowly coming to accept both, without trying to change or deny what I am feeling as I go through this.
February 26, 2009 at 10:09pm

Drenda Lane Howatt is counting the days until she goes to Los Angeles to see Anna perform at Azusa Pacific University! Can't wait to see her baby.
February 26, 2009 at 8:30am

Andi Pedersen Jordan at 9:07am February 26, 2009
Any word on the "randomization"

Drenda Lane Howatt at 9:47am February 26, 2009
Just now...randomized into the third arm of the study...I will receive both drugs! That means treatment is on for today! First the Herceptin (proven drug) for twelve weeks along with the chemo, then a six week break. After the break, the trial drug Tykerb (laptanib) for the remainder of a year. Good news!

Andi Pedersen Jordan at 10:04am February 26, 2009
Excellent! Good! Thinking of you.

Sally Park at 12:13pm February 26, 2009
Wonderful!

Chemo on Track Again...
How Odd to be Excited for Poison

Thursday, February 26, 2009 at 6:47pm

The call came this morning. I had been randomized. Into the third arm of the clinical trial. Good news, because the third arm uses both the proven drug (Herceptin) and the trial drug, lapatanib --Tykerb) in conjunction with Taxol (which is the chemo drug). I'll have 12 weeks of Taxol and Herceptin. Both of these drugs are administered through my port -- another good thing. The fewer injections the better. After the twelve week cycle, there will be a six week "wash out" period with no drugs. After those six weeks, I'll start the daily lapatanib pill and will take that for the remainder of a year. Radiation treatment will be after the 12 weeks of chemo. If all goes "well", I should be done with chemo and radiation by early July. Oh, that seems so very far away.

I was surprised to learn that the nurse from Legacy Oncology Research will come to each of my chemo appointments. Today, she had me fill out the initial "Quality of Life" survey. Some of the questions were difficult to answer, some not so difficult, and some of the questions I refused to answer. There is still personal privacy, and I am not interested in sharing some aspects of my life with cancer with the research team, or with you, for that matter, thank you very much. Now, I realize that you may be reading this and thinking "what??? She is worried about privacy? Has she read her own notes on Facebook? She already shares too much information!" Surprise! I am NOT telling you everything. Nor will I begin to. And I am not sorry about keeping some things to myself. I know you're all in a twitter with curiousity. You'll always wonder....

Interesting interaction with Dr. Segal today. He called me before my appointment to tell me about the randomization. When I answered my phone "Drenda Howatt", he said, "Hi, Drenda, this is Jerry". Ok. So we're on a first-name basis now. No more Mrs. Howatt or Dr. Segal. I knew we'd get to be great friends.

Drenda Lane Howatt: nuts. I forgot to write that today's treatment lasted 5 1/2 hours. They promise the next ones will be shorter...
February 26, 2009 at 6:56pm

Sally Park: So you aren't supposed to get so sick with this new round?
February 26, 2009 at 8:44pm

Drenda Lane Howatt: Nausea is not an expected side effect. Good news. And so far, so good. Cumulative effects include neuropathy in fingers and toes, extreme fatigue, aches in bones
February 26, 2009 at 10:05pm

Susan Rasmussen Lane: Oh, dear. I hope the neuropathy is temporary.
February 26, 2009 at 11:10pm

Amanda Lane: still sending you all my love.
February 27, 2009 at 8:24am

Who Am I?

Friday, February 27, 2009 at 8:37pm

More good news. I have not been nauseated from the new chemotherapy drug I received yesterday. What a relief! I was so hoping that this would be the case. I could not fathom the idea of being sick for 12 weeks with no break in between treatments. Thank you, God!

This evening, I have been reflecting on the last few months. As I looked at my body in the mirror, I thought "my body is a carved~up mess now". Two surgeries and three incision scars, two of which are quite prominent, hardly any hair on my body. But I am not my breasts. I am not my hair. I am not cancer. I am ME.

I am not the same "ME" that I was before the evening of November 8, 2008. That was the night that I felt the lump in my breast and I KNEW. The next hours, days, and weeks were filled with sheer terror. How does a Mom tell her daughters that she has breast cancer? Two of those precious girls are away at college and had to hear the news over the telephone. What wrenching calls to make, and, I am sure, even more wrenching to receive. Telling our third daughter, only 12 at the time, was just as difficult. Only instead of just hearing the tears, she had to watch them. After explaining to her the diagnosis, Don asked "Ellie, do you know what cancer is?" "Yes. It's the virus that kills people." Oh my goodness. Moms are supposed to protect their babies, not scare them.

The old "ME" had things under control. Life was planned. Had to be -- lots of responsibilities and not enough time in each day.

No more control apparently. But there is more time in each day because circumstances require more "no" answers to requests.

As I have journeyed through the trials and tribulations of breast cancer, I have thought more about death than ever before. I have re-examined my faith in the true and everlasting God. I have questioned Him beyond what I could have imagined. I have experienced triumphs and failures over panic attacks and illness. I have known such true love and support from my amazing family and my dear friends.

No, I am not the same. I am weaker. I am stronger. I am more fearful. I am more courageous. I am scared. I am bold.

But I am not my body. And I am not cancer.

Andi Pedersen Jordan: Hooray! No nausea ... amazing. Hopefully, you can enjoy the weekend!
February 27, 2009 at 9:14pm

Susan Rasmussen Lane: Oh, that's wonderful! Hope the rest of the treatments go so well!
February 27, 2009 at 10:59pm

Karen Buehrig: Drenda- I am so glad to hear that the treatment went well. hopefully you were able to get out and enjoy the beautiful day yesterday.
February 28, 2009 at 7:53am

Ginger Clausen: You are so transparent- letting your weakness reflect His work in your life! I always know- there but for the grace of God go I- I just hope I would be as brave as you have been (not in going through it- you have no choice), in going through it with GRACE!
February 28, 2009 at 9:25am

Wendy Ackley: You are you. I love your not being defined by what is fleeting and scary.
February 28, 2009 at 10:33am

Sandy Hagstrand: Drenda - You are a woman of grace and courage, reflecting HIS life in you! Your walk is inspiring to many of us, even when you may not think it is. Thank you for all you've given....
February 28, 2009 at 7:05pm

Zachary Lane Koval: You are also incredibly insightful and a beautiful writer.
March 1, 2009 at 3:33am

Drenda Lane Howatt is attending the Breast Cancer Issues Conference at the Convention Center today because she is a breast cancer survivor.
February 28, 2009 at 7:15am

Attending the conference was a mistake. Too early. I was overwhelmed by the number of women who have battled breast cancer multiple times. I was overwhelmed by the amount of information on the long lasting side effects of cancer and its treatment. I was overwhelmed by cancer. And when I arrived home, I went in my bedroom and cried.

Drenda Lane Howatt attended the conference and now knows that even when cancer is over, it is not over. oh my goodness.
February 28, 2009 at 4:53pm

> Maureen Gatens Thompson at 7:14pm February 28, 2009
> True...but it slowly starts to not occupy your every thought or fear, at least that's how it is for me. It's a part of what contributes to being a "Survivor" which is intensely personal. And you are well on your way.
> Your Bosom Buddy, Maureen
>
> Linda Waggoner at 8:17pm February 28, 2009
> Drenda, Thanks for joining Dustine, Jessica and me today between sessions. I really felt good about the conference and all of the information provided -- and I love the hat! I wore it all the way home on MAX!

Drenda Lane Howatt is home for the evening, and has lots to do, but is not sure anything on the list will get done.
March 2, 2009 at 4:45pm

Drenda Lane Howatt is down to 3 days to L.A., 4 days to Anna!
March 2, 2009 at 8:37pm

Drenda Lane Howatt has a sibling provided frozen dinner in the oven, so it is time for the hot bath.
March 3, 2009 at 4:55pm

Drenda Lane Howatt has chemo tomorrow...#2 Of 12, or #6 of 16...either way, 10 more to go after tomorrow.
March 3, 2009 at 4:56pm

Drenda Lane Howatt is off to work for a few hours, then to cancer war for a few more. Watch out Los Angeles, she'll be there in the morning.
March 4, 2009at 6:51am

> Jennifer Stady at 7:31am March 4, 2009
> Have a great time in LA!!
>
> Linda Waggoner at 12:00pm March 4, 2009
> Have fun!
>
> Kris Howatt at 12:53pm March 4, 2009
> Bring some warm sunshine back in your suitcase

Drenda Lane Howatt is, to quote a famous oncologist, “the perfect patient”. No kidding.
March 4, 2009 at 4:53pm

Perfect and Fat: That's Me!

Wednesday, March 4, 2009 at 5:08pm

A note I must write.

During my time today with Dr. Segal, (or Jerry, as he is now known to me), he was quite in awe of me.

Awe.

Of me.

Because, it seems, I am "the perfect patient".

You may now be shaking your head and asking "why is that?" My reaction, too! And, why am I the perfect patient? Because I "am well educated" and "ask questions about things" that he, Jerry, forgets to tell me.

Now, lest my pride swell at the wonderful label of "perfect", Don did point out that Jerry also called me fat. Well, not a quote exactly. In response to my question about one of the long term side effects of chemo causing loss in bone density, Jerry's response was "well, for someone like you who is a, hmmm, bit overweight (picture here a small nervous smile from him)...." and then "bigger women tend to have better bones than smaller women"...That is a positive, right?

Despite what it may appear to you, the reader, I do not usually keep a tally of compliments. However, the ones that have come my way during cancer treatment are too precious to let go. Let's see -- I use big words ("cumulative"), I have "amazing bone marrow", I am "so impressive" (because I continued to work through the four nasty, vile, A&C chemo treatments), and now, drum roll please,...I am "THE PERFECT PATIENT"!

But, I also lead the research nurse for the clinical trial to believe that Jerry is "in collusion" with me (because I had planned to refuse the trial if I didn't get into the part I wanted), and I am, "hmmm, a bit overweight". Ok. I am fat.

But I get good bones!

Elizabeth Lundquist Calhoun: Congratulations on being the perfect patient! And it just goes to show there is a bright side to everything. Your way of looking at things always cheers me up!
March 4, 2009 at 5:21pm

Kortney Stewart: Mrs. Howatt you are Absolutely Adorable! :)
March 4, 2009 at 5:43pm

Drenda Lane Howatt: Thank you both! Adorable and cheering are good things.
March 4, 2009 at 8:58pm

Faith Jossi Lichtenberg: Drenda, I love your storytelling!!!! You are the best! And I am quite sure I would be told I too have good bones! Thanks for the great new spin on that.
March 5, 2009 at 2:26pm

Hollace Howatt Chandler: I think good bones are beautiful!
March 5, 2009 at 9:59pm

ilities. where do they come from?

Thursday, March 5, 2009 at 3:37am

I heard an ad on the radio yesterday that really made me stop and think. The ad was for a college that was advocating it was "the" place to get ility. Yes, ility. As in capability, ability, flexibility, responsibility etc. As I listened, I thought "where did I get my ilities?" The answer was immediate and resounding: My parents.

I have a large "family of origin" -- eight siblings. My parents had babies over 18 years. Really, two families in some senses. I am child number seven, but there are almost six years in between me and the next oldest. Children number eight & nine followed me rather closely. My Dad told me once that I was an accident, Becky was to keep me company, and Janette was "oh well, what the hell!"

We didn't have a lot of "things" growing up, but we did have family, and we did have love. There were no entitlements at our house - we worked. Ok, I have realized as I have gotten older that the pay for summer berry picking may have been subsidized depending on our age, but work was still expected. We each had to earn enough to purchase our school clothes for the coming year. How's that for learning how to budget?!

Mom was home always. Always. Dad working the land, and always other jobs, too, providing for his family. Dinners together every night. I remember my childhood as happy. Good. Not perfect, of course, but safe. Stable. Carefree.

Traditions. Sunday dinner after church. Popcorn and top-of-the-stove cookies Sunday night. Christmas Eve cookie deliveries to the neighbors while Santa came to our house. Having to wait for Mom to come to the car on Easter Sunday...that was the one Sunday she was always late getting ready. Coming home from church to find Easter baskets hidden throughout the house.

Mom and Dad provided a firm foundation. A foundation that gave us stability and the freedom to explore. From that foundation, we each have been able to grow. My parents raised nine children into caring, creative, capable, and contributing adults.

I am hopeful that I can honor my parents by striving to continue their tradition. The tradition of providing a firm foundation for my children that will allow and spur them to continue their growth into caring, creative, capable, and contributing adults.

I am filled with thankfulness to my parents for all that they gave to me. I realize the gift of that strong foundation did not come without great personal sacrifice and cost to them.

But I am even more thankful for them. As people. Not just what they did, but for who they are.

I miss my Mom. Tremendously.

I love my Dad. Tremendously.

Sally Park: Oh my goodness...you have brought tears, not easy to do. Your note has queued memories. I too miss Mom so much. Seems like a lifetime ago. She would be proud of you Drenda Mary!
I have NEVER tasted fried chicken like hers. Sage was the key ingredient; take a whiff of sage and it will take you back!

The nine of us all have good kids with good hearts, making their way.
Can you imagine how tickled Mom would be?
March 5, 2009 at 5:28pm

Amber Lynn Montgomery Lane: "My parents raised nine children into caring, creative, capable, and contributing adults." In the relatively short time I've known the Lane family, I would have to agree 100% Caring? YES! Capable and contributing? Absolutely. I could easily go on and add to the list of positive attributes you all share. I love your Dad, too... and am sorry to have missed knowing your Mom.
March 5, 2009 at 8:16pm

Sally Park: Amber she would have loved you.
March 5, 2009 at 8:41pm

Linda Waggoner: Oh, Drenda. What a wonderful stroll down memory lane! My childhood was, obviously, different from yours (being so much older than you!!) but I do remember many of the same things -- Christmas Eve deliveries to the neighbors, Sunday afternoon dinners with delicious fried chicken, picking berries.... thank you for taking us back to those days for even a few minutes!
March 6, 2009 at 11:11am

Laurie Lane: Do you remember the "stick horses?" They were so much easier to handle than our horse Chockie ever was! Then there was playing in the barn filled with hay, licking the salt licks (ugh), and playing soft ball in the cow pasture using dried (and sometimes fresh) manure for our bases. Well, we didn't use the fresh manure for our bases exactly, it's just that it was present...

We worked hard and had LOTS of Fun! Thanks for the walk down memory "LANE!"
March 7, 2009 at 2:24pm

Drenda Lane Howatt is in Azusa, California. She will see Anna's performance tonight!
March 6, 2009 at 5:45pm

> Gail Hilderbrand at 9:59am March 7, 2009
> Well its raining here...and cold! Have a fabulous time!

Drenda Lane Howatt is home.
March 8, 2009 at 9:46pm

> Kris Howatt at 9:52pm March 8, 2009
> Did you bring some warm weather? Snow forecast for the morning - welcome back

Drenda Lane Howatt is settling in for the season premier of Dancing with the Stars. Oh yeah!
March 9, 2009 at 8:03pm

> Faith Jossi Lichtenberg at 8:28pm March 9, 2009
> Me too!!

> Robin Reilly at 10:02pm March 9, 2009
> Melissa & Tony!

Drenda Lane Howatt is getting ready to meet with the Market Mavens.
March 10, 2009 at 5:38pm

Drenda Lane Howatt is surprised to have her finger tips and part of her tongue numb from the chemo...Jerry said it would take 4-6 weeks to occur. It's only been 2. Harumph.
March 10, 2009 at 9:11pm

Andi Pedersen Jordan at 10:28pm March 10, 2009
love that you and the doc are on first name basis...

Laurie Lane at 7:04am March 11, 2009
Have you checked into acupuncture?
That might help lessen the neuropathy.

Drenda Lane Howatt is preparing herself for chemo treatment tomorrow...3 of 12 or 7 of 16. She likes 7 of 16 better -- that statistic makes it seem like she's almost half done.
March 11, 2009 at 5:44pm

Kris Howatt at 6:36pm March 11, 2009
3 of 12 reduces down to 1 of 4 - nice odds - I was thinking of you today and hope Thursday goes well

Drenda Lane Howatt has one extra ticket to the Broadway play "Wicked" for Saturday evening. Wanna go? Send her a message if you're interested.
March 11, 2009 at 7:55pm

Christina Elford at 8:05pm March 11, 2009
AAAAHHHHHHHHHHHHHHHHHh I want to go so bad!!! But this is one of my LAST Saturdays I have to work in the evenings!!!

Drenda Lane Howatt at 8:05pm March 11, 2009
any way you can get the night off?

Christina Elford at 8:09pm March 11, 2009
Hmmm I will call tomorrow and ask! But if someone else knows they can go... you don't have to hold the ticket, but I can possibly get it off now that I think about it.

Kayleen Hagstrand at 11:29am March 13, 2009
Have you found a taker on the Wicked Ticket? If not let me know.

Drenda Lane Howatt at 6:01pm March 13, 2009
Yes...the ticket was gone almost immediately! Popular show! Sorry

Drenda Lane Howatt is preparing to go have cancer-killing drugs injected into her body. Cancer war continues, and Drenda is winning!
March 12, 2009 at 8:54am

Milt Buckelew at 9:00am March 12, 2009
GO DRENDA!!!

Andi Pedersen Jordan at 9:01am March 12, 2009
Strong and Courageous...

Drenda Lane Howatt has discovered that, in an odd twist of fate, most people, herself included, actually gain weight while on chemotherapy. Oh my goodness. How does THAT happen?
March 12, 2009 at 7:36pm

Maureen Gatens Thompson at 11:08pm March 12, 2009
That happened to me as well. They said it was from the steroids they gave me along with the chemo drugs. The steroids were used to calm my veins down so they could

pump the chemo drugs into me...a necessary evil. Hang tough, strong one!

Drenda Lane Howatt is getting ready to have her house cleaned -- WONDERFUL gift from her co-workers. Big (old) house, 4 hours, where to start? Woo Hoo!
March 13, 2009 at 6:42am

Andi Pedersen Jordan at 7:21am March 13, 2009
Cool co-workers!

Gail Hilderbrand at 10:49pm March 13, 2009
That is wonderful! Enjoy!

Kris Howatt at 4:42pm March 14, 2009
That's it - the wreath on the front door is coming down

Drenda Lane Howatt has all thee of her girls home for the weekend. Wicked, here we come!
March 13, 2009 at 6:05pm

Wendy Ackley at 11:02pm March 14, 2009
Loved Wicked and the whole evening!

Kim Burns at 6:53am March 15, 2009
Wow I did not know Wicked was in Portland. I would love to see it. Hear it is wonderful. It has been years since I have seen a Broadway Production. There are perks to living near a big city. Tell us all about it. Great all your girls are home. How long will Anna and Rachel be in town?

Drenda Lane Howatt at 8:28am March 15, 2009
Wicked was wonderful! It was great fun. Anna and Rachel are both leaving this evening; Anna via plane (!), and Rachel via train. Came home to see Wicked. Family

night out. We purchased the Wicked tickets last summer, so we'd been looking forward to the play for a looooong time. I organized a group of about 55 people who all went last night -- seats in different places throughout the auditorium. Our seats were in the 3rd and 4th rows. AMAZING!

Drenda Lane Howatt had a wonderful evening last night with family, friends, and co-workers at Wicked!
March 15, 2009 at 8:36am

Drenda Lane Howatt is getting ready for her annual date with Ned Devine.
March 15, 2009 at 3:16pm

Drenda Lane Howatt is going to have a normal Monday.
March 16, 2009 at 6:31am

Amber Lynn Montgomery Lane at 10:17am March 16, 2009
Ambiguous... could be good being normal (not sick), could be bad as people often don't like Mondays. I'm rooting for good, for your sake. :)

Kris Howatt at 10:22am March 16, 2009
I usually like Mondays - the house is quiet after the hustle/bustle of the weekend - Happy Monday!

Drenda Lane Howatt at 5:47pm March 16, 2009
In my world, normal is now "good". Absolutely.

Karen Buehrig at 7:10pm March 16, 2009
And life at the office wasn't too bad either. Back to the routine.

Drenda Lane Howatt is having a good week. Good spirits, good sleep (perhaps they go together?), and good aches.
March 17, 2009 at 6:18am

Drenda Lane Howatt almost, almost forgot today that she is battling cancer. Then the leg, hip, and other bone aches reared their ugly heads. Yikes
March 17, 2009 at 8:34pm

> Andi Pedersen Jordan at 8:45pm March 17, 2009
> Tell it to go away!
>
> Drenda Lane Howatt at 8:46pm March 17, 2009
> I keep trying! Actually, I'll take the bone aches over the nausea any day. I can power through pain much easier than through urping...
>
> Maureen Gatens Thompson at 9:51pm March 17, 2009
> Oh my dear, Drenda...it was great seeing you today. I remember when I first got the "bone pains" and I was convinced I had bone cancer. The docs hadn't prepared me that this was normal and part of "the journey." I cheer because you almost forgot about your BC...that is great spiritual progress. You will go back and forth like a see-saw but you've experienced the beginning of the healing process. Cheers to you and your progress. Hugs!

Drenda Lane Howatt is preparing herself emotionally for another chemotherapy appointment tomorrow.
March 18, 2009 at 5:08pm

> Sally Park at 7:56pm March 18, 2009
> What time? I will be thinking good thoughts ~
>
> Sally Park at 8:00pm March 18, 2009

I am the advisor for NHS at the high school and one of our new spring projects is the Relay for Live Rally in June, also one in April for the "teen" population. We are collecting for each team we sponsor and promoting donations for the luminarias. Taken on a project close to my heart!

Gail Hilderbrand at 9:50pm March 18, 2009
Lots of prayer coming your way:)

Kim Burns at 3:13pm March 19, 2009
You will have courage because you will have hope... Job

Thursday Regulars

Thursday, March 19, 2009 at 5:35pm

Today was another chemo treatment, preceded by a visit with Jerry. Unfortunately, he was not quite himself today.

No awe of me.

No compliments.

I was expecting something, needing something, really. But, alas, just a normal dr./patient exchange. I asked him about a few issues I am having and then asked "would these be caused by the taxol?" He responded "probably. Yes. I think the taxol." Did not do much to inspire my confidence, I must say. Then, when I went upstairs for the infusions, I had to wait quite awhile because Jerry had not sent up the drug orders. Odd.

Some good news, though. First is that, according to Jerry, the doctors like to give at least three weeks between the end of chemo and the beginning of radiation. That will mean a later finish date, but a break will be good. Also, when I asked him about the port in my chest and how long it will have to stay, Jerry said the port can come out as soon as chemo is done. WOO HOO!

But let me tell you about the waiting room. The Thursday regulars were there. Eleanor came in with her son. She is an old(er) lady who wears a bright blue turban...every week. I would guess she is in her late 70s (sorry, Eleanor. If you are by some remote chance reading this, I apologize if I am way off on your age. So hard to tell, isn't it?) Silky man was there, too. I can't quite figure out if he is a patient or if he comes with someone else. He is "silky man" because he is obviously wearing a wig, but it is most definitely a woman's wig/hairstyle. And it is very silky. The bangs are a bit short, though. I am tempted to bring my wigs for him.

In the infusion room, there is a very sweet old lady getting her treatment with her adult son at her side. Seems the classic. Her son may be the one who never leaves home and can't keep a job. But he is there supporting his Momma.

I had "dancing legs" today. The benadryl made me very antsy. Couldn't keep my legs still. I asked the nurse about feeling so edgy, and she explained it was probably the benadryl. I had assumed it was caused by the steroids, but apparently not. She said that next time they'll cut down on the benadryl and see if that helps. Antsy is not good when you have a 1 inch needle in your chest.

To pass the time, I made it through Metro's 20 - 50 year population and employment growth prediction summary, AND Congressman Schrader's federal stimulus package summary. Great reading. End result of both: lots of people coming, not so many jobs coming, and the U.S. Government bleeding dollar bills.

Time to leave treatment...3 1/2 hours start to finish. As we left, Eleanor and her son were playing a rousing game of cards.

Jerry still not on track. My orders for the next treatment(s) had not been entered into the computer, which meant I could not get the appointment for next week scheduled. Perhaps scheduling can be done tomorrow.

So the whole afternoon leaves me wondering what the "regulars" think of me.

Do they think it odd that I am the only patient in the room

without a wig or a hat? (I do. Think it is odd that, in a cancer/chemo clinic, no one is comfortable being bald. Where else should it be more normal?)

How do they describe me in their blog? Perhaps they don't even know I am there...it has taken me a number of weeks to recognize the "regulars".

Weeks to come out of my miserable world and notice others. Weeks to process the routine and almost get comfortable with it. Weeks to know which nurse is the one to I want to be assigned to. Weeks of counting. Weeks of crying. Weeks of dread. But now, weeks of hope. Because my God is a God who offers hope for the hopeless.

4 of 12 treatments done. 8 to go.

Hope
Strength
Courage

Because He commands it.

And He provides it.

Barb Van Dusen Butler: was thinking of you today as you went for treatment. What do they give you and how long does it take? How are you feeling?
March 19, 2009 at 6:15pm

Drenda Lane Howatt: I receive taxol and herceptin. Today's treatment took just under 4 hours start to finish -- labs, vitals, dr., infusion. These drugs don't make me nauseated, just strong bone aches and extreme fatigue.
March 19, 2009 at 6:18pm

Barb Van Dusen Butler: glad there's no nausea. Enjoy your "good eats".
March 19, 2009 at 6:25pm

Danielle Becker: Drenda- I have to tell you that every time I read your notes I am teary-eyed. You are one amazing woman and I envy your strength in the LORD. I know that I should trust him that much but I am afraid that I fall short in that area. Thank you for being such an amazing example to me and so many others! You are such a great example for the rest of us! Praise God that he will always be there to take care of you... and me! :-)
March 20, 2009 at 12:35am

Barb Van Dusen Butler: I had not read your full account till just now - after seeing Danielle's comment come up on my e-mail (not sure I like the new Facebook). Anyway, you are an amazing example to me as well. I really appreciate you letting us in on your journey. I feel like I am getting to know you a bit better. Thanks
March 20, 2009 at 10:00am

Hollace Howatt Chandler: Thanks for sharing, Drenda. I hope the week (starting Thursday) is going okay.
March 2, 20091 at 4:04pm

Elizabeth Lundquist Calhoun: I love your description of the regulars. Sounds like the makings of a good character-driven movie...
March 23, 2009 at 6:37am

Drenda Lane Howatt has killed cancer cells for this week, and will plan to attack the laundry tomorrow. If the pain in her bones allow.
March 19, 2009 at 10:40pm

> Hollace Howatt Chandler at 8:26am March 20, 2009
> I'll be in the basement, too, throwing in loads of laundry between sorting bins. Arrgh.

Drenda Lane Howatt is going to learn from the new "Coupon Queen" how to slash grocery bills with little effort...
March 21, 2009 at 8:21am

> Sally Park at 9:37am March 21, 2009
> Great! Share what you learn, ok?
>
> Don Howatt at 9:54am March 21, 2009
> I think I have a coupon for Guitar Center! You didn't throw it away did you?!

Drenda Lane Howatt is wondering what happened to the weekend?
March 22, 2009 at 8:47pm

> Abbi Howatt at 8:48pm March 22, 2009
> You and me both!
>
> Drenda Lane Howatt at 8:49pm March 22, 2009
> It went by too fast! I am not ready to go back to work/routine tomorrow. You, Miss, make sure to enjoy your vacation -- rest up and soak in family!
>
> Abbi Howatt at 8:52pm March 22, 2009
> I'll do what I can.

Drenda Lane Howatt had a great day at the office. Now, dinner, hot bubble bath and bed. Wondering about the odds of staying awake for Dancing with the Stars...
March 23, 2009 at 5:13pm

> Sally Park at 5:19pm March 23, 2009
> I have the same problem...what's my excuse though?
>
> Drenda Lane Howatt at 6:29pm March 23, 2009
> Your excuse is that your sister is battling breast cancer, and it is emotionally exhausting to be supportive of her...

Drenda Lane Howatt is home from work, and refusing to let the bubble bath win right now...because she is sure that her husband will want to take her out to dinner tonight.
March 24, 2009 at 5:29pm

Drenda Lane Howatt is, once again, preparing emotionally for tomorrow's battle in the cancer war.
March 25, 2009 at 5:11pm

> Zachary Lane Koval at 5:50pm March 25, 2009
> You can do it! Love and strength! :)
>
> Sally Park at 7:08pm March 25, 2009
> Go Get It!!!
>
> Amanda Lane at 8:22am March 26, 2009
> You are in my thoughts today. Sending you all my love.

Drenda Lane Howatt must grocery shop prior to deploying to the war zone. Daily life collides with combat.
March 26, 2009 at 9:26am

Popular? Not Me.

Thursday, March 26, 2009 at 7:16pm

I was not a popular mother today.

I insisted that Ellie and Rachel accompany me to my chemo treatment this afternoon. Neither one of the girls was very happy with me. Rachel had been to the clinic one other time when I went to get my neulasta injection. I was hopeful that they would be able to meet Jerry, even though I did not have an appointment with him. Jerry is gone all week on vacation, so that didn't work out.

It is important to me that my daughters are aware of at least some of the day to day aspects of my cancer treatment. If they never see the clinic, or the "infusion" room, I fear their imaginations may be worse than the reality. Perhaps, in their minds, the imaginations were safer. But I wanted them to know that the reality is o.k., too. That the weekly treatments are not awful physically. That the people who care for me there are nice, gentle, and concerned. I don't want my daughters overcome with fear when they think of breast cancer. That is why I had Rachel and Ellie feel my tumor/lump before surgery. That is why I have shown them my scars. Ellie asked me a few weeks ago if my breast will always be so flat. "Don't know...just have to wait and see!" I want my journey to be an open and transparent one for them.

I had Ellie come in with me to the lab and to the"vitals" area today. She got to see the one-inch needle put into the port. She was able to see the "model" port, and have a visual of what is inside my chest. She knew what it felt like under my skin, but now she knows what it actually looks like. She knows what really happens when my blood is drawn out of the port. She knows that I walk back to the waiting room with tubes hanging out of my sweater. She knows that there is a lot of waiting involved!

Don and the girls and I then headed upstairs to the infusion room. It was a ZOO! Lots of cranky little kids there with their parent or grandparent. Weird. More patients than normal. No normal patients (as in the regulars...) There were only three nurses working instead of the usual five, so it was crazy. Luckily, I got my treatment started fairly quickly.

My nurse described Jerry to the girls as "kind of a nutty professor. Very very smart. Looks like Jerry Garcia, or Osama Bin Laden". Great descriptions! Made us laugh. Ellie and Rachel stayed just until the i.v. fluids were started, then we let them leave to go home.

At one point, while we were waiting, Ellie asked me if there has been cancer in my family. "No, not before me". "Did your Mom have any cancer?" "No." "Could I get breast cancer because you have it?" "Yes, it can be inherited, but you'll have early and regular check-ups when you become a grown woman." "I don't want cancer...."

I wonder to myself, again, what God's purpose is in my babies having to confront cancer at 13, at 18, at 21. How can there be good out of this? They're too young. They're too sweet. They're too precious. Oh, how I want to protect their hearts. But I cannot. And that makes me sad. And, some days, that makes me mad.

The fact that I question the purpose does not negate that there is a purpose. I do believe. Actually, I KNOW there is a purpose.

And I generally know what it is.

That, through this, God will be glorified. But I want the details....I want that scroll that says "Drenda, by going through this, your family will be __________. " And I want the blanks all filled in with good things. Great things.

A dear friend sent me a verse from Jeremiah today. It is sweet. "Call to Me, and I will answer you, and I will tell you great and mighty things which you do not know." Jeremiah 33:3

I continue calling. I am trying to listen. I am waiting for the great and mighty things which I do not know.

Andi Pedersen Jordan: Way to go, Mom. The rest of us have your back.
March 26, 2009 at 11:57pm

Hollace Howatt Chandler: What you are teaching the girls is not that they might get cancer, but if that day ever happens to them (or anyone), they will be given strength for the day, grace to bear it and courage to believe God's promises.
March 27, 2009 at 12:20am

Amanda Ouellette: Drenda,
I am so encouraged by what you write. I think it's a wonderful gift that you are giving your girls by making sure they see the realities of living in a fallen world, because your desire seems to be that they know who God is, and that even through something as devastating as this, He can- and should be praised and glorified. I hope that as my family goes through our trials, that Keith and I will follow your example to use the opportunity to keep the kids involved, and to teach them how to face reality with a God-centered perspective. Thank you.
March 28, 2009 at 6:04pm

Psycho vs Physical

Thursday, March 26, 2009 at 7:44pm

Which comfort is more important?

I have discovered that, for me, it is definitely physical. I am willing to be bald in public because the physical discomfort of a wig and sometimes of a hat is too much for me. Not that I couldn't bear the discomfort. But the question has become, for me, "why should I bear the discomfort?"

It is becoming, really, ALL about me.

Pride? No. In fact, I hear often, now, how beautiful my head is. "So round!" "Not knobby!" "No bumps!" (And what if there were knobs and bumps? What then?)

Other people's obvious discomfort being in a room with baldy me? Sometimes.

The discomfort of others has been the most difficult. But I am slowly helping people I live with, work with, play with, come to terms with my baldness. Men are finding that they don't have to look at the floor or the walls when they come into my office to talk to me and find me at my desk without a hat. They can still look at my eyes and I don't melt! And neither do they! Amazing. School teachers are done with their second glances. Almost normal.

So, the usual decision point is temperature. If my head is cold, I wear a hat. If my head is hot, I don't wear a hat. I want physical comfort.

But this process, in retrospect, is fascinating to me. I realize how much we all bear sometimes very difficult physical discomforts in order to “fit in”. Me too, still, in many ways. There is freedom in deciding it is all about me.

Selfish? Perhaps.

But that’s o.k.

Because I am worth it!

Laurie Lane: It’s time to be SELFISH!
I found this quote by Dr. Doug Sawin:
“I have found it useful to break the word selfish down into its two components self and –ish and look at the meaning of these two parts. Self refers to me, the person that I am. –ish is defined as “of, related to, or being”. Combining these, we can see that selfish is “of, related to, or being the entire person of an individual”. That is, pertaining to, or focused on, ones entire being. Thus, to be selfish is to be conscious of one’s self, one’s whole self, one’s being.”
March 27, 2009 at 5:33am

Drenda Lane Howatt is now caught up on work e-mail, so she can go enjoy(!) Costco. whoop.
March 27, 2009 at 10:12am

Amanda Graber at 1:10pm March 27, 2009
oh Costco :)

Drenda Lane Howatt has a clean house (HUGE THANK YOU to her co-workers for financing such a tremendously wonderful gift!), a full refrigerator, full gas tank, and is now completely ready for the coming week. And, it is only Friday! How cool is that? When reality hits, she will know that cleanliness, food, and gas will be seriously depleted by Sunday evening....
March 27, 2009 at 2:27pm

Drenda Lane Howatt is having a wonderfully lazy Saturday. A little laundry, a little 7th grade Math and English, a little coffee, a little nap later.
March 28, 2009 at 9:48am

Sally Park at 9:59am March 28, 2009
Simple pleasures!

Elizabeth Lundquist Calhoun at 1:28pm March 28, 2009
Sounds perfect

Cindy McElmurry at 3:10pm March 28, 2009
Hope you had a good week. See you Sunday.

Drenda Lane Howatt has a new blog page...for all her non-Facebooking friends!
March 28, 2009 at 5:45pm

Linda Waggoner at 6:02pm March 28, 2009
I enjoyed your blog so much! You inspire me to be a better person -- I am so proud of you!

Drenda Lane Howatt at 6:13pm March 28, 2009
Thank you, Linda. Not my intent, to inspire people, but if that happens through my trials and triumphs, so much the better! I write because I have to.

http://iamstrongandcourageous.blogspot.com/

Drenda Lane Howatt just made cookies...1977 Orient Community Club recipe book..."Coconut Diamonds". Recipe submitted by the wonderful Becky Lane!
March 29, 2009 at 5:34pm

Drenda Lane Howatt at 6:53pm March 29, 2009
They're winners! Even Don, who has a strong dislike for coconut, thinks the cookies are good. Thanks, Becky!

Maureen Gatens Thompson at 8:33pm March 29, 2009
I LOVE coconut. I'll trade you some yummy Baskin Robins chocolate chip ice cream cake for some cookies. It's Rachel's BD cake but she won't mind. *s* Just leave the cookies by our front door, I'll get 'em when I sneak in tomorrow morning.

Gail Hilderbrand at 10:18pm March 29, 2009
Coconut is my favorite and I never get it because Jeff hates it. Interesting both men in brown dislike coconut.

Drenda Lane Howatt is up late.
March 30, 2009 at 9:27pm

Drenda Lane Howatt gets to have stroganoff for dinner...compliments of her family!
March 31, 2009 at 5:55pm

> Sharley Massman at 6:37pm March 31, 2009
> Yummy, what time is dinner?
>
> Drenda Lane Howatt at 6:50pm March 31, 2009
> :-)
> Sorry, you already missed it! I love having the frozen dinners ready to go in the freezer...take one out and put it in the oven in the morning, set the oven timer, and, viola! Dinner is ready when I get home from work.

All About Me? Not Really.

Tuesday, March 31, 2009 at 7:53pm

It has been less than a week since my last two entries, and I have not been able to stop thinking about what I wrote. Because, in some senses, my writings were wrong. Everything is NOT all about me. Not breast cancer, not breast cancer treatment, not life.

I wrote about wanting to know the purpose of this trial called cancer. I wrote that I knew it is ultimately for God's glory.

That IS true.

But I also wrote that I wanted the scroll to show me the good things, the great things, that would come from this. As I have mulled over my thoughts, I realized that my words could be misconstrued. Because it is quite possible that the outcomes that I will see and know about are not good in my estimation. Or the estimation of my family. My definition of "good" may not be the true definition, or God's definition. I am hopeful that we can see how the purpose of bringing glory to God has short-term good for us.

But what if I can't see good? What if the outcome is different than I want it to be? What then? Will God not be glorified because I don't like the outcome?

NO.

I KNOW that good will come from this journey. What that good will be, and what it will look like, may remain a mystery for a long time. Perhaps forever in our timelines. Good WILL come. "And we know that in all things God works for the good of those who love him, who have been called according to his purpose." Romans 8:28

Of course, I want, hope, that the good is complete healing. Normal routine and life back in place. Health. Happiness. The American Dream. My ideas. My definition.

I am slowly understanding, in my heart, that my "good" and true "good" may not be the same. So I am praying that my definition and understanding of "good" will be redefined to align with "true good".

I also wrote about being selfish in deciding whether or not to be bald or wear hats. No apologies for being selfish, or for being bald. Nope. Not sorry. My selfish-ness in this particular situation is more of a "sense" of self. Awareness of what I am willing or unwilling to deal with.

But, again, everything is NOT all about me.

All of which leads me to these next thoughts: so many of us wonder "what is God's will (or plan) for my life?" "What does God have for me to do?"

I believe that is backwards. Because it is NOT about us.

I believe the real question is "How do I fit into God's plan?" It is all about HIM.

He tells us in His Word what He has for us to do.

"He has showed you, O man, what is good.
And what does the LORD require of you?
To act justly and to love mercy
and to walk humbly with your God." Micah 6:8

I wrote that I want to protect my babies' hearts. I do. So very much. I wrote that I am sad that I have no power to protect those precious hearts through the battle, or war, of cancer. I wrote that some days I am mad about being unable to protect them.

Most days, though, I realize that their Protector, and mine, is oh so much more able than I to protect, and heal, the hearts of my babies.

And my husband's.

And mine.

No matter what happens.

Sally Park: Although I would never EVER wish the cross you bear upon anyone, I see the good. It's in the sharing and opening up that is happening in the family, it's in the cross generation cooking days, it's about the "strong and courageous" modeling. There is Good happening right now. Maybe we just need to share it with you more.
March 3, 20091 at 9:21pm

Amanda Lane: I agree with Sally, though I have been totally remiss on the cooking days... the sharing is contagious and has been a big help with my life these days.
April 1, 2009 at 8:42am

Robin Reilly: Although I whole-heartedly agree with everything that you said (can't identify with the "bald" part), how hard it is to live it. Only by the grace of God...Drenda, I can already see the "good" that I'm sure is God's "good". I do not envy you at all, but I know that He chose YOU, not me, because of the "good" that has already come. You know what you believe and

you LIVE what you believe. That is the good. Some of the rest of us would have curled up into a ball and given up. You go girl! By the grace of God.
April 1, 2009 at 9:28am

Amber Lynn Montgomery Lane: Also, there is a difference between selfISHness, and self awareness. I believe you are self aware, and that is nowhere near a bad thing.
April 1, 2009 at 1:03pm

Gail Stempel Hilderbrand: We will not know Gods purpose until we can ask him first hand. Witnessing to people through your grace and strength is good. Just sharing with people in the chemo room, making them feel a little more lighthearted is good. Instead of asking God "Why me"? Ask "Why not me"? Should it be the child down the street going through this, or maybe a family member? I say no way to that. Maybe some of the good was simply drawing you closer to him. That alone is eternally worthwhile.
April 1, 2009 at 3:49pm

Linda Waggoner: It is so difficult to believe that anything good could come from such a horrific diagnosis -- but --- in a strange way I really do think that, as a family, and, as individuals, we have become better because of what you are teaching us. Your journey, as a faith filled person, through one of the most challenging of battles and your reflections as you embrace parts of the journey and rail against others has helped me (who is selfish? - not me!!) so much on my own journey. I know you said you write because you have to and not to inspire but your writings are truly a ministry. I, as your sister, am becoming a better person (not quite as self absorbed) because of your example. Bet you never expected to become so admired by so many people!! Stay strong!! I love you!
April 1, 2009 at 4:13pm

Drenda Lane Howatt knows that it is that time of the week again...prep for poison. Gotta keep killing those cancer cells. Gets to see Jerry tomorrow, too!
April 1, 2009 at 7:22pm

> Jennifer Stady at 7:56pm April 1, 2009
> Go get em! Argggggg...
>
> Janette Wilkinson at 8:03pm April 1, 2009
> Not that it is all about me but...could you ask your friend and mine, Jerry, about the hair situation? I am kind of getting used to no "do" although preparation for what is to come is a good thing...
>
> Andi Pedersen Jordan at 11:02pm April 1, 2009
> Big step? Ahhh . . . you are just the strong and courageous one!

Drenda Lane Howatt has a busy and diverse day. First, driving dogs to Beavercreek. Then, Stimulus Team meetings in Oregon City, next, Jerry and poison at the Rose Quarter. Busy and diverse.
April 2, 2009 at 4:55am

Fuzzy Semblance

Thursday, April 2, 2009 at 5:03pm

I got to see Jerry today.

What a guy.

He is back to his usual self. I am doing "outstanding". Blood counts are good -- still a bit of anemia, but nothing bad enough to treat.

I was in a quandary. Because there are a number of people, objective ones among the group, who tell me my hair is starting to grow. So here's the quandary: If I AM receiving Taxol (chemo), and a side effect of Taxol is total hair loss, how is it that my hair is GROWING? Am I *really* receiving Taxol? And if I am, can it be working against the cancer cells correctly if it is allowing my hair to begin to grow?

I am sure you can understand my confusion.

I asked Jerry. "How is it that my hair can be growing while I am on Taxol?" His answer? As he peers over his glasses and looks closely at my scalp, he responds "well, it is not uncommon for a semblance of hair to appear while on Taxol. What you really have there is fuzz".

Semblance?

Fuzz?

Perhaps Jerry should now be known as a "joy robber". I will add that Don joined right in with Jerry and agreed. "That's what we have at our house...'semblance of hair'".

Not that I was exactly *joyous* over the possible beginnings of hair growth, but it would be an encouraging sign, don't you think? A sign that I am, indeed, nearing the end of chemotherapy and preparing for the next phase of my cancer treatment.

The sad part is that I had to text my sisters Linda and Janette and relay to them that my "fuzz" is but a "semblance" of hair. And that they'll need to keep buzzing their heads. And that we've got a long way to go.

I am not sure they had a clear understanding of the words "we'll shave our heads and stay bald until your hair grows back".

I think they're starting to get it now.

I was wrong to let them get their hopes up that my hair was coming back already.

Because it is just a semblance.

Fuzz.

Janette Wilkinson: Drenda I have had some experience with "semblance". "Semblance" is what I had when I "thought" I had some natural red in my hair. Now that I have "stubble" my sense of "semblance" has changed. There is NO "semblance" of red. There is only salt and pepper and it is definitely more than "semblance"! And by the way...ever think of the word semblance? Say it out loud. It is a strange sounding word.
April 2, 2009 at 8:03pm

Linda Waggoner: I also have salt & pepper -- unfortunately more salt than pepper but what's a person going to do?
April 3, 2009 at 10:07am

Hollace Howatt Chandler: I have hair, too. A hair. Right on the crown of my head. It's about 1" long but it's neither a semblance or fuzz. If I weren't so excited to have it I would pull it out for uniformity's sake.
April 6, 2009 at 4:02pm

Drenda, Linda, and Janette met for dinner and a 'hair check'. (May, 2009)

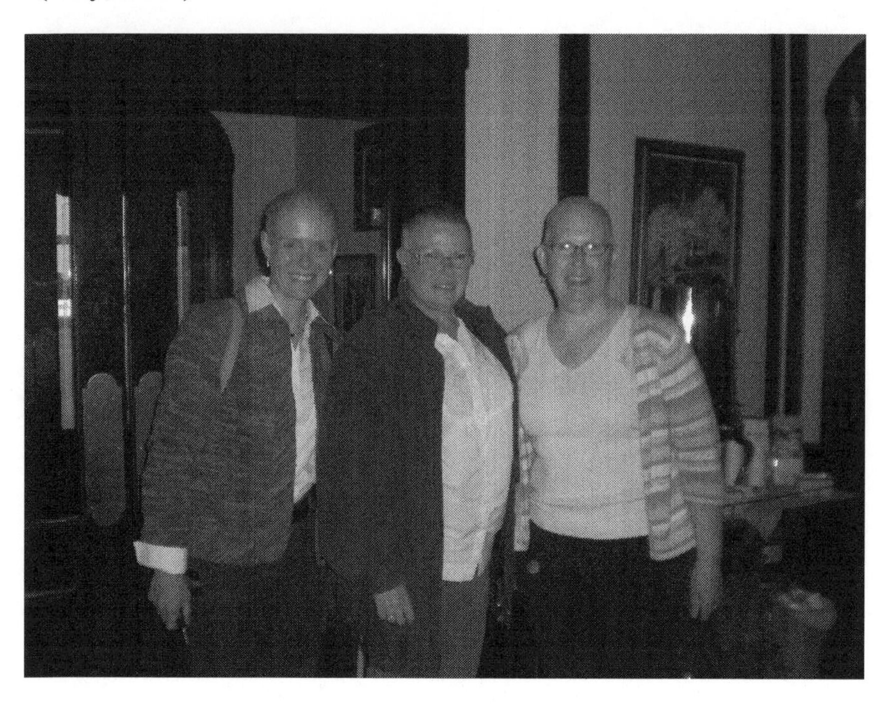

Drenda Lane Howatt is happy to have six down, six to go. And...thrilled to learn that she can take a one-week break in chemo to celebrate Anna's college graduation in Azusa, California! Now THAT is good news!
April 2, 2009 at 6:10pm

> Amber Lynn Montgomery Lane at 6:24pm April 2, 2009
> Happy Hump Day!

Saturday, April 4, 2009

Rachel's Perspective

The following note was written by my daughter, Rachel:

"Philippians 1:27

New quarter! I am excited for Spring Quarter.

Lots of things have changed.

Cancer update -
Spring break at home was refreshing, but, as I have come to expect, going home is hard. Sometimes I am completely prepared to walk into my kitchen and see my baldy-mommy and other times I need to do a double take. Wait? What? Oh yeah... she has breast cancer. You know, I have to tell you that I feel stupid sometimes making a big deal out of my mom being bald. But picture your mom bald... yeah, it's pretty different, now isn't it?

Life is the same, and life is so so different. Schedules are just as demanding, probably even more demanding than they were before. Mom still goes to work, Dad commutes too. Ellie has school. As if life isn't busy enough without chemo, dr. appointments, etc. etc.

Over break I went to the cancer center with my mom, dad, and Ellie for chemo. I had a bad attitude about going. I had already gone there before, over Christmas break. I was a brat about going, and made it pretty clear I didn't want to have to do it again. My mom said "do you think I want to have to come here again, Rachel?"

I can handle my mom being bald, I can handle the emotional turmoil (with help), I can handle the sick and twisted effects breast cancer has on my family, but for some reason... I can't handle being in the building where the cancer is treated. I hate it. I just cannot stand it. But, it was good for me to go again, and good for Ellie to go and understand what happens when mom goes in for treatment. Ellie needed to see it, I think. It's bad and scary and twists your stomach into knots, but it's good because it teaches you.

When people ask me how my mom is doing I am flattered and touched that they care. But, honestly, when most people ask me how my mom is doing I usually just use the cop-out and say: "fine." That is mostly because I don't like going into the detail of how much breast cancer disgusts me. It is evil, it is sick, it is bad. I say fine because part of me doesn't want to overwhelm someone, part of me doesn't want to be pitied, and part of me just doesn't want to talk about it. Also, in the back of my head I always wonder if the person will think I'm just being dramatic and wish I would just get over it. But, I do talk about it with some people, which is good. As a general rule I keep it to myself. I don't bring it up unless someone asks me about it, which is true of the people I do and don't share with. This isn't to discourage anyone to ask me how my mom is doing, it is really encouraging actually. Just don't expect me to always gush about it. Gushing is hard sometimes, even for me. There are just some days that I don't want to think about breast cancer, and I think I am entitled to that. I don't know if that's right or wrong. After all, my mom can't ignore it. She can't choose to be healthy one day and then go back to fighting cancer the next. But I do know that when I try not to think about my mom being a cancer patient it's not me living in a dream world, it's not depriving myself of the truth... it's giving myself a break. Letting loose. Let me have that.

Another thing that I've noticed is that now, like a turkey is drawn to shiny things, I am drawn to the pink ribbon. Out of compulsion, I look at merchandise - no matter what it is - if it is flaunting Susan G. Komen or Breast Cancer Awareness. Support the Cure reusable grocery bag? Absolutely. Pink highlighters with the pink ribbon on it? Yes, please. Post-its. Give them to me. Buttons. How can I resist? Jewelry. Wrap it up. It's actually not that bad. I don't usually buy it, but if I had the money on me... I would. I usually just look at the packaging like it is the coolest thing in the world. Did you know that I have even been crocheting pink ribbons for people to put on their back packs? It's true. I have a condition.

This is a long battle. After my mom's first surgery, when they removed the lump from her breast, it annoyed me when people gave me books or breast cancer information. I was like... hello? She's done with surgery. It's over. Wrong! Not over, it won't be over for a long time.

BUT this is amazing. This is great. I am EXCITED. My mom is strong and courageous and a fighter. She is shining Christ's light through this situation. I remember that when I was getting ready to go home for her first surgery I was PUMPED! I was so excited because I believed God was going to kick this situation in the butt because I knew there would be people we loved surrounding us who don't know Jesus. If one person, just one, can see Jesus in this situation it will be more than worth it. I want to see lives changed for Christ and my mom is living her life for Him and I know that people are seeing that. She would have no hope, I would have no hope, my family would have NO HOPE if it wasn't for Jesus Christ. Because we know He has a plan for us and that we have placed our faith in the one who knows us better than we know ourselves."

Scott Lane said...
Rachel Howatt is an amazing young woman and Drenda is lucky to have her as a daughter. Lucky, not really. I don't think luck had anything to do with Rachel being who she is and who she is becoming. I do think her parents can accept some of the credit for her strength, sense of humor, intellect, and don't

forget, awesome writing ability. When Rachel writes, I'm with her. When Rachel writes, I'm with Drenda as she responds to this thing called cancer. Scott
April 5, 2009 9:47 PM

Drenda Lane Howatt once again, in the midst of cancer treatment, realizes how fleeting life here on earth really is. Praying for the Dyal and Silva families as they walk through the fire of losing loved ones.
April 6, 2009 at 7:22pm

Drenda Lane Howatt sending a message to Linda and Janette...Jerry may indeed be wrong. Fuzz is looking (and lengthening) much like hair...
April 7, 2009 at 5:41pm

> Linda Waggoner at 11:37am April 8, 2009
> Oh my gosh! Fingers are crossed!!

Drenda Lane Howatt is going to have a hot bath and then go to bed...all in preparation for tomorrow's battle against breast cancer. The war continues.
April 8, 2009 at 7:11pm

> Sally Park at 7:29pm April 8, 2009
> Go get it girl!

Perspective: Contrast and Comparison are Great Helps

Wednesday, April 8, 2009 at 7:50pm

I am told that I look "so good!"

And that I look like "all is going well".

And that I am "doing great!".

I do.

And it is.

And I am.

But only because it is in contrast to how I looked and how I was doing in December, January, and February. No contest about which chemo drugs are harder to "tolerate" (as Jerry would say). There are reasons that one can receive those first drugs only once in one's lifetime...and I happen to think one of those reasons should be the nasty side effects.

It is true, my life goes on. I still get up in the morning and switch out the laundry, fix lunches, get something underway for dinner (ok -- usually I have only to pull something out of the freezer and put it in the oven and set the timer, but still...), make sure Miss Ellie is ready to go, and then it's out the door by 7:10. Drop off Ellie at school, and then head to work in Oregon City. Leaving Oregon City in time to pick up Ellie from track practice, and back in through our kitchen door by 5:15 if we're lucky. Dinner, bath, bed.

But, there are side effects from the current chemo that threaten to sideline me.

Fatigue. Fatigue sometimes so severe that I truly think I will melt into the floor if I don't hold on to something. Fatigue that comes so fast and is so overwhelming that staying awake for afternoon meetings is a gamble.

Aches. I now know, I think, where EVERY bone is in my body. Trust me. This is not a good discovery. I know because EVERY bone aches. Finger joints. Elbows. Tailbone. Toes. Hips. Heels. Feet. Ankles. Wrists. Neck. Shoulders. Not every bone all the time. Some bones some of the time. But I never know when. Or what. Usually at least one severe ache going on always. Jerry gave me vicodon for the pain, but I haven't used it. Scared of those darn narcotics.

Skin loss. The skin on the bottom of my feet is peeling away. Large amounts. Down to bleeding in a number of places. All damage from the taxol. So much skin loss that it is painful to walk. Good thing my white blood count has remained fairly stable. Bad place to get an infection. Jerry is checking my feet every time I see him. Wants to keep "an eye" on them. Some skin loss on my finger tips and the palms of my hands, but nothing severe there. Sores on my gums and roof of my mouth -- as if I have had burns. Skin loss there, too.

I am not complaining. No siree. Because I'd rather these side effects over the nausea any day. I can power through fatigue and pain. Or I can sit down and rest for a minute. I can deal. I can "tolerate".

Yep.

It's all in the perspective.

This is tolerable because the previous treatment was not.

Lynn Peterson: Drenda-unimaginable. All I can say is that while you are in Oregon City tomorrow, you will receive a hug!
April 8, 2009 at 9:07pm

Drenda Lane Howatt: Thank you, Lynn...hold the hug for me because I won't be at work tomorrow. Chemo day. See you on Monday, though!
April 8, 2009 at 9:09pm

Lynn Peterson: Hug holding...does that come with elevator music?
April 8, 2009 at 9:13pm

Drenda Lane Howatt: I would think so.
April 8, 2009 at 9:17pm

Andi Pedersen Jordan: :-) Ya know ... you ARE so Strong and Courageous. Yes siree, you ARE!
April 8, 2009 at 10:00pm

Drenda Lane Howatt Hi Ho, Hi Ho, it's off to chemo I go. Hi Ho Hi Ho Hi Ho. Hi Ho. Hi Ho. (is that enough hi ho's? or did I leave one out?)
April 9, 2009 at 7:00am

Hollace Howatt Chandler at 3:52pm April 9, 2009
How did it go?

Kim Burns at 4:56pm April 9, 2009
How do you feel this afternoon? How long were you there?
You are in my thoughts today.... and prayers.
What are you doing for Easter this year?

Drenda Lane Howatt at 8:23pm April 9, 2009
Thanks for asking~ treatment was fine. Didn't see Jerry today - just lab work, vitals, and infusions. Almost 4 hours start to finish. I did have a little nap while the drugs were dripping. Five more to go...I am on the downhill side of chemo. Yeah!

Drenda Lane Howatt has been up since 4 a.m. and awake even earlier...please tell her again why steroids are her friends?
April 10, 2009 at 4:51am

Andi Pedersen Jordan at 7:20am April 10, 2009
There needs to be a "don't" like button.

Drenda Lane Howatt at 8:07am April 10, 2009
If only...

Gail Hilderbrand at 12:45pm April 10, 2009
I was hoping you could tell me! Tylenol pm doesn't even help! Hang on:)

Drenda Lane Howatt at 1:54pm April 10, 2009
I have had the steroids every week...but this is the first time that I have had such trouble with being antsy and unable to sleep -- or even really sit still for very long. I only have 5 more chemo treatments left, but I am really hoping that the steroids' effect is not cumulative.

Janette Wilkinson at 2:56pm April 10, 2009
There you go again using those big words!

Getting Punched Hurts

Saturday, April 11, 2009 at 4:22pm

I have had a busy day today.

Up early to work on projects -- Don had a recording session scheduled for the office, so I had to be in and out before 9 a.m.

Laundry.

Then inspiration!

A bit of yard work -- really just cleaning up the weeds and moss growing up alongside and in the middle of our front sidewalk. While I was outside working, Richard came by. Richard is one of our tenant-neighbors. He asked me how I was doing. I told him that I was doing ok, still in the middle of chemotherapy, with more and different treatments ahead.

As I answered him, I heard my voice and listened to my words, and thought "who is she talking about?"

It was one of those surreal moments. Like when you analyze a word you use all the time. You see a word like "semblance" and it all of a sudden looks weird. You think "isn't that an odd spelling?"

So, who was I talking about?

Who is battling breast cancer?

Chemotherapy?

Other treatments?

It COULDN'T be me!

Ohh. It IS me.

Another "punched in the stomach by cancer" moment.

I hate being punched.

Because it hurts.

Amber Lynn Montgomery Lane: Yuck yuck yuck yuck! Don't forget... you're Strong. And Courageous. PUNCH BACK!
April 11, 2009 at 7:14pm

Susan Rasmussen Lane: Ditto!
April 12, 2009 at 12:48pm

Kim Burns: Drenda sometimes when I am praying for you and your family I also find myself pausing and wondering.... No not Drenda. This is not real. I can only imagine how it feels to be the ONE getting hit in the stomach... the one fighting the battle first hand. Keep punching back!
April 13, 2009 at 11:32am

Drenda Lane Howatt Jesus Christ is risen from the dead! O death, where is your victory? O death, where is your sting?
April 12, 2009 at 8:54am

Drenda Lane Howatt is wondering why the Easter Bunny did not, as is his usual custom, leave extra robin's eggs in the candy dish for her.
April 12, 2009 at 7:48pm

> Amber Lynn Montgomery Lane at 7:53pm April 12, 2009
> Check for blue-lipped suspects.
>
> Drenda Lane Howatt at 8:47pm April 12, 2009
> That is one reason I LOVE the robin's eggs...great lipstick in colors that are otherwise hard to find!
>
> Anna Howatt at 11:26am April 14, 2009
> Did the Easter Bunny leave anything for me and Rachel?
>
> Drenda Lane Howatt at 8:02pm April 14, 2009
> Guess you'll have to check your mailbox...nothing here. Sorry

Drenda Lane Howatt and family had leftovers for dinner...each enjoying a different menu. Thanks to Chef Janis for sharing the Easter dinner bounty.
April 13, 2009 at 7:50pm

> Maureen Gatens Thompson at 9:06pm April 13, 2009
> We had leftovers as well. Almost as good as the original dinner. YUM!

Drenda Lane Howatt is not quite sure how April 14th arrived so quickly...with April 15th looming on the horizon. Time for

taxes, and wouldn't you know, the printer won't work! yikes. May have to try e-file afterall.
April 14, 2009 at 7:56pm

Andi Pedersen Jordan at 11:07pm April 14, 2009
huh??? You don't e-file?

Drenda Lane Howatt at 6:49am April 15, 2009
I haven't...and I didn't this year -- the site indicated that it could take up to 48 hours to receive confirmation that the IRS received the info. When I worked for Congress, I learned not to mess with the IRS~

Drenda Lane Howatt is attending an "Effective Writing" class at work today...
April 15, 2009 at 6:50am

Jennifer Stady at 7:30am April 15, 2009
That sounds like a fun thingy.

Gail Hilderbrand at 8:50am April 15, 2009
I don't think you need a class for that, you are already accomplished!

Hollace Howatt Chandler at 9:16am April 15, 2009
You should be teaching it.

Anna Howatt at 12:55pm April 15, 2009
Sounds cool.

Drenda Lane Howatt at 6:04pm April 15, 2009
I learned a lot! Some great grammar reminders, a "blueprint" for writing (it really helps!) and more. Too bad none of you will get to read my memos, letters, or "professional" writings. You poor Facebook friends only get to read my rants and emotional upheavals. Sorry~

Maureen Gatens Thompson at 11:13pm April 15, 2009
I took that class too...I thought it was good. :-)

Drenda Lane Howatt just heard the phone message reminding her that chemo #8 is on tap for tomorrow. She is very slowly starting to realize that yes, indeed, chemotherapy will come to an end.
April 15, 2009 at 6:06pm

Elizabeth Lundquist Calhoun at 6:15pm April 15, 2009
Yes, it will! Keep kicking that chemo's butt!

Stephanie Fiskum at 1:48pm April 16, 2009
Agreed! And, you are prayed for by so many.

Drenda Lane Howatt is going to have a great day! A bit of laundry, a bit of cleaning, a bit of shopping, and a lot of killing cancer cells.
April 16, 2009 at 7:39am

Kim Burns at 2:16pm April 16, 2009
You are on the downhill stretch. I hope things went well today and that you feel good. Nice to come home to a clean house. Do you still have dinners in the freezer?

Jennifer Stady at 6:15pm April 16, 2009
All bits in moderation.

Honestly? (Rachel Howatt)

Thursday, April 16, 2009 at 8:26pm
Here's my mom's latest note. After reading it, I am pissed! Livid. Angry. Unsettled. So annoyed. Who does this woman, and anyone like her, think she is? That is so rude and I am so disgusted. I would like to see her go through what my mom is going through and still praise Jesus everyday, still go to work (and do her job *well*), still take care of her family, still keep up with her responsibilities, still look gorgeous!, and still have a smile on her face! So rude.

~~~~~

Endowed Ear-Rings

Thursday, April 16, 2009 at 7:44pm

Today was treatment day. I have now finished 8 of the 12 Taxol/Herceptin treatments. Yeah!

Before we went to see Jerry and have the poison, Don took me to Kohl's so I could do a little shopping. One unwelcome side effect of chemo (aren't they all unwelcome? Yes.) is weight gain. I do not have many casual clothes that fit me right now. The problem comes with planning a trip to Southern California to celebrate Anna's graduation from Azusa Pacific University. A Mom needs decent clothes to go on vacation.

So shopping.

A successful trip!

I managed to find capris that fit and were actually comfortable.
~~~~~

And two cute tops. All in less than an hour. I was feeling good. And looking good -- make-up on, ear-rings in, hair growing, ready to face cancer killing. I was on a roll.

Until.

Until I went out to the car to wait for Don.

It was a beautiful morning. Sunny, warm, gorgeous. I was standing there holding my shopping bag. I watched as a woman that I had seen shopping near me through-out the women's department came out of the store. She walked in my direction, and as she neared, I smiled.

Too soon.

Because, as she approached me, her words were shocking.

"Good thing you're wearing ear-rings."

I apparently didn't comprehend her words initially. I chuckled.

Then, to myself, "WHAT DID THAT WOMAN JUST SAY TO ME?" "OH MY GOODNESS!".

Shocking.

Now, I do realize that I am bald.

And I do realize that I am not "overly-endowed" -- but there *is* endowment.

I have never rested my understanding of my femininity on my hair. And the rest of my body is the same.

Well, not exactly the same.

But pretty close.

Just a bit lop-sided...

But ear-rings?

Seriously?

Don Howatt: Yeah, it's a good thing cuz men don't wear ear-rings, right?!
April 16, 2009 at 7:48pm

Drenda Lane Howatt: exactly!
April 16, 2009 at 7:49pm

Rachel Howatt: This pisses me off! Who does that woman think she is saying something like that?!!?!??!?!?!?!?!??!?!?!?!?!? I'd like to see any other woman look as great as you do, Mom.
April 16, 2009 at 8:23pm

Kim Burns: I am shocked... Unbelievable...I want a chance to tell that woman off.
April 16, 2009 at 8:49pm

Drenda Lane Howatt: Rachel, you're a dear. Thank you.
I am glad that it took me a moment to register the words...that way I didn't have time to respond negatively. But it is a reminder to me about the power of words. It left me wondering, later, whether that woman was thinking of what to say to me as she watched me shopping, or if she even noticed me in the store...
April 16, 2009 at 8:58pm

Drenda Lane Howatt: and I did think of some great replies later!
April 16, 2009 at 8:59pm

Ginger Clausen: How could anyone doubt your femininity (did I spell that right?) if you flashed them your smile! Hair or no hair, God has given you a beautiful heart that shines through your eyes and your smile! Brush it off, girl!
April 16, 2009 at 9:05pm

Sally Park: Drenda, I am sorry that you had to be subjected to such an ignorant (you know what i want to call her) !
April 16, 2009 at 9:51pm

Gail Stempel Hilderbrand: I feel sorry for that woman. She obviously has a closed off, angry heart. It would have been so easy to say "Look hard this is the face of cancer". That would have made her feel like...but what good would it do. You are beautiful and you know it!!!
April 16, 2009 at 10:57pm

Cindy McElmurry: You are beautiful my friend. I think that person is always grumpy. Seriously, who would say something like that?
April 18, 2009 at 8:13am

Drenda Lane Howatt is going to celebrate with new brides and new mommies!
April 18, 2009 at 10:13am

Drenda Lane Howatt is wondering what her new hair will look like. Will it have any curl like before? Will it be red? Or white? Does it matter? hmmm. No. Doesn't matter. Still fun to wonder!
April 20, 2009 at 6:56pm

> Amber Lynn Montgomery Lane at 7:43pm April 20, 2009
> Would still like to take your picture while you're baldy... is there a time that's good for you?
>
> Sally Park at 8:12pm April 20, 2009
> You sound light hearted, music to hear. How long is your hair?
>
> Drenda Lane Howatt at 8:30pm April 20, 2009
> Amber, I don't work on Fridays...
>
> Drenda Lane Howatt at 8:31pm April 20, 2009
> Don says my hair is not long...it's short. harumph.
>
> Jennifer Stady at 8:04am April 21, 2009
> That is a fun thought. Maybe you will be blonde and you will have to buy some ugg boots! Maybe you will have jet black hair or black and white...when will you get to start seeing it?
>
> Drenda Lane Howatt at 5:10pm April 21, 2009
> Now! It is growing. Really soft, like baby hair.
>
> Sally Park at 5:51pm April 21, 2009
> Lane/Lampert genes! Strong!!!!!

Drenda Lane Howatt at 6:15pm April 21, 2009
Something like that...

Maureen Gatens Thompson at 8:58pm April 21, 2009
My hair was straight as a board and grew in curly...go figure? Same color though...

Touched

Tuesday, April 21, 2009 at 8:51pm

"Eventually, cancer touches everyone."

That is the t.v. ad line to sell the Providence Cancer Center.

Obviously, I am "touched".

As is my immediate family.

And my extended family.

And my friends.

My co-workers.

But does my "touching" affect others? People I may never know? The woman in the parking lot?

I wonder about the effect of the affect on all these people, known and unknown?

What is the effect of the affect in me?

In some real ways, I want the "touching" to be merely a "brush"...just a fleeting encounter with sickness, terror, and inconvenience.

But if that is all it is, if the only effect is a fleeting brush, wouldn't touching be wasted? Shouldn't I be different for all I have experienced? Shouldn't there be lessons I learn really well?

I want to be a better person for the cancer. I want to be a better wife, mother, daughter, sister, friend. A better staff assistant. A better landlord. A better Drenda. I want my first responses to be compassion, understanding, love, laughter.

And, if those things happen, I will be able to say that the effect is a strong and lasting change. I will never forget having cancer. And I hope I never forget my lessons learned from going through the sickness, terror, and inconvenience. Especially the terror.

I would love to hear the effect of the affect my cancer has had on you. Good, bad, or ugly! If you are unwilling to make a public comment on this note, please send me a private message.

Because hearing from you will encourage me.

Because hearing from you will "touch" me.

Elizabeth Lundquist Calhoun: Your cancer has put me back in touch with a family member I probably would never have gotten in touch with otherwise...
Your cancer has made me appreciate EACH day for the gift that it is...
Your cancer has allowed me to see the beautiful character of your sisters and daughters as they support you...
Your cancer has encouraged me to write and express my feelings (just about life) on paper more, reviving a long-dormant passion...
Your cancer has given me hope that if I ever have to go through anything even somewhat as terrifying as this disease, maybe I can get through it too...
April 22, 2009 at 5:41am

Zachary Lane Koval: Your cancer has put life in perspective for me. I never really dealt with my own cancer. I went through the surgeries, and all that, but psychologically I still don't think I have actually acknowledged what happened. Reading what you're going through strikes a chord and is forcing me to face my own experience.

It's also odd being on the other side. Funny- my cancer I could handle, yours is not so easy.

Your words and essays have inspired me. They are beautiful and insightful. Your courage and strength amazing. It's been said before, but I'll say it again- thank you for sharing this experience with all of us. I don't think anyone could read it and not be touched.
April 22, 2009 at 6:40am

Susan Rasmussen Lane: It still takes my breath away thinking it's real. I'm not dealing with it well.
April 22, 2009 at 8:09am

Linda Waggoner: You are my LITTLE sister. You should not have cancer! You should not have to deal with the pain, the terror, the rude, inconsiderate remarks. My LITTLE sister should not have to deal with all this! But you ARE dealing with it - in a brave, thoughtful, generous way. When Janette and I discussed shaving our heads in support of your "baldness" I had no idea what that would really mean in my life. In my selfish vanity I wanted to hide under hats or look away if anyone looked at me with I thought was disdain or revulsion (my perception - probably not real!). But as time has passed my lack of hair has turned my thoughts to the path you have been forced to travel. I think about you every day and I thank God that He gave me such a wonderful sister! Having said that I, selfishly, love not having to style my hair -- if it weren't for Ron I might consider... oh, well...
April 22, 2009 at 10:35am

Rachel Howatt: Your cancer has made me strong. I believe what the Bible says - to rejoice when there are trials in your life (James 1). When you called me that night in November and told me you had cancer I did not want to rejoice. I cried and cried. But looking back at how far our family has come through this, I do rejoice! I know that Christ is at work and He is able to use something so terrible as breast cancer to bring about good. Cancer sucks, but you rock! You are not defined by your cancer, you are defined by how you react to it. I am defined by how I react to it. I don't want to be the girl whose mom has breast cancer. I want to be the girl whose mom has breast cancer and yet is strong and courageous. You are strong and courageous, so it makes me want to be that way, too.
April 22, 2009 at 11:53am

Amber Lynn Montgomery Lane: Your stories here, make me feel like I can empathize with all cancer victims just a tad better.

They make me feel like I'm getting to know a little more about my Grandmother, who I never knew because she died from Breast Cancer... after a fifteen year battle with it. (Long enough to raise her youngest child.)

You cancer makes me feel like I know you better, but still feel awkward and at a loss of words when physically in your presence.

I'm worried for you. I'm worried for all my family. What would I ever do if I lost my mother? If my children faced the possibility of losing me?

I'm grateful for you. For your stories. For your STRONG approach... especially in sharing your vulnerabilities.

I am touched. In so many ways.
April 22, 2009 at 5:49pm

Laurie Lane: Isn't that a question we all ask; has my life touched someone else in a positive way? Have I made their journey through life a little brighter, a little easier, a little more humorous because I connected with them? But to ask the question, "How have they touched my life?" is a question I rarely ask myself because I generally focus on my impact on others. Drenda, you have touched my life in many wonderful ways and your cancer is just one small part of the story. You are part of my story, an important part and you have touched me just by being one of my wonderful, caring sisters.
April 26, 2009 at 6:54pm

Drenda Lane Howatt Emergency Declaration Training. Today.
April 22, 2009 at 6:52am

Drenda Lane Howatt Dog the Bounty Hunter: "Listen. You don't need nothing but friends and God."
April 22, 2009 at 8:18pm

> Tina Stinson at 9:06pm April 22, 2009
> I love that show!!!! I love his quotes too!!
>
> Shannon V Fleming Means at 10:09pm April 22, 2009
> Such a good show! I saw Tiff's post on your wall so I thought I'd say hi too. :) How're you doing? I really liked how you wrote your note about the ear-ring lady. Dumb person, but good writing.
>
> Drenda Lane Howatt at 6:21am April 23, 2009
> Yes, Dog makes me laugh. A lot. Every week. And Beth.... Thanks, Shannon, for the compliment on my writing~I just have to get those words out, sometimes.

Drenda Lane Howatt has a quiet house this morning...father/daughter weekly breakfast date today. Then it is off to the battlefield...going to kill those cancer cells DEAD.
April 23, 2009 at 6:35am

> Andi Pedersen Jordan at 7:28am April 23, 2009
> Strong and courageous. You go, girl!
>
> Denise Lane at 7:52am April 23, 2009
> I will be thinking about you, as I do quite often through your struggles. You give me inspiration. I admire your courage and your relentless smile. Keep it up and those stupid bleeping cancer cells have no chance!

Love coming your way, especially today as you face another batch.

Sally Park at 6:56pm April 23, 2009
How did it go?

Drenda Lane Howatt at 8:27pm April 23, 2009
Uneventful...except I should have taken ear plugs with me. One nurse is very loud and crass, and add to her a few patients who do not know the meaning of "inside voice". Makes napping a tad bit difficult. And one needs to nap while getting chemo drugs. It's in the breast cancer manual. Required.

Drenda Lane Howatt Ace of Cakes. Amazing. Check it out now on the Food Channel.
April 23, 2009 at 10:03pm

Chelsea Plover at 10:23pm April 23, 2009
I love that show!

Tayler Younge at 10:02pm April 24, 2009
OH MY GOODNESS! That is my most favorite show ever!

Napping. Required.

Friday, April 24, 2009 at 8:28am

Yesterday was chemo #9 of 12 (13 of 16). An uneventful day...except I was, in retrospect, quite crabby.

The "infusion suite" was very quiet when we arrived. Hardly any patients in the suite. Cold, cold. Choosing my recliner (back against the wall so I have a good view of the surrounding area). Making the trip to the bathroom (I don't want to have to get up and walk around pushing an I.V. pole in front of me, so I go to the bathroom early in an attempt to prevent that necessity). Then, because of the apparent presence of air conditioning, I need two, yes TWO, hot blankets. But I chose bad blankets. Because as I sat in my recliner and tucked myself in, the blankets were only warm! not hot. drats. Don to the rescue -- he brought me a third hot blanket, and that one was perfect. Put the hot blanket directly on me, and then tuck it in with the other two blankets on top.

So this is where my upset starts to come in. The first drugs that are "infused" are anti-histamines. They make me drowsy. I am dozing off, and things are good. However, business is starting to pick up in the suite, and more patients are coming in. LOUD patients. Patients who, I think, have never been instructed in the use of their "inside voice".

And why is it that the old men who come in feel it their duty to flirt with the nurses? Loudly? And what are their wives thinking as they sit and have to observe such behavior? And the one nurse who is loud as well -- and so often replies to the flirting inappropriately. I mean, really. No one attempting to kill cancer cells needs to hear sexual innuendo. Please, guys, I am trying to rest here. Even Don crunching ice cubes is loud in my ears.

But, no resting. Because the guffaws and chortling seem to go on and on. Oh my goodness. Irritation.

Obvious irritation, I am afraid.

Then, with no napping in sight, I start to listen.

I hear one older gentleman talking to Bubba (remember Bubba? He's the son bringing his Momma to treatment who I surmise lives at home and doesn't/can't work). I hear the older man tell Bubba that the doctor said that he had 10 weeks to live. "And that was in January. Those doctors don't know a damn thing."

10 weeks to live? And I'm irritated because I can't nap?

I had written yesterday, in response to my sister Sally asking how chemo went: "uneventful...except I should have taken ear plugs with me. One nurse is very loud and crass, and add to her a few patients who do not know the meaning of "inside voice". Makes napping a tad bit difficult. And one needs to nap while getting chemo drugs. It's in the breast cancer manual. Required."

And, in my last post, "Touched", I had written that I want my first responses to be compassion, understanding, love, laughter.

There is no "breast cancer manual" -- except the one I have written in my head. But I know better. Because my head is not always right.

Because the manual I have written on my heart makes it clear that napping is not required.

Compassion, understanding, love, and laughter are.

I flunk.

Robyn Honeycutt: You have been transparent and authentic. This definitely does not represent "flunking." As I read your account of chemotherapy I thought of my friend (you) who is genuinely connected with her feelings yet still able to let God teach her about His feelings. It's a blessing to know you Drenda and I hope you get a nap today!
April 24, 2009 at 8:53am

Amber Lynn Montgomery Lane: Drenda, I didn't forget that you said you were available today... but our car died last week and is not done getting fixed. My camera and I still want to come visit you soon...
April 24, 2009 at 9:46am

Drenda Lane Howatt: Amber,
We'll find a time - but the hair IS starting to grow! Here's a thought...you could come with me to treatment on Thursday if you're interested. Or, next Friday would work, or pretty much any evening next week. Whatever, or not, that works for you.
April 24, 2009 at 10:01am

Shannon Swope: Hello friend. It's difficult to imagine you being crabby. (smirk) But yeah, things do get put into perspective don't they. But that teachable attitude and humility is where it's at. Good girl! :) I'll have to remember NOT to be flirtatious whenever I get a job! The getting 'hit on' thing is definitely an ongoing thing. I think it makes light of difficult situations-whatever they may be. I interviewed at Adventist on Wednesday; will not hear 'til next week. Meanwhile, it's nice outside and although the weeds are yelling at me the hammock is louder! Later dear...remember, you have a lovely smile and it warms people's hearts!
April 24, 2009 at 1:25pm

Gail Stempel Hilderbrand: I remember looking forward to talking and listening while in "the recliner". It always made my problems seem so small. Especially the last time when the nurse who had been missing for awhile was back. When I asked her if she was on vacation she said no, her husband had just died of Lou Gehrig disease. He was only 36. God always finds a way to remind us, and teach us. Remember sometimes you can't help being crabby, it's not you but rather the steroids.
April 24, 2009 at 7:03pm

Drenda Lane Howatt is not nearly old enough to be the Mom of a college graduate. Not nearly.
April 28, 2009 at 5:41pm

> Sally Park at 5:59pm April 28, 2009
> ummmmm.....ya huh ;)
>
> Drenda Lane Howatt at 6:20pm April 28
> no. NO. no.
> well...o.k., yes.
> But 22 years have just flown by.
>
> Annette Mattson at 12:21am April 29, 2009
> I know...How does it happen so fast?
>
> Maureen Gatens Thompson at 12:27am April 29, 2009
> And at 54, I still have one in high school! They do keep you young and best of all laughing.

Drenda Lane Howatt and Eleanor are home from 31 cent night at Baskin Robbins. Yum.
April 29, 2009 at 8:18pm

> Kris Howatt at 9:39am April 30, 2009
> We were there too - double yum.

Drenda Lane Howatt If this is Thursday, it must be Paris. No. Wait. It's chemo day.
April 30, 2009 at 6:07am

> Kris Howatt at 9:36am April 30, 2009
> Tuesday it must be Belgium

Clarke J. Howatt at 9:42am April 30, 2009
Suzanne Pleshette's (sp?) finest role. She looked great in his shirt didn't she . . .

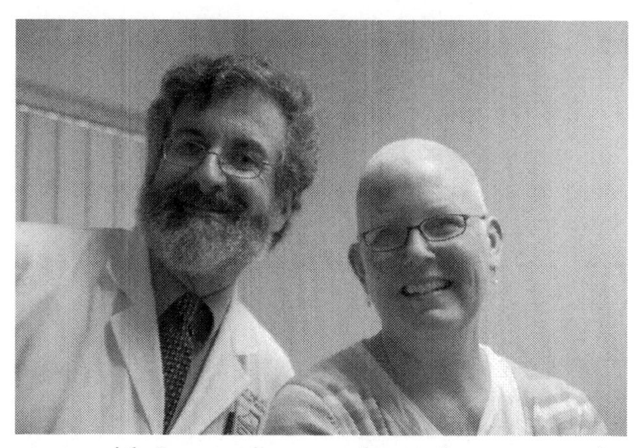

Drenda meets with Jerry prior to a chemotherapy appointment.
Photo by Amber Lynn Montgomery Lane

Drenda as she waits for chemotherapy to begin.
Photo by Amber Lynn Montgomery Lane

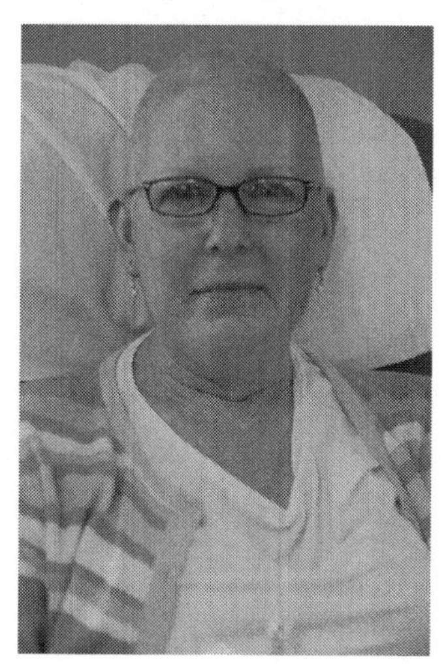

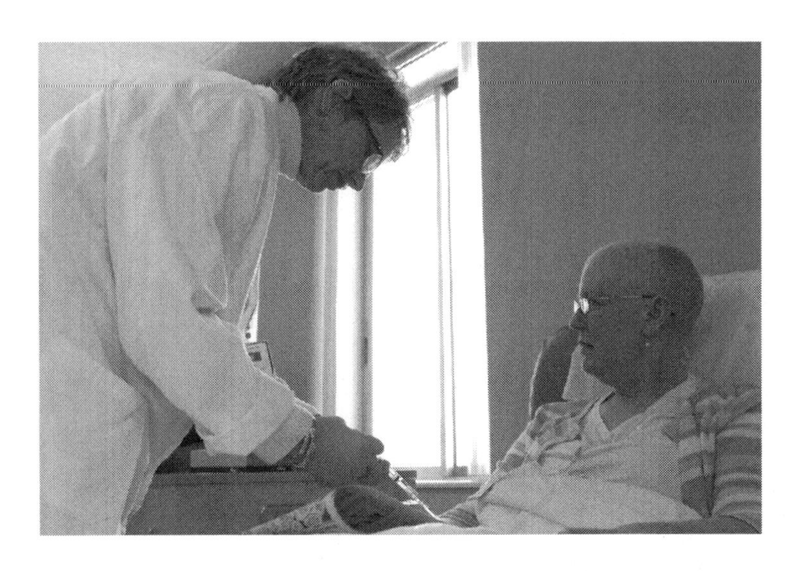

Chemotherapy I.V. line preparation.
Photo by Amber Lynn Montgomery Lane

Drenda watches IV line as the drugs are injected.
Photo by Amber Lynn Montgomery Lane

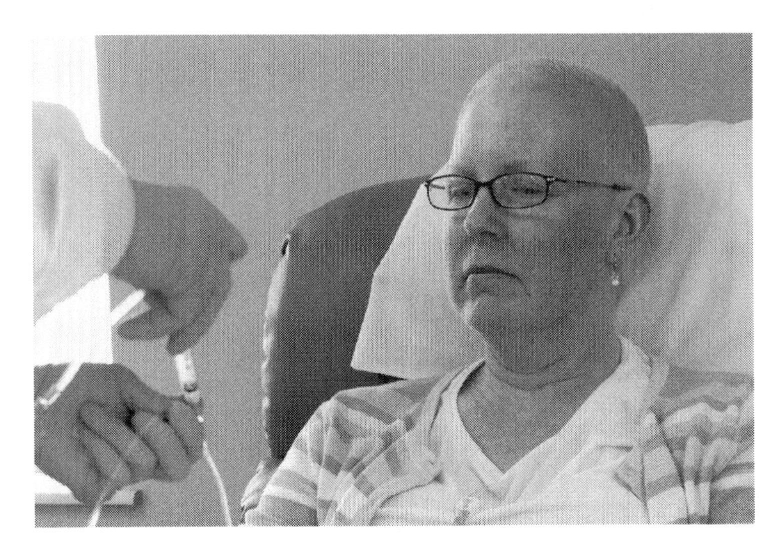

Drenda's husband Don watching as the chemotherapy begins.
Photo by Amber Lynn Montgomery Lane

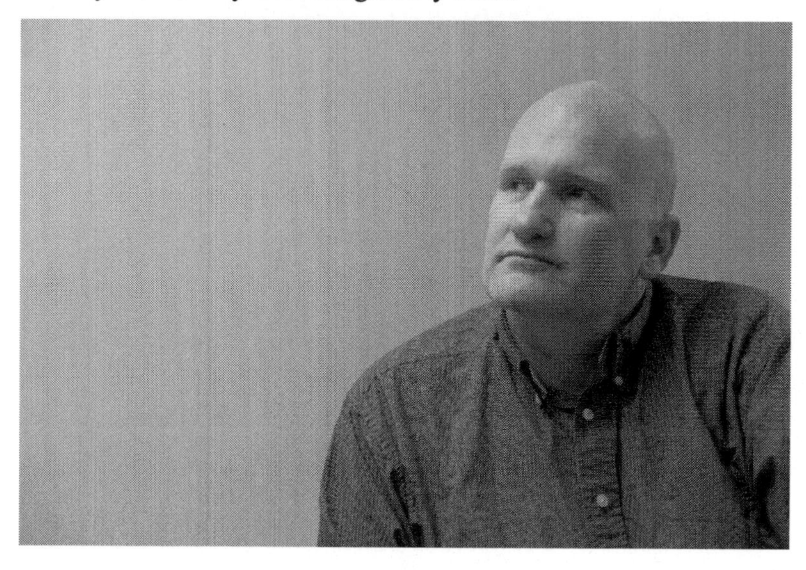

Drenda works on suduko puzzle while receiving chemotherapy.
Photo by Amber Lynn Montgomery Lane

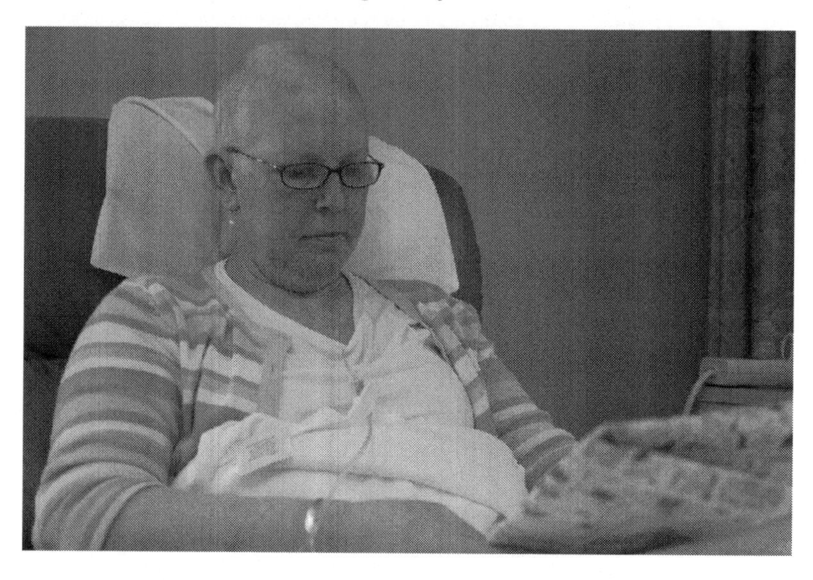

Drenda Lane Howatt is home from Paris and is going to leave again to go to dinner and, just maybe, shoe shopping.
April 30, 2009 at 6:19pm

> Gail Hilderbrand at 6:39pm April 30, 2009
> I am so glad your "flights" are getting easier:)
>
> Drenda Lane Howatt at 9:51pm April 30, 2009
> Me too! Only two more to go...

Drenda Lane Howatt thinks she is in the process of losing some of her fingernails. Not good. Not good at all. Thank you, Chemo.
May 2, 2009 at 10:00am

> Susan Rasmussen Lane at 10:24am May 2, 2009
> Oh, no. It wouldn't be permanent, would it?
>
> Drenda Lane Howatt at 1:50pm May 2, 2009
> Not permanent...just as long as it takes to grow new nails. Nothing lost yet, but they are progressing towards being gone...lifting up from the nail-bed. Very painful!
>
> Susan Rasmussen Lane at 1:53pm May 2, 2009
> Eeewww, so sorry!
>
> Gail Hilderbrand at 5:38pm May 2, 2009
> That is just not fair:(
>
> Sally Park at 9:47pm May 2, 2009
> I am sorry Drenda. So much you have to deal with!
> I love you.
>
> Linda Waggoner at 11:10am May 3, 2009
> NOT FAIR!!!!
>
> Drenda Lane Howatt at 9:21pm May 3, 2009

Absolutely not fair! Fingernails should not be painful to touch. But I think I am finally, after 47 years, starting to give up on "fair". Not completely, but starting.

Drenda Lane Howatt has, after 12 hours and 700 miles, lost her ankles. They are nowhere to be seen.
May 3, 2009 at 9:27pm

Bradley Ruhl at 9:31pm May 3, 2009
Heavens! It's the kankle lady

Linda Waggoner at 11:53am May 4, 2009
Not good - take care of yourself!

Drenda Lane Howatt at 7:55pm May 4, 2009
Thanks, Linda. I'll take it easy.
Still no ankles, though. Maybe they'll come back soon?

Linda Waggoner at 12:46pm May 5, 2009
Probably - if you stay out of the car for long enough!

Drenda Lane Howatt looked all over Disneyland...Mickey couldn't be found. How odd is that?
May 4, 2009 at 7:46pm

Amber Lynn Montgomery Lane at 8:10pm May 4, 2009
Ugh, they have him way in the back (Toon Town) in this house and you have to wait in line to see him. I guess it's more fair for those who really want to, but ugh!

Tom Turnbull at 8:56pm May 4, 2009
He does a Main Street drive by every once in a while.

Janette Wilkinson at 9:13pm May 4, 2009
Enough already! Who cares?! So what! You ARE in Disneyland! NOBODY cares! Do you hear me?

N-O-B-O-D-Y C-A-R-E-S!!!!! by the way dland had so many cut backs they cut Mickey's position. Check for him at unemployment office in Anaheim.

Andi Pedersen Jordan at 9:25pm May 4, 2009
Where is thumbs down when you need it?
Ha, Janette, funny!

Amber Lynn Montgomery Lane at 10:28pm May 4, 2009
Drenda... you have a green sister. Mouse envy.

Robin Reilly at 3:19am May 5, 2009
He's in Orlando. =}

Drenda Lane Howatt at 7:26am May 5, 2009
Yes, a very green sister. Janette protests too much, me thinks.

Don Howatt at 7:57am May 5, 2009
Ahh, excuse me! We did see him!, Mickey is the personification of D-Land. He is all around us. DUH!!

Ginger Clausen at 12:51pm May 8, 2009
Did you look for the hidden Mickeys? They are everywhere, if you look!

Drenda Lane Howatt at 4:32pm May 8, 2009
Yep. We've found some.

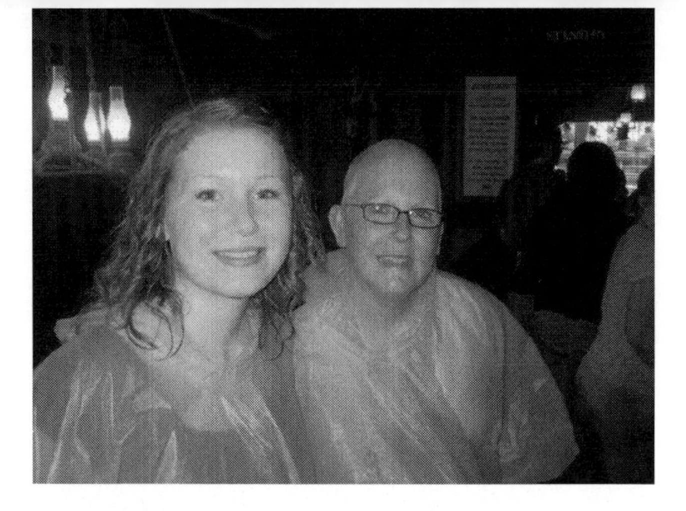

Drenda and daughter Rachel enjoying Disneyland. (May 2009)
Photo by Don Howatt

Drenda Lane Howatt spent the afternoon resting in the hotel room. Now about dinner...
May 5, 2009 at 6:47pm

Drenda Lane Howatt is convinced, after a day at California Adventure and an evening at the hotel pool, that there is a parenting crisis in America. Crisis. Pandemic of screaming parents and disobedient children. Oh my.
May 5, 2009 at 8:44pm

> Drenda Lane Howatt at 8:55pm May 5, 2009
> Or perhaps it is the "whine" flu...
>
> Maureen Gatens Thompson at 9:29pm May 5, 2009
> LOL...but I absolutely agree with you. When Jim and I go out we are amazed at the behaviors on both sides. Our kids never pulled that stuff in public not because they were afraid of the consequences but because they knew it was w-r-o-n-g. I still wonder, what changed?!

Gail Hilderbrand at 10:26pm May 5, 2009
That can ruin an evening by the pool

Drenda Lane Howatt has, FINALLY, laid eyes on Mickey, Minnie, Donald, and her very own ankles. Woot.
May 7, 2009 at 7:58am

Drenda Lane Howatt RACE FOR THE CURE - Walking for Drenda
STRONG AND COURAGEOUS is looking for walkers of all ages! Join the team "STRONG AND COURAGEOUS" on September 20, 2009 in an untimed 5k walk to help raise money for the cure. (We're listed as a friends and family team.)

The Susan G. Komen Breast Cancer Foundation: Oregon and SW Washington Affiliate - Race for the Cure®
Source: www.komenoregon.org
Thank you to the more than 45,400 participants and 1,200 volunteers who joined together September 21, 2008 for the 17th Annual Komen Portland Race for the Cure®. Thanks to your efforts we raised ...
May 7, 2009 at 6:25pm

> Drenda Lane Howatt at 6:33pm May 7, 2009
> Looks like we have 11 team members so far...
>
> Christina Elford at 9:19pm May 7, 2009
> 12!
>
> Drenda Lane Howatt at 9:41pm May 7, 2009
> Excellent! Thank you, Christina, for being part of the Strong and Courageous.

Stop Talking Already

Friday, May 8, 2009 at 4:56pm

Disneyland.

The Happiest Place on Earth.

I was riding as a single rider on Toy Story - the arcade ride/game. As soon as I got in the "car" and sat down, I took off my hat. Whew. It was hot and sunny out, so my head was hot and sweaty. The woman I was sitting with immediately asked me if I had cancer.

"Yes."

"Breast cancer?"

"Yes."

"I am a three year survivor!"

Turns out her cancer was later stage, but the same type as I have. She was so happy that I was in Disneyland... "I came here in mid-treatment, too! But my husband had to push me around in a wheelchair".

She asked about my treatment, and this is where I gave too much information. Too much scary information.

I told her about the clinical trial with lapatinib. I told her about the HER-2 neu cancer going to the brain. I told her herceptin doesn't cross into the brain.

I told too much.

Because she was obviously shaken.

Because she didn't know about the brain connection.

Because she didn't want to be scared by cancer again. I could tell.

Too late.

As I walked away and lost sight of her in the crowd, and ever since, I have felt terrible. Here this woman reached out to encourage me, and I frightened her.

Shut up, Drenda.

Close your mouth.

Stop talking already.

Hollace Howatt Chandler: Hey, Drenda, don't beat yourself up. You may have just given her life-saving info. It may have been a divine appointment that will get her to seek medical help.
May 8, 2009 at 5:02pm

Drenda Lane Howatt: Oh, Holly! Thank you. That is a great thought, and one I hadn't considered. Her face has haunted my thoughts for the last few days.
May 8, 2009 at 5:06pm

Erin Frazier Miller: "Someone" may have been working through you. You said all the right things.
May 9, 2009 at 7:10am

Kris Howatt: I agree with Holly - and she saw you having fun at Disney - encouragement.
May 9, 2009 at 10:34am

Drenda Lane Howatt is getting ready to help Anna move out of her apartment; next is attending Anna's graduation. From college. Oh my goodness. Not sure how this graduation thing came so fast, but it sure is exciting! Anna is wonderful!
May 9, 2009 at 6:55am

> Elizabeth Lundquist Calhoun at 10:04am May 9, 2009
> I haven't seen her since she was just a little girl! Time sure does fly... Congratulations on this milestone!

Drenda Lane Howatt and Ellie are home, Rachel is back in Seattle, Anna and Don are en route to Portland somewhere along I-5. We are officially "graduated". woo hoo!
May 10, 2009 at 3:40pm

> Maureen Gatens Thompson at 11:07pm May 10, 2009
> Another major milestone for you and your family. What a great Mother's Day weekend for you. *s*

Drenda Lane Howatt is late...already missed part of Dancing with the Stars. Oh my goodness. Gotta go...
May 11, 2009 at 8:18pm

Drenda Lane Howatt is attending the Villages of Mt. Hood annual meeting and then the grand opening of the Multipor overpass.
May 13, 2009 at 6:03am

Drenda Lane Howatt is home from having dinner with dear friends. Now it is time to go to bed. Tomorrow is a big day.
May 13, 2009 at 9:04pm

Good Days and Bad Days

Drenda Lane Howatt is weary. Heart weary. Body weary. Mind weary. Completely and utterly weary.
May 14, 2009 at 10:35pm

> Andi Pedersen Jordan at 10:47pm May 14, 2009
> I want a dis-like button now. Maybe that's what you get from going to Disneyland? :-/
> I know . . . strong and courageous you are, ever so strong and courageous.
>
> Drenda Lane Howatt at 10:51pm May 14, 2009
> No strength or courage here, not tonight...
>
> Andi Pedersen Jordan at 10:53pm May 14, 2009
> I'm sorry. I'd take some for you. You can do it, Drenda. You have to. Beat it girl... Just ask for more . . .

Drenda Lane Howatt is feeling a bit less weary this morning...everything is always a tich better when the sun is shining.
May 15, 2009 at 9:38am

> Kim Burns at 2:53pm May 18, 2009
> I will say Amen to that....

Scared

Friday, May 15, 2009 at 12:42pm

"Courage is being scared to death -- but saddling up anyway." John Wayne

"You gain strength, courage, and confidence by every experience in which you really stop to look fear in the face. You must do the one thing you think you cannot do." Eleanor Roosevelt

Oh my goodness. Is it possible to be courageous and be "saddled up", but still scared to death?

Yes.

Scared of death?

Yes.

Is it possible to gain strength, courage and confidence by looking fear in the face, and still being scared to death?

Yes.

I know.

Because I am.

I am "saddled up"...on the breast cancer bucking bronco.

I am stopped and looking fear in the face.

I am doing the one thing I thought I could not do. I am fighting cancer.

I am gaining strength, courage, and confidence.

But I am still scared to death.

And scared of death.

Looking fear in the face is a daily process. A moment to moment process.

I have learned that just because I look fear in the face, stare fear in the face, glare at fear in its face, it doesn't go away for long. Sometimes not at all.

I will keep staring at that monster called fear.

I will keep glaring at that monster.

And I will win.

Amber Lynn Montgomery Lane: Yes. You WILL!
May 15, 2009 at 12:58pm

Sally Park: You will look back on this last year and know that you can face anything, tackle and conquer. And ... that most of life's ups and downs are just popcorn compared to what real stress is.
Soak up some of this beautiful sun, this afternoon!
Love you.
May 15, 2009 at 1:31pm

Andi Pedersen Jordan: That's more like it. Yes, you will win, Drenda.
:-)
May 15, 2009 at 5:54pm

Drenda Lane Howatt has a clean house and most of the laundry done...ahhh. Oh, what to do, what to do? How about a shopping trip to Trader Joe's with Ellie for dinner ingredients. Gotta love those 7th grade Home Ec assignments! Menu planning and cooking. Ellie is a great cook already.
May 16, 2009 at 7:51am

Drenda Lane Howatt has scones in the oven, sun shining through the windows, and a fresh breve on the way. Perfect!
May 17, 2009 at 8:13am

Drenda Lane Howatt is reflecting on the last six months...surgery #1 was six months ago today. Just a few short months, but, oh, it seems like a lifetime.
May 18, 2009 7:14pm

Six Months

Monday, May 18, 2009 at 7:53pm

Six months.

One half of a year.

Six short months.

A lifetime.

And yet, just a few short weeks, really.

In some ways, I have come so far.

In other ways, I have not progressed at all.

Some days, it is two steps forward, one (or three) steps backward. But I AM stepping. There is something to be said for that. I did not completely curl up in a ball and retreat. Not completely.

I just read my cousin Hollace's blog. One entry in titled "Good words are good things". She stresses that we should focus on the positive, on the good, and not be weighed down by the negative.

So, I will list the good of the past six months, the things and people I am eternally grateful for:

I have been overwhelmed.

Overwhelmed with love.

Support.

Care.

Prayers.

Concern.

My God. I call Him "my" God because He is known to me. Not because I have "my" God and you have "yours". There is only One. And it is He.

My husband. He is amazing. Cancer has only proven, again, what a great and wonderful man he is.

My family.

My friends.

My church family.

My work friends.

Acquaintances that follow my journey through my blog, on Facebook, or through others.

Fellow cancer survivors, some complete strangers, who speak words of encouragement just because they remember.

The Palm Spring Girl Friends. None of whom I have ever met.

Jerry.

So, there is a common thread through most of the good.

That thread is people.

People who take time to put action to their care and concern. Action of calling. Sending a card. Praying for me. Crying with me. Lifting me up. Encouraging me. Cheering me on. Propping me up when I am collapsing. Cooking dinners for my freezer. Leaving a comment or short message on Facebook.

This is not a journey I would ever want to take alone. O.k....it is not a journey I would ever want to take at all.

But I didn't get to choose, and I am on the journey. And so very thankful that I am accompanied along the road by people who love me and care for me and have made the effort, some over and over, to make sure I remember that they are there.

Thank you.

Because I hate being alone on road trips.

Gail Stempel Hilderbrand: You are a "positive" in my book. You encourage me so much with your words. What a blessing you are to everyone you touch:)
May 18, 2009 at 8:58pm

Andi Pedersen Jordan: No, I think it's "thank you".
I think you are teaching the rest of us a thing or two.
May 18, 2009 at 11:08pm

Linda Waggoner: Even though you might not have met her you have already given comfort to Ron's sister-in-law, Janet. She is at the very beginning of her breast cancer journey. Her husband told me last night that she didn't know it yet but after the mastectomy it was decided that she will need chemotherapy in addition to radiation therapy. He also told me that Janet felt comforted by my conversation with her the night before -- I

just shared a bit of what your journey has been like. Your willingness to reach out to us and share your struggle has lifted us all up.
May 19, 2009 at 10:17am

Shannon Swope: Lovely words dear friend. Thank you for sharing~ :)
May 19, 2009 at 3:33pm

Kim Burns: Thank you for sharing your heart. Thank you for your life long friendship. It is a treasure that grows more valuable through time (good and tough times). I love you my friend.
May 19, 2009 at 5:37pm

Drenda Lane Howatt two baldies in the library, each with a breve. No, wait, one of the baldies is growing hair! "Unkempt" even. Cool.
May 20, 2009 at 6:18am

Hollace Howatt Chandler at 9:46am May 20, 2009
I wish it were 3 baldies with 3 breves.

Don Howatt at 8:53pm May 20, 2009
Swirls of white fluff

Drenda Lane Howatt at 8:54pm May 20, 2009
Not white...golden

Don Howatt at 8:55pm May 20, 2009
Wouldn't golden be gold?

Chemo Coming to an End

Drenda Lane Howatt is going to war again today, full of excitement and anxiety...today is chemo treatment #16...FINAL and LAST chemotherapy. So happy and excited to be done with this segment of the journey. So anxious that, after this week, no more chemo in her blood to kill cancer.
May 21, 2009 at 6:34am

> Bethann Westfall at 6:50am May 21, 2009
> Love and prayers to you today! You are AMAZING! Cling to our Father and He will carry you today.
> Love you tons,
> Bethann
>
> Andi Pedersen Jordan at 7:00am May 21, 2009
> Hooray!
>
> Annette Mattson at 7:09am May 21, 2009
> I am sending you courage and hugs through this time...
>
> Elizabeth Lundquist Calhoun at 7:59am May 21, 2009
> Wow, this is a milestone. Congratulations! And I will be praying for extra helpings of peace and strength for you today.
>
> Gail Hilderbrand at 8:30am May 21, 2009
> YES!!! You did it, you made it through! You're a rock star! (not Don, you):)
>
> Adrienne Fajen at 9:44am May 21, 2009
> Sounds like cause for celebration--another breve?

Drenda Lane Howatt at 11:55am May 21, 2009
Yes, celebration! Dinner out tonight!

Hollace Howatt Chandler at 5:01pm May 21, 2009
Thank goodness IT'S OVER

Laurie Lane at 5:23pm May 21, 2009
Yes! Two treatments down, one to go. There is a huge light at the end of the tunnel!!!

Sandy Hagstrand at 7:23pm May 21, 2009
Congratulations!

Abigale Mary Lane at 8:50 pm May 21, 2009
woo hoo!

Jumbled Hurdles

Thursday, May 21, 2009 at 10:29pm

Jumbled.

Conflicted.

Emotional.

Happy. No, ecstatic. Giddy, even.

Scared.

Relieved.

I could list even more emotions -- all of which I have felt today.

I knew my last chemo treatment would arrive and that it would bring with it the conflict of feelings.

I knew it.

And yet I was totally unprepared.

Unprepared for the shakiness as I sat in the lab chair waiting for my port to be accessed.

Unprepared to have tears as I talked with nurse Katherine.

Unprepared for the panic rising. Literally rising.

Unprepared for the sadness as I realized I won't be able to

follow Denny, the man who, -- in January, was given 10 weeks to live. Or Eleanor. The Russians. The young girls, both of whom are probably barely 20.

Unprepared for the surprise of the nurses -- "what? today is your last treatment? You're not doing more herceptin? Aren't you coming for the weekly 1 year herceptin treatment?"

Unprepared for the second guessing of my decision to participate in the clinical trial.

Unprepared for more tears. After treatment was finished, nurse Katherine said to me "o.k., when you get up and get your things together, I am going to give you a hug". So, I get up, hobble to the bathroom, go in and shut the door, and immediately burst into tears.

Unprepared to deal with myself and all this crying. Oh my goodness. Wipe away the tears, give myself a verbal lashing -- "pull yourself together, Drenda". Go back out, hug nurse Katherine, and more tears. Not sobbing, but the silent tear rolling down the cheek type of crying. Those eyes/tears ducts are not under my control apparently.

Since December 18th, my life has been chemo.

Chemo and its side effects.

I now move on into another unknown. Knowledge, good and bad, in some ways equals safety.

But now I feel unsafe.

Unsafe and unprepared.

Unprepared, even though the consent form for the clinical trial was 24 pages of possible side effects. That is, supposedly, preparation. That is a lot of side effects, I must say.

I am still unprepared.

But I am just as happy and excited.

Because I have stayed the course.

I have jumped one of the major hurdles of breast cancer treatment -- and I didn't fall. I clipped that hurdle a few times, I hit it with my feet or my legs as I jumped. But I did jump, and I cleared that hurdle.

There were times that I didn't think I'd make it. I didn't think I could continue one more day, one more hour, one more minute, one more hot flash or one more night laying awake with severe bone aches.

But I did.

I made it. And I think it is fair to say that I came through chemotherapy with flying colors.

Jerry would agree. I know he would.

God has protected me. My immune system is compromised due to the chemo. And yet, there have been times when Ellie was very ill, times when Don has been quite ill, people at work sick with coughs and colds, and I have been protected. No colds. No illness. Even with all that illness around me, my blood counts have remained in the "safe" low levels.

I will focus on the excitement.

I will focus on the achievement.

I AM stronger because of chemotherapy.

And I WILL be courageous as I face the next steps.

"HAVE I NOT COMMANDED YOU? BE STRONG AND COURAGEOUS. DO NOT BE TERRIFIED; DO NOT BE DISCOURAGED, FOR THE LORD YOUR GOD WILL BE WITH YOU WHEREVER YOU GO." JOSHUA 1:9

Andi Pedersen Jordan: And I remember your first posting when you wrote you were "strong and courageous" . . . I thought you were mocking your boss ... SW. Yep. That's what I thought.

Strong and courageous . . . no matter which boss suggested it ... sounds good in my book. You go, girl. You go.
May 21, 2009 at 10:34pm ·

Drenda Lane Howatt: oh! No, no mocking. Not even. That first posting was as I waited for test results.
Thank you so much, Andi, for your on-going encouragement. It really means so much to me.
May 21, 2009 at 10:43pm

Andi Pedersen Jordan: Turn around is fair play, "my friend". (extra points for who likes the phrase "my friend".)

well ... not even really mocking ... but didn't you ever say "hey, SW, how are you today?"

"Strong & Courageous" ... was the reply
... have you ever had that exchange with him?

More importantly ... has someone burned sage in that darn office? kind of kidding.
May 21, 2009 at 10:47pm

Tina Stinson: Drenda, you are amazing!!
May 21, 2009 at 10:57pm

Amanda Lane: I have hit the wall myself, completely ready to give up and walk away from the house and everything. Don't think I can possibly last another day (especially with cramps coming on strong and shooting pain down my legs). But damn it, you made it through so much more, and I know I can and will go on.
In short, you are an inspiration. Sending you all my love.

p.s. sorry, I didn't say so earlier, but you are definitely part of the not sucking family
May 22, 2009 at 8:36am

Drenda Lane Howatt: Amanda,
I've found that the walls we hit end up crumbling...sometimes after we crumble, but they do break into small pieces -- pieces that we will kick out of our way, or walk on top of. And if we walk on top of those pieces of the wall we will end up higher and we will be better people for it. And the walls force us to re-evaluate what is important. Is the house important? Yes. But how much? Only you can answer that. We both know, now, that physical pain combined with emotional pain is incredibly overwhelming, but we WILL (and do) get through. Keep going, my dear. It is only making you stronger, whether or not you realize.

I am SO glad that I am part of the not sucking family.
I love you, and happy to have you as a friend and niece!
May 22, 2009 at 9:24am

Amanda Lane: Unfortunately with the house, I can't really walk away. When I looked into apartments, none anywhere near me would rent to a dog over 40lbs. (even though most advertise as having "no breed restrictions). I can't take my babies with me many places at all...
May 22, 2009 at 10:46am

Sally Park: Wow! Hope Floats!!!! You are amazing. I can only believe that if I am faced with what you have encountered I can

be so strong. When you first wrote months ago on FB (before you revealed your challenge) that you were “Strong and Courageous” I wrote back that we were from good stock and that indeed you had it in your blood (paraphrasing). Well, it looks to me like that was a true-dom. I believed that then, and you have proven me true. I know that fear is harder then anything. We take one day, one minute at a time and that is truly how we should live. I love you dear Sister, love you dearly and think about your mountains every day.
May 23, 2009 at 5:56pm

Amanda Graber: Drenda-
You absolutely amaze me and have amazed me every single time I have read one of your notes. You are a fighter and a wonderful woman. I am very happy to hear that you have come through the chemotherapy and have such a good attitude, especially when it comes to your faith. You are an inspiration to me. Knowing that you have stayed strong going through this battle helps me stay strong going through little things that seem like molehills compared to the mountain that cancer is. Thank you so much for that. I will keep you in my prayers.
-Amanda Graber
May 25, 2009 at 5:07pm

Drenda Lane Howatt: Thank you, all, for your kind and encouraging words! Sally, I do remember that FB posting....”strong and courageous” and I was so praying that I wouldn’t have to be strong and courageous through cancer. But then, the diagnosis. I have come far. Far to go, but I am up for the trek...I think.
May 25, 2009 at 6:12pm

Drenda Lane Howatt is happy to be home after a relaxing long weekend in Central Oregon.
May 25, 2009 at 6:09pm

Drenda Lane Howatt is off to work this morning, then to Providence for yet another echo-cardiogram. Be still my heart. No. Wait. Don't be still...work well. Pump that blood.
May 26, 2009 at 6:35am

> Gail Hilderbrand at 11:09am May 26, 2009
> Has your ejection fraction stayed the same throughout?
>
> Drenda Lane Howatt at 6:23am May 28, 2009
> I think so. I'll get the results today. How are you, Gail?

Drenda Lane Howatt is going to get up out of her chair in the library and proceed to the kitchen and stare in the refrigerator looking for inspiration for lunch and dinner. Oh, yes. And breakfast, too.
May 27, 2009 at 6:40am

> Clarke J. Howatt at 8:39am May 27, 2009
> Heard you went shopping in Sisters. That's enough to wear out anybody.
>
> Drenda Lane Howatt at 4:23pm May 27, 2009
> Yes, it did wear me out. Still in recovery. But so worth it!

Drenda Lane Howatt is confused. Today is Thursday...but no chemo? OH YES! CHEMO IS DONE! OVER! Okay. Now she is calm. She is happy to see Jerry this afternoon, have an EKG, and find out the results of Tuesday's echo-cardiogram. Also, making a list of questions for the good Doctor.
May 28, 2009 at 6:25am

Hollace Howatt Chandler at 9:05am May 28, 2009
Yay!

Drenda Lane Howatt was pleased to learn that her heart is normal...but she wonders how that can be possible after the lab tech removed 13 vials of blood. Blood, another somewhat renewable resource. God knew what He was doing when He created the human body.
May 29, 2009 at 6:54am

Milt Buckelew at 7:14am May 29, 2009
Hey, your body is green:-)

Carolyn Kempf at 12:12pm May 30, 2009
We are just big bags of water and skin...well and a spirit/soul too. Yeah! Glad you are doing well!

~Saying "NO" Feels So Good~

Sunday, May 31, 2009 at 8:15am

Last Thursday was another appointment with Jerry.

First, though, to the lab to have blood drawn. The clinical trial called for lots of blood that day. Thirteen vials. Yikes. This was the first time that the lab tech has had any problem with drawing blood from my port...seems the needle was trying to suck up my vein. So I ask the tech "which needle are you using?" Response: "3/4 inch". "hmm. That's is why my chart says to use the 1 inch needle...3/4 inch is too short."

After weeks of going for blood work and always asking to make sure the 1 inch needle was used, the one time I don't ask/remind, the short needle is used. This is the kind of thing that is so tiring. Rhetorical question here, but must I always tell them how to do their job?

After a bit more fiddling around, the lab tech was able to get the short needle to draw blood.

All 13 vials full.

Good news at vitals. Lost 3 pounds since the previous week. Fluid retention is slowly relenting.

My time with Jerry went well. Everything seems fine…echo-cardiogram results unchanged and completely normal. No detectable heart damage from chemo-therapy. EKG results also normal. I am a normal girl...except that I have breast cancer. Go figure.

I asked Jerry if I can get back to normal life now. Yes. Manicures and pedicures? He chuckles. I chuckle. Don shakes his head at me. As if my normal, before cancer, life held time for such pleasures. Then Jerry responds, "oh, well wait a few weeks on those..." Shaving? "wait a few weeks on that, too". Occasional glass of wine? Yes.

Jerry tells me that I'll come back for more blood work, and start the clinical trial drug lapatinib on July 9th. I asked Jerry what happens if I decide to quit the trial. Can I go back to the regular treatment of herceptin? "Oh. Why do you ask?, But, yes. If you stop the trial, you can finish out the treatment schedule with herceptin. Most people tolerate lapatinib quite well, though." I feel better knowing that I still have the option, but I think my question made Jerry nervous.

I won't see Jerry again until July 16th. Oh my goodness. That is a long time from now. Good news and bad news. Jerry makes me feel safe.

He says I will also need to come in sometime between now and July 9th to have my port flushed. And then he tells me to "keep up the good work."

Wait!

How, exactly, do I do that? It's his good work, not mine.

Or maybe it's His good work.

As we leave, I stop at the front desk to make my appointments.

The woman at the desk is very friendly and we get the lab appointment and the appointment to see Jerry all set.

And then I say "I need to come in to get my port flushed." "Oh, I can't make that appointment here. You'll have to go upstairs to the Infusion Suite to make that appointment."

"Excuse me?"

"You have to go upstairs."

"No, thank you, I'm done upstairs and am not going back." She looks at me, quite confused.

I say, to myself, 'you're confused? Really? Surely I am not the first patient who refuses to go upstairs?'

But I just repeat my first response to her.

"I am finished upstairs and am not going back there."

Pause.

"Oh. I guess you can call in to get the appointment."

Okay.

I'll call.

And then I may send that cancer office some of my thoughts...like a little primer in customer service and patient emotional care.

In retrospect, I may have gained a bit of insight into two year old children.

Saying "no" feels good.

It is empowering.

And I didn't even stomp my feet.

Ron Chandler: Stomping is good.
June 2, 2009 at 11:21am

Sally Park: Spunky! Love it!!!!
June 2, 2009 at 9:24pm

Drenda Lane Howatt is looking forward to the coming week...no doctor or medical appointments...no, not even one! It will be her last week completely free until at least the second week in August. And it will be only the second week free since, umm, November?
May 31, 2009 at 4:53pm

> Sally Park at 10:23pm May 31, 2009
> Enjoy it!
>
> Marie Pestalozzi at 10:34pm May 31, 2009
> Yeah Drenda!!! A Nice Sunny Week (hopefully) to enjoy being away from DOCTORS and Clinics :)
> Thinking about you!!
>
> Hollace Howatt Chandler at 5:39pm June 1, 2009
> Have a great week Drenda

Drenda Lane Howatt is up late. Yes, 7:54 is LATE when one's alarm goes on at 5 a.m. and when one is fighting cancer. Time for bed.
June 1, 2009 at 8:01pm

> Kris Howatt at 9:43pm June 1, 2009
> I don't set my alarm that early, but the birds seem to think 5 a.m. is getting up time.

Drenda Lane Howatt is waiting for that handsome man in brown to arrive...
June 3, 2009 at 5:54pm

Radiation, Oh My!

Wednesday, June 3, 2009 at 6:27pm

Don and I visited the radiation oncologist, Dr. Alice Wang, the Friday before Memorial Day. May 22nd.

That day, she outlined the radiation trek ahead.

Oh my goodness. It is a trek. Not as arduous as chemotherapy, but it will still be intrusive.

I will see her on Monday, June 8th for "mapping"...and my tattoos.

Sorry to say that the tattoos will be only dots. But I may connect them in the future.

Then, Dr. Wang will need a week to "plan" my treatment. That means doing the math and computer work to map the best shot at my breast. Trying to hit as little of my lungs as possible. Good for me that the cancer was in the right breast. That saves my heart.

Dr. Wang said radiation treatment should begin on June 15th.

I asked for a slight delay in treatment -- two days. Don is off of work that week (yeah! for finally getting some vacation time in summer!), and we'll have all three of our girls home until Wednesday. I want some all-family fun!

I am slated to begin the radiation on Wednesday, June 17th. By my calculations (and my calculations could be off - I've never been great at math), I will finish radiation on August 4th. Yikes. That is A LOT of radiation. And many days. 33 treatments in all...every day, Monday through Friday. Holidays off.

We leave Dr. Wang's office with the understanding that someone on her staff will call to schedule the follow-up appointments. That was May 22nd.

Today is June 3rd. No call yet. I am starting to get a bit nervous. So I call the office. "Oh. Drenda Howatt. We've got you scheduled for 9:30 a.m. on Monday, June 8th." "Really? I didn't know." "What? No one called to tell you?" "Nope."

Then I say "I am supposed to start treatment on June 17th." "Oh yes! We have you scheduled for 11 a.m. on the 17th." Great. Good to know they're taking care of business. Just wished they'd have thought to tell me.

During our visit with Dr. Wang, she discussed radiation side effects with us. (I am really beginning to hate those words. "side effects". As if they are just by-standers. Let me just say that some of them are not really on the "side". They are sometimes "front and center". Often, they have not been by-standers, but involved in the game....and sometimes winning. I understand that "front effects", or "front and center effects" doesn't really sound right either. But I do hate "side effects".)

Anyway, back to what Dr. Wang told us. Fatigue is a big issue with radiation. Apparently, I will probably feel fine for the first two weeks or so, but then "it hits". And the fatigue will (I shall tell myself that it "can"...not "will") last for quite some time after radiation is over. What does that mean for me? No telling at this point.

I am liking the date of August 5th.

Loving it already.

And, if we can get passports in time, I am thinking that Don and I will have to celebrate its arrival with a little trip to Victoria sometime that month.

Yep.

I may not be good at math, but I can make a plan!

Hollace Howatt Chandler: You've passed one huge hurdle. Good for you! You can do this too, but looking ahead at it all at once is daunting. Just take one step at a time, one day at a time. His mercies are new every morning; great is His faithfulness
June 3, 2009 at 9:56pm

Amber Lynn Montgomery Lane: I always said that if I ever got a tattoo, I would want tiny numbers next to my moles so I could play connect the dots. However, in context of your experience... it just doesn't seem so funny any more.
June 4, 2009 at 11:03am

Kim Burns: Some seasons in life we have to take "one moment" at a time. It is too overwhelming to look tomorrow in the face. Yet you do keep moving forward with such grace and faith. You do ask the hard questions and prepare yourself as much as possible for each battle. You are AMAZING!
The day is coming when you will not center your days or weeks around doctors. The day is coming when they will write on your chart, "Cancer Free."
June 4, 2009 at 4:47pm

Drenda Lane Howatt: oooh. How I long for that day. But in my longing, I do not want to miss what God has for me in these days. But "Cancer Free" will sound so wonderful.
June 4, 2009 at 5:01pm

Drenda Lane Howatt thinks kankles are bad. Even the "fat" shoes don't fit. Something wrong with having to purchase bigger clothes AND bigger shoes. Not gonna do it. No sir.
June 3, 2009 at 7:40pm

Drenda Lane Howatt is happy that today is Ellie's last day of school! Woo Hoo for summer!
June 4, 2009 at 6:21am

> Becky Annus at 9:39am June 4, 2009
> wow! They are out early!
>
> Sally Park at 8:12pm June 4, 2009
> Summer!

Drenda Lane Howatt yeah for 7th graders and pizza at the Howatts'!
June 5, 2009 at 4:51pm

Drenda Lane Howatt is, once again, amazed that parents she has never met are willing to drop their child off at the Howatt home without coming to the door to make sure that there will be adults present during the party... "Dear Parents: Please love your child enough to check out the party home and meet the host parents..."
June 5, 2009 at 6:44pm

> Tina Stinson at 8:07pm June 5, 2009
> Isn't it AMAZING!!!
>
> Maureen Gatens Thompson at 8:25pm June 5, 2009
> I would meet the parents w/ both of our kids and, of course, they were humiliated but I left feeling that they

were in a safe environment. Now they don't even remember. LOL

Rachel Howatt at 9:01pm June 5, 2009
How exciting for Ellie to have a party with all her friends!
You know, mom... I didn't have a co-ed party until freshman year.

Drenda Lane Howatt at 9:03pm June 5, 2009
I love her more

Andi Pedersen Jordan at 10:47pm June 5, 2009
ouch. don't take that Rachel.

Milt Buckelew at 11:05pm June 5, 2009
Explains a lot about some of the problems in our culture, doesn't it.

Drenda Lane Howatt at 7:53am June 6, 2009
Rachel, who said anything about co-ed?

Rachel Howatt at 8:25am June 6, 2009
You did.
"I have to go, rowdy jr. high boys"

Drenda Lane Howatt at 8:33am June 6, 2009
Oh yes, I did not remember that little note. Chemo brain...

Amber Lynn Montgomery Lane at 9:57am June 6, 2009
Just to stir the pot, perhaps these particular parents have children that are so trustworthy that they believe their choice of friend to be good, and assurance that parents will be there to be true.

Drenda Lane Howatt at 12:19pm June 6, 2009
Amber, I think that is EXACTLY the case here. But I

believe we need to protect our children, and even when we trust them completely (as I do with my girls), it is important to follow-through with checking in. Sometimes, teenagers can be caught unaware ("Mom, they told me their parents would be there...") and sometimes, even in trust, it is good to let our kids know that we do check on and care about their welfare no matter what. No matter what. And, I want my kids to know that parents communicate with each other! Especially in jr. hi and high school.

Don Howatt at 8:28pm June 6, 2009
I certainly wouldn't leave my kids with a man with a 22' X 18' room full of Batman toys!

Drenda Lane Howatt is enjoying her morning coffee in the library whilst playing on the computer.
June 6, 2009 at 7:55am

Sally Park at 8:09am June 6, 2009
Have enough on your plate already?!!

Chemo Brain

Saturday, June 6, 2009 at 8:57am

Chemo Brain.

An actual condition.

One I've claimed to have on a number of occasions.

But those claims were just examples of me being a "cancer user".

As in using cancer as an excuse for my own, normal, lapses.

But no more.

Because I have experienced Chemo Brain for real this week.

And it is REALLY frustrating. Really.

I was upset with my daughter and "lecturing". But I couldn't supply the right word. She had to do it for me.

It went something like this (although typing the conversation leaves much to be desired. Hard to hear the emotion.) "Ellie, you MUST get your room cleaned. You MUST clean it so that the carpet can be seen. I am going to run errands, and when I come back, you better have...have...have...made.

...um....um..." "Progress? Do you mean progress?" "YES! YOU BETTER HAVE MADE PROGRESS!"

(and, o.k., I realize that is not a great example of good parenting...before you even start to point out how I could have handled room cleaning better, please know I realize I could have been a better parent. I have lots of room to improve, and understand that I won't really "get it" until I am a grandparent...)

Not funny at the time, that my little girl has to help me find the words for her own lecture, but I can almost see the humor now. Not sure she does, or will ever, see the humor. She was just mad at me that she had to clean her room.

Another 'real' example of Chemo Brain: I was at work, and writing an email to a number of people regarding grant requests that the County will be submitting for federal stimulus dollars. In the email, I was asking for draft language that could be sent to our Congressional Delegation that they could, in turn, use to send support letters on our behalf.

I was spelling out what the draft language should include. I couldn't think of the word I was looking for, "hmm, no, not 'important', 'profound?' 'something like propelling, but WHAT is it?"....so I went out in the hall and asked a co-worker to help me.

"Karen, I am looking for a word but can't think of the right one..."

She looked at me blankly. I realize that I did not give her much to go on. But she stood there listening patiently to me as I talked it out.

And then the word came to me.

"COMPELLING"

Yes! That was the word. The draft language should include compelling reasons that the County should be awarded the grant.

It is very disconcerting to have these brain lapses. I am not usually at a loss for words.

Luckily for me, and for all of you, Chemo Brain is not supposed to be permanent.

That's what I am telling myself...when I can find the right wordage.

Milt Buckelew: Yep, you're not alone...it is real:-)
June 6, 2009 at 10:18am

Laurie Lane: I do the same thing but don't have the "chemo brain" excuse. It's just me.
June 6, 2009 at 10:54am

Kristi Smith: I don't have chemo brain. But I hate it when I suddenly can't think of the word I want, but it's there right on the tip of my tongue. Yesterday I finally remembered a word I have been trying to think of for 13 days ("hedonistic" was the word). I'm sorry that your treatment is making it happen frequently for you!
June 6, 2009at 12:16pm

Drenda Lane Howatt: Me, too. But these last episodes were much more pronounced. Disconcerting
June 6, 2009 at 12:20pm

Maureen Gatens Thompson: Rest easy, my dear. This too shall pass. Hugs!
June 6, 2009 at 1:47pm

Stephanie Fiskum: I too do not know what it is like to have

chemo brain. But I have 40 plus something brain and teenagers who regularly finish my sentences...and it frustrates me when they do it.
June 6, 2009 at 3:14pm

Amber Smart: Drenda, I appreciate how open you are with your cancer and treatment and laughed when I read that you were a cancer "user" because I remembered our conversations about it.

I, too, suffer from brain lapses all too often! I think there is a "mom" brain. When you are always thinking about your kids there isn't room for those all important words!
June 6, 2009 at 5:00pm

Drenda Lane Howatt ...that which was lost has now been found. And he who was driving that which was lost is now in the slammer.
June 6, 2009 at 11:47pm

Erik Lane at 11:47pm June 6, 2009
Yay!! Did he screw it up at all?

Drenda Lane Howatt at 11:51pm June 6, 2009
just a bit...ruined the lock mechanism on the trunk; not sure what else. Everything that was in the car is gone, except the high school musical pillow...(!), clothes, cds, car emergency kit, etc. Arrested at a gas station in Vancouver as he went to get gas.

Kristi Smith at 11:51pm June 6, 2009
Wow! Not just the car found, but some actual justice. That's unheard of.

Drenda Lane Howatt at 11:53pm June 6, 2009
Not justice yet...but at least he was apprehended!

Erik Lane at 11:55pm June 6, 2009
How'd they know at the gas station, or was a cop just there?

That's great, though! Seems like stories like this usually have worse endings...

Drenda Lane Howatt at 11:58pm June 6, 2009
Must have been a slow night...the officer said they just did a routine plate check..."it's a Honda...we run Honda plates all the time". So, yeah! We're so happy to have the car back and in drivable condition, too.

Drenda Lane Howatt enjoyed a wonderful graduation party for Anna last night...so great to have friends and family all together! Today is 'full-up' with doctor appointments.
June 8, 2009 at 6:48am

Drenda Lane Howatt thinks everyone should get summer vacation...as in June through August. Yes.
June 8, 2009 at 7:02am

> Linda Waggoner at 11:40am June 10, 2009
> Works for me - as long as the money continues to arrive!

~ 30 Minutes ~

Monday, June 8, 2009 at 6:09pm

Today I had my upper torso mapped.

3-D imaging.

I didn't get to see the map, but I am guessing it is pretty cool.

When I arrived, I was given "some more paper work to fill out".

Except I didn't fill it out. It was for the social worker. Asking personal questions. Sorry. Thanks but no thanks. I am not interested in filling out a form about my emotional well being, and my sex life, that is then reviewed by office staff and probably entered into a computer. Nope.

Next was the tour and instructions on how the radiation treatment regimen will unfold. No need to check in, just go to the treatment waiting room. Go change into a gown and robe. The waiting room has cameras, so the staff will see me when I arrive and come get me.

Today, I had to identify myself by my birthdate, as the technicians could not tell if I was me. The photo they had of me (taken on December 3, 2008) is of a woman with red hair and terrified and sad eyes. I tell myself they couldn't recognize me from the photo not just because my hair is gone, but because my eyes are no longer terrified and I do not look sad. Yes. That must be why. Not sad and terrified, but strong and courageous. I ask the technicians to take a new photo -- and they cheerfully agree.

I had two technicians helping me today, a man and a woman. Both very friendly and helpful.

Then into the mapping room. The doctor came in and marked my chest with a pen. As she was looking at my breast, which has one big incision scar across the breadth, she asked, with uncertainty in her voice, "is this the lumpectomy site?" Well, hello, yes. There is only one scar; where else would it be?

The technician must have seen some response on my face, because he said "doesn't even look like a scar! Just a red line on your breast!" I think "really? how odd is that? A woman with a red line across her breast. Is that better than a scar?" But I said nothing.

After the CT scan mapped my chest, it was tattoo time. The male technician did the tattooing because the woman tech had just painted her nails (at work? what?), and didn't want to put gloves on her hands quite yet.

I have four little dots now forever on my upper body.

And a recognition that my initial opposition to tattoos is renewed.

I have given serious thought (much to my husband's chagrin...) to getting a tattoo once this cancer stuff is done. But after today, and the four little dots, I doubt I am brave enough to proceed.

Because tattoos hurt -- feel like bee stings.

And I am guessing that the pain (not unbearable, but certainly uncomfortable) will be enough to keep my head on my shoulders and prevent any craziness of subjecting myself to repeated pin pricks... Just imagine a bee sting over and over and over in a small area. Ouch.

Ok, now for the last part of my mapping adventure...here's where you may want to stop reading if you're wary of too much information. Because the next paragraph will certainly be too much information.

One of the last things the male technician did was snap a few photos..."ok, Drenda, we need to get a photo to show the position of your arms". I think, ok, that sounds reasonable.

"Ok, great. Now I just need to get a photo of your breast straight on."

WHHAAATTT?

Before I could say anything (not that it would have mattered), snap! The photo of my breast is now a digital memory. OH MY GOODNESS!

After having babies, and cancer surgery, and repeated exams, and, and, and..., I am pretty good about letting the medical professionals see parts of my body that they need to. BUT A PHOTO? Are you kidding me?

I am thinking that in any other context, that photo would be considered pornography. Not even a chance it would be considered art. But now a part of my chart, apparently.

What a day. I am exhausted.

This appointment actually only took 30 minutes; I am learning that lots can transpire in 30 short minutes.

Gail Stempel Hilderbrand: That was a very interesting/moving post as usual. Although I am still stuck on the gal painting her fingernails at work! No warning letter there, I would have fired her, geez.
June 8, 2009 at 8:49pm

Drenda Lane Howatt: I was surprised about the nail polish as well! So weird.
June 8, 2009 at 8:59pm

Linda Waggoner: WOW! The fun just keeps coming! Ron said your new name should be Drenda Rooney (you know, like Andy Rooney only Drenda) because your writing is not only very powerful but it is also very funny!
June 9, 2009 at 10:56am

Sherri Detweiler Purcell: The writing is funny, but informative, from a patient's point of view. Often we on the otherside of the medical "task" see it as just that. Sometimes in a hurried work world, enough compassion and attention may not be given to our patients. This could be material for training of new doctors and nurses...food for thought.
June 9, 2009 at 11:50am

Shannon Swope: Appreciate your perspective. It IS sobering to me to read from your (patient) eyes and encourages me to be kinder and gentler even if I am rushed. Thank you!
June 9, 2009 at 7:41pm

Drenda Lane Howatt: During cancer treatment, some things have just been 'loud' to me...comments made on the side, or the questionnaire, or the sound of a digital camera. Part of the 'memory making moments' I think. Little things to the technicians or doctors, but those little things can make a big impact.
June 10, 2009 at 6:58am

Drenda Lane Howatt has a quiet house...Don is on his weekly breakfast date with one daughter (this is Ellie's date week), Anna is asleep, and Rachel is in Seattle.
June 11, 2009 at 6:24am

Drenda Lane Howatt loves Fridays and pilot projects.
June 12, 2009 at 7:44am

Drenda Lane Howatt is happy to have all her girls home. Yeah!
June 12, 2009 4:55pm

Drenda Lane Howatt believes that Sunday afternoon naps are a requirement. Yep.
June 14, 2009 at 2:43pm

> Abigale Mary Lane at 6:47pm June 14, 2009
> I agree. And there is nothing like watching loved ones sleep. Love that.

~Normal, I Love You~

Sunday, June 14, 2009 at 6:03pm

"Normal day, let me be aware of the treasure you are. Let me learn from you, love you, bless you before you depart. Let me not pass you by in quest of some rare and perfect tomorrow. Let me hold you while I may, for it may not always be so. One day I shall dig my nails into the earth, or bury my face in the pillow, or raise my hands to the sky and want, more than all the world, your return"-Mary Jean Iron

I have lived that quote. So many times, I have buried my face into my pillow, sobbing, wanting to return to "normal life". Life as it was before November 8th, 2008. Life before cancer.

But, in reality, even November 7th, 2008 was not life before cancer. Or June 2008. It was just life before I knew I had cancer. Life in ignorance of cancer.

But now, in the last two weeks, I have had some "normal" days.

Almost.

I am loving "almost normal".

Loving it.

Because I am starting to feel good.

GOOD!

Still tired. But not so much.

I can almost stay awake until 9 in the evening. That is late for me.

I still am watching and feeling my fingernails separate from my nail beds.

The bottom of my feet are still numb.

When I get up to walk somewhere, I must stand still for a few seconds to get my balance and my footing before putting one foot in front of the other and walking out the door.

I still have kankles. You know, where there is no definition from knee to ankle.

I still have weight gain and fluid retention.

And episodes of 'chemo brain'.

But....

I don't have severe bone aches.

And I don't have severe nail pain.

And I am not melting into the floor nearly as often.

And I have had two weeks without treatments.

Normal days.

Working.

Being a wife.

Being a mother.

Just normal stuff.

I love it.

No cancer war until Wednesday.

Bethann Westfall: You are an inspiration, a hero, a survivor. You are a living, breathing example of God's love and faithfulness to the world around you. You are blessed and loved by our Father. Thank you for sharing your journey.
June 14, 2009 at 6:16pm

Sally Park: Raise it to "normal"! I am so happy for you!
June 14, 2009 at 9:08pm

Zachary Lane Koval: :)
June 14, 2009 at 11:19pm

Laurie Lane: You've come so far on this journey!
June 15, 2009 at 6:48am

Amanda Lane: love it! Normal, here we come...
All my love, and does the radiation have any fun side effects (glowing extremities, setting off airport security, super powers?)?
Always thinking of you
June 15, 2009 at 11:10am

Amy Hickman: Thank you for sharing, Drenda. It certainly puts things into perspective. I have a few of your same symptoms being pregnant, but that is for such a more joyful reason... May the Lord continue to hold you up and keep you close to His side as you wait for 'normal' to return.
June 17, 2009 at 2:29pm

Drenda Lane Howatt is just about finished with her morning coffee...then it's time to start the day! Well, time to go figure out breakfast, lunch, and dinner, and then head to wonderful OC.
June 15, 2009 at 6:18am

Drenda Lane Howatt wondered, for a quick moment, whether 7:20 p.m. was too early to go to bed. But then the wondering ceased and the fatigue was completely in charge. Good night.
June 15, 2009 at 7:21pm

Gail Stempel Hilderbrand at 10:21pm June 15, 2009
Sweet dreams:)

Drenda Lane Howatt thinks there must be a better way that doesn't add 1 trillion dollars to our debt. That's my debt. And yours.
June 16, 2009 at 6:54am

Gail Stempel Hilderbrand at 1:36pm June 16, 2009
I am with you on that!

Drenda Lane Howatt is fighting sore throat and sickness. Somehow, the virus didn't get the memo that Drenda CAN'T be sick...radiation treatment starts tomorrow.
June 16, 2009 at 5:03pm

Abbi Howatt at 5:18pm June 16, 2009
Blah :(

Becky Annus at 5:28pm June 16, 2009
Don't forget what Mom always had us do...gargle with salt water....

Laurie Lane at 7:36pm June 16, 2009

Weren't we to add a little bit of apple vinegar? It always made me gag...

Hollace Howatt Chandler at 9:36pm June 16, 2009
Oh, no! I just was reading about your normal day!

Amanda Lane at 11:24am June 17, 2009
Apple cider vinegar does help and so does cayenne (both of which you can get in capsule form, which does go down easier, but should take with milk or something else soothing in your stomach as it can get a bit upset...) plus your basics like C and zinc and i also depend greatly on oil of oregano (which is also amazing on mouth sores, but can burn a little. also available in softgels)
I hope you get better right away!

Drenda Lane Howatt is hopeful that illness doesn't delay radiation treatment...she wants this phase of the cancer war started so that it will end. At least some summer without treatment would be a good thing.
June 17, 2009 at 6:45am

Drenda Lane Howatt one down, 29 to go.
June 18, 2009 at 7:50am

Lori Buckelew at 8:37am June 18, 2009
Remember to get rest...the fatigue sneaks up on ya! And talk with your radiologist about something to put on your skin...your gonna need it!

Drenda Lane Howatt at 8:49am June 18, 2009
What did you use? I am a bit nervous about the fatigue...is it "can't function" fatigue, or just "I am tired" fatigue?

Lori Buckelew at 12:35pm June 18, 2009
I used Lama Oil...but my doctor wasn't real happy with me. It worked though...the fatigue with the radiation was harder than the Chemo...make sure you get lots of rest and keep the area being radiated moisturized

Lori Buckelew at 12:36pm June 18, 2009
Remember…the burn is happening 24/7/365 not just on the day you are getting the radiation...

Lori Buckelew at 12:37pm June 18, 2009
Well, maybe not 365, but definitely during your treatment time and a week or so after your last one...

Drenda Lane Howatt at 5:28pm June 18, 2009
yikes

Maureen Gatens Thompson at 7:51pm June 18, 2009
Use aloe vera...it worked great for me and my Radiologist approved. :-) Also, 100% cotton shirts whenever possible. I would wear Jim's t-shirts. Yes, the fatigue slowly catches up to you but it's not "I can't function" fatigue. For me, it was more like "I need a 2 hour nap" fatigue. I went Monday through Friday at the end of my workday for 6 weeks. I would go home, take a nap, eat dinner and go to bed at my regular time. I did this while working full-time. It was a piece of cake compared to chemo.

My, How They Love Cameras

Thursday, June 18, 2009 at 9:19am

Yesterday was the trial run on radiation.

I started things off wrong.

Who would know that they want the gown on with the opening in the back? My goodness, one would think (I think) that the opening would need to be in the front if one's breast were going to be radiated.

But, no. Opening in the back. So I take off the gown and turn it around. The technicians (two women this time) hold up a robe in front of me for "privacy". This action makes me chuckle to myself. Modesty? Really? I do appreciate their care - so thoughtful and sweet.

The 'treatment room' is so high tech it makes me think I am in a movie. Laser beams shooting out of the walls and ceiling. The lasers are used to line me up according to my tattoos. Pretty darn amazing.

As I lay there with my arms above my head, I have an itch.

On my collar bone.

And it is a pretty intense itch..."can I move my arms?"

"NO! We need you to stay still."

"But my collar bone..."

The kindness comes again. The technician comes over and itches my collar bone for me. And she is good at it! Follows my directions quickly and precisely. "up just a bit. over towards my chin. yes yes you got it. Thank you!"

Before Dr. Wang came in to check and make sure all was well, the markers come out again. One more large circle on my chest and onto my back. Something makes me think that perhaps these technicians are the ones who only wanted to draw in kindergarten...Reminds of me of Miss Rachel who would (and did) draw on everything and anything (sheets, Camille's lamp, walls, etc. etc. etc.)

Then the camera came out.

Again.

I had to wonder, just how many photos of my breast does one radiation center need to have? More than they do currently, it seems.

I ask "what do you need the photos for?"

Chuckle. (The chuckle only made me more wary...) Dr. Wang responds "the photos only go in your treatment chart. They aren't used for anything else". Good. Good.

Then one of the technicians says "we don't take any photos of your face, so no one who ever sees these would know it is you..."

Ok, then. I feel much better.

Not really.

So the test run begins.

And it is all well and good. Because all went well, I get the first treatment.

Done!

Dr. Wang has changed the treatment plan, according to the technicians. Only 30 treatments instead of 33. Higher dose of radiation, so fewer treatments. Not going to argue with that!

I will report at 3:00 p.m. every day, Monday-Friday, for the next six weeks.

And get my picture taken every week or so.

I may be completely camera shy by the time I'm done.

John Lynch: Thank you for letting us walk through this journey with you, precious sister of God.
June 18, 2009 at 9:49am

Laurie Lane: When I was pregnant with Nathan and had a utrasound, I was asked if I would give permission to have the pictures used as advertisements for the ultrasound machine in medical journals, to which I agreed. Somewhere there are pictures of my insides, minus any identifying personal characteristics so you wouldn't know it was me, hanging out in medical journals.

Thanks for taking us along on your continuing journey.
June 18, 2009 at 9:56am

Milt Buckelew: Oops:-) I hate those gowns...and to call 'em gowns is quite misleading! Who would go to a ball in one of those?
June 18, 2009 at 10:03am

Elizabeth Lundquist Calhoun: Glad it's only 30 treatments instead of 33. And one down already! You are amazing.
June 18, 2009 at 10:55am

Drenda Lane Howatt is still sick...Dr. Wang says that a weakened immune system will allow the illness to linger longer. Yuck.
June 19, 2009 at 7:21pm

Gail Stempel Hilderbrand at 8:15pm June 19, 2009
Boy do I know how that goes! This too shall pass:)

Sally Park at 8:55pm June 19, 2009
Sorry to hear that... take the weekend to rest and pamper yourself. You deserve it!

Karen Buehrig at 9:04pm June 21, 2009
If you have what I had, it took over a week before I started to feel better. Lots of sleep and cough medicine seemed to do the trick for me.

Drenda Lane Howatt Old Navy $2 tank top Saturday
June 20, 2009 at 9:49am

Sally Park at 9:50am June 20, 2009
Oh my goodness, on line too?

Tina Stinson at 9:51am June 20, 2009
Thanks Drenda…

Sally Park at 11:49am June 20, 2009
yeah!! 20 tanks later....

Drenda Lane Howatt at 12:19pm June 20, 2009
20 tanks????? Oh my goodness. We just returned from the store...between three of us we purchased 14...

Sally Park at 1:14pm June 20, 2009
Some for me, some for Merlie. They didn't enforce the #5 per rule.

Tina Stinson at 1:56pm June 20, 2009
Thanks for the Heads up on the sale!!!! Had a rewards card…Just went school shopping and got a ton of stuff for $24.00... WOO HOO!!!

Drenda Lane Howatt at 3:21pm June 20, 2009
I am glad that I mentioned the sale! I just happened to see the Old Navy commercials on t.v. last night. I thought it would be a zoo at the store, but it wasn't bad at all. Good shopping, Tina and Sally!

Drenda Lane Howatt is scheduled to 'boat along' on the Sheriff's River Patrol tomorrow...but she is not sure if that is a good idea.
June 21, 2009 at 5:36pm

Karen Buehrig at 9:28pm June 21, 2009
Stay home and rest up!

Drenda Lane Howatt did 'boat along' with the Sheriff's River Patrol...up the Clackamas River to Carver, back to the Willamette, and then up to the Falls. The Clackamas County Sheriff's Department does great work!
June 22, 2009 at 6:03pm

Drenda Lane Howatt is 16% done with radiation. Good. Good.
June 23, 2009 at 5:08pm

Abigale Mary Lane at 5:35pm June 23, 2009
Very good.

Wonder Away

Tuesday, June 23, 2009 at 5:41pm

Hair.

Over-rated.

Under-rated.

I am learning.

My hair is growing...and it is DIFFERENT.

No surprise.

Lots of people have told me about someone they know who went through cancer treatment and their hair grew back curly, or straight, or an odd color.

Mine is white.

In places.

And, in someplaces, there is a twinge of red. ish.

But mostly white.

AND I DON'T CARE.

Nope.

Because I am comfortable with who I am, and if the person I am has white hair, or no hair, or straight hair, or hair that stands on end, I am comfortable.

Ok. Almost comfortable.

I really wouldn't want to be bald for ever.

And I may decide, later, that white hair is not what I desire. I may decide to have a bit more of the 'ish', as in red, back.

But I have learned over the past 7 months that there are other, more important things. Like life. And family. And friendships. And my relationship with my Creator. I am learning -- even these things I already knew.

I am learning anew.

I have learned that other people, friends even, are not comfortable with what I look like.

"Are you going to color your hair when it gets longer?"

"No"

"Oooooh....are you sure?"

NO! I am NOT sure.

Because I am learning to try and not say "I will/would 'never'".

Slowly learning, but I AM learning.

But I am happy, right now, with white hair.

With curly hair.

With straight hair.

And the ease that that happiness provides, that that acceptance provides, is priceless. That ease allows me to be me. Not my hair. Not my body (ok, another caveat...I am not entirely comfortable with my body...not the weight gain, not the new body that does not fit into my clothes, etc. -- but I am not going to obsess about it.)

People who know me, know me. Whether my hair, or my body, is 'normal' or odd. And they either love me or they don't.

People who don't know me probably wonder.

That's ok by me.

Wonder away.

Abigale Mary Lane: I know your post goes deeper than your hair, but I love your hair! It is beautiful.
June 23, 2009 at 5:48pm

Drenda Lane Howatt: You're so sweet! I love it too! Thank you.
June 23, 2009 at 5:49pm

Cindy McElmurry: You are amazing! Can I have your autograph? You know I might have one around here somewhere. Ebay here I come!
See you soon. Hope you are feeling better!
June 23, 2009 at 7:31pm

Sherri Detweiler Purcell: Well written Drenda. You do have a gift...now if I could just get comfortable with all my white hair (and it would almost ALL be white)....
June 23, 2009 at 8:00pm

Drenda Lane Howatt: White is the new 'black'. Lots of freedom

in white. Lots.
June 23, 2009 at 8:09pm

Drenda Lane Howatt: and thank you!
June 23, 2009 at 8:10pm

Amy Tuttle: I actually can't wait til most of my hair is white!! I'm gaining new white ones daily... then I'm going to dye it ALL white!

...maybe :)

Thanks Drenda for writing this post. What a process the Lord is taking you through. Isn't He amazing? I am so encouraged by your outlook.

Yep, my mom had the exact same thing happen with her hair, it came back really weird and went through several stages, but now, seven years post-treatment it is pretty normal again :) whatever normal is... heheh. ;)
June 24, 2009 at 12:17am

Bobbi Mapes: Drenda this is amazing...You are AMAZING!!!!! White is very becoming to everyone. I said that I would never dye my hair…well I did and now I can say never will I again. I love my white hair.
Beautifully written.
June 24, 2009 at 6:22am

Amanda Lane: I definitely recommend dying the hair. Not because it's white, and definitely not because of what anyone might think, but because I love changing my hair color!

Besides, after making bald the new hot, just imagine what you will do for white hair...
June 24, 2009 at 8:36am

Linda Waggoner: Drenda,
You are wonderful!! I love your hair too - it is so pretty - different from before-- but that's not a bad thing. I saw a look of dismay on my husband's face when I told him this morning that I have decided to keep my hair short - at least for the near future (it's about 1/2 inch long). The convenience and freedom very short hair allows (like no blow dryer, no expensive beauty shop visits) is wonderful. I will probably decide to let it grow out eventually (maybe) but for now I'm staying short and gray! I love you and I continue to be so proud of you!!
June 24, 2009 at 11:44am

Adrienne Fajen: yes!!
June 24, 2009 at 9:56pm

Stephanie Fiskum: I love how open and honest you are. You are my kind of gal!
June 30, 2009 at 2:40pm

Drenda Lane Howatt 20% down.
June 24, 2009 at 5:00pm

Drenda Lane Howatt 23%...well, actually, it is 23.333333333333%...not that she is keeping track or anything.
June 25, 2009 AT 6:40 PM

Drenda Lane Howatt had a little shopping time, a little family time, and now a little culture time.
June 27, 2009 at 5:14pm

> Ginger Clausen at 9:28pm June 27, 2009
> Does Facebook count as culture?!
>
> Drenda Lane Howatt at 10:30pm June 27, 2009
> Oregon Bach Festival

Drenda Lane Howatt viewed a very small part of a large stand of old growth trees...450-500 years old! And right in Clackamas County's very own Eagle Fern Park. Cool.
June 29, 2009 at 5:50pm

> Amber Lynn Montgomery Lane at 7:32pm June 29, 2009
> We're looking for the best Clackamas park to use our passes. Would you suggest Eagle Fern?
>
> Drenda Lane Howatt at 7:46pm June 29, 2009
> No camping there...I'll do a bit of investigating tomorrow and see about recommendations!
>
> Amber Lynn Montgomery Lane at 8:26pm June 29, 2009

Thanks, that would be great!

Drenda Lane Howatt is thankful for a beautiful day, a good job, and most of all, life!
June 30, 2009 at 6:39am

Kimberly Roberts at 10:40am June 30, 2009
Life is good. Glad you are doing good.

Drenda Lane Howatt is happy to be exactly 1/3 of the way to the end of radiation.
June 30, 2009 at 3:21pm

Sandy Hagstrand at 8:54pm July 1, 2009
Yeah!!!! Rest up for the final push...

Drenda Lane Howatt 's man in brown isn't home from work yet...this is NOT the Christmas season. What's the story?
June 30, 2009 at 8:12pm

Tom Turnbull at 8:18pm June 30, 2009
Something about an Appalachian Trail hike is what I heard :)

Drenda Lane Howatt at 8:21pm June 30, 2009
Appalachian Trail is not on his route...and he doesn't have his passport.

Wendy Ackley at 8:26pm June 30, 2009
4th of July?

Drenda Lane Howatt at 8:27pm June 30, 2009
He just walked in the door. Long day!

Gail Stempel Hilderbrand at 8:36pm June 30, 2009

It was probably chit chat in the parking lot after his shift

Drenda Lane Howatt received her clinical trial drugs today via certified mail. They are, umm, quite large.
July 3, 2009 at 7:45am

Cindy McElmurry at 8:31am July 3, 2009
More likely to kill the cancer cell my pretty!

Milt Buckelew at 9:28am July 3, 2009
Did they accidentally sign you up for equine clinical trial?

Drenda Lane Howatt at 9:43am July 3, 2009
perhaps...

Gail Stempel Hilderbrand at 1:20pm July 3, 2009
As long as it can be swallowed it sounds good to me.

Milt Buckelew at 9:25pm July 3, 2009
Missed you at the wedding today:-(

Drenda Lane Howatt at 9:48pm July 3, 2009
I was there...I was the blonde in the new short "hip" hairstyle...

Milt Buckelew at 11:27pm July 3, 2009
...but I still missed you:-(

Drenda Lane Howatt at 6:45am July 4, 2009
And I missed you. I did see you, though...sitting up in the front in the sun. Poor guy. I was in the shade.

~Pride~

Sunday, July 5, 2009 at 8:17am

Pride.

In the first weeks after I learned that I had breast cancer, I actually said (a number of times, even) "I am not saying 'why me, God?'." I said "why shouldn't it be me?".

Oh, those words sounded so good.

So noble.

So mature.

Strong and courageous perhaps.

I wasn't going to be the Christian who questioned God. No. Not me.

Instead of asking "why me?" I was asking "how did this happen?". Those were my actual words.

"HOW DID THIS HAPPEN?"

How DID this happen?

I don't know.

And it doesn't matter, really.

Because it DID 'happen'. And there is no alternative but to walk forward through the 'happen'.

Then I realized that "how did this happen?" can be translated to mean "why me?".

Really.

I WAS asking God "why me?"

And I was doing the asking in a very prideful way.

The question was not, and is not, the problem.

The pride is.

I had my life planned out.

Well, not completely or really planned out, but the outline did not include breast cancer.

My outline did not include suffering.

Or pain.

Or emotional turmoil.

Or anything difficult or negative.

Time to scrap the outline.

And live by God's outline.

Really, it is living by God's leading. He has my hand.

And, remember, He has promised to go into the foreign land with me.

Funny that I have never asked God "why me?" when I receive good news, or something I consider a blessing. Perhaps because

I expect good things? Because I think that I deserve good things?

Suffering can be a blessing, too.

I am starting to see that.

God tells us to consider it pure joy when we face trials.

Pride must be pushed out of the way.

God knows my questions.

He knows my emotions.

He knows my sin. But He won't remember it. That is the promise of the cross.

And He loves me anyway.

Cindy McElmurry: You are my Amazing friend. You humble me. Thank you for putting yourself out there and sharing with us. I love you my friend.
July 5, 2009 at 3:20pm

Kimberly Tibbetts Roberts: You are an inspiration to me. God is good. He is amazing. He doesn't let us just walk alone, but carries us through. He won't leave us in our times of pain, hurt or suffering. He is with us every step of the way.
July 5, 2009 at 5:51pm

Shannon Swope: Humility is a good thing my friend. Not easy...but good and right. Thank you for the words. The best- "He loves me anyway." We are merely weak humans totally dependent on our Almighty Father although I often forget that

part! :)
I miss you...won't see you tonight or Sunday...bummer!
July 7, 2009 at 12:15pm

Drenda Lane Howatt is, let's see...doing the math...well, never mind. Just know that 13 of 30 done and over. Getting there. Slowly but surely.
July 6, 2009 at 9:54pm

Sharley Massman at 9:56pm July 6, 2009
Why are you doing math?

Drenda Lane Howatt at 10:02pm July 6, 2009
Percentage...13 of 30 is what percentage? I'll blame my unwillingness to do the math on chemo brain...

Sharley Massman at 10:04pm July 6, 2009
hhhmmm i'm the most un-math person on the planet so i can't really help...sorry good luck w/ that...lol

Susan Rasmussen Lane at 10:26pm July 6, 2009
13/30=.4333333333... so 43-1/3% done. Yep, getting there.

Andi Pedersen Jordan at 10:36pm July 6, 2009
Almost half sounds MUCH better...NEARLY 50%

Nancy Newton at 12:47pm July 8, 2009
You've been amazing through this process. The goal is in sight now...

Drenda Lane Howatt strongly believes that marking milestones is important...she just passed the halfway point of radiation. Well, umm, yahoo.
July 8, 2009 at 5:22pm

Susan Rasmussen Lane at 5:51pm July 8, 2009
Hooray!

Amber Lynn Montgomery Lane at 6:04pm July 8, 2009
Happy hump day.

Jennifer Stady at 7:35pm July 8, 2009
I believe in it too so happy halfway point to you!

Sally Park at 7:54pm July 8, 2009
Indeed ~ !

Adrienne Fajen at 8:54am July 9, 2009
That is a big deal! Good job!

Drenda Lane Howatt starts the trial today. Not sure if she'll be able to swallow the big, as in quite large, orange pills. Hopeful that the long long long list of possible side effects is pure fiction, and not even one of those nasty possibilities will camp at her doorstep. But, if nasty possibilities can keep her brain cancer-free, they may not be so nasty after all.
July 9, 2009 at 6:13am

Drenda Lane Howatt at 6:16am July 9, 2009
I am working on my perspective...how bad can bad be if it does good?

Bradley Ruhl at 8:25am July 9, 2009
I hope the verdict is "not guilty"

Nancy Newton at 12:11pm July 9, 2009
I guess after chemo a pill isn't too bad by comparison? Maybe if you had a really good treat afterward.

Drenda Lane Howatt has good news. First try with the "quite large orange pill" was easily successful. Easily. She realizes that this post may qualify in the "too much information" category, but then reminds herself that her fb friends do care about her,

no matter what she shares.
July 10, 2009 at 6:11am

Cindy McElmurry at 6:45am July 10, 2009
I am so glad! We are sharing this with you as much as we can.
I love you my friend!

Linda Waggoner at 8:16am July 10, 2009
Hurray!

Kimberly Roberts at 11:35am July 10, 2009
Pills aren't fun but they do their work. Would love to get together with you some day for lunch or coffee. Let me know. Joy (Jesus over you). Kim

Susan Rasmussen Lane at 8:21pm July 10, 2009
How are you doing? Is the large pill giving you side effects? Or is it being nice?

Drenda Lane Howatt at 9:32pm July 10, 2009
One pill down...no side effect noticed at this point. Another pill tonight. Have to be taken at the same time each day...one hour before food, or two hours after food. Decided bedtime is the best time to 'imbibe' with lapatinib; maybe I'll sleep off side effects!

Susan Rasmussen Lane at 9:44pm July 10, 2009
Well, that would be great!

Drenda Lane Howatt is starting to notice discomfort at the radiation site...Dr. Wang says all is normal for "this early in the radiation treatment". "Still healing from surgery, and radiation causes inflammation of the tissue"...which causes discomfort and swelling. Oh yes. Some areas of one's body should not be inflamed.
July 10, 2009 at 9:37pm

Susan Rasmussen Lane at 9:43pm July 10, 2009
Oh, darn. Sorry to hear that you're normal in this.

Erik Lane at 9:58pm July 10, 2009
Not that it's a good thing, or any fun, but I would think that knowing it was normal would be more of a relief.

I'm sorry that you have to go through this, Drenda!!

Lynn Peterson at 10:11pm July 10, 2009
How many weeks left?

Drenda Lane Howatt at 6:38am July 11, 2009
Thank you. I am just complaining...this radiation treatment stuff is absolutely better than chemo. Lynn, I have just under 3 weeks left...go to the end of July I think.

Maureen Gatens Thompson at 10:35am July 11, 2009
This too shall pass...cotton, cotton, cotton.

Drenda Lane Howatt is waiting for the man in brown to arrive...just about sure he wants to take her out to dinner. July 14, 2009 at 5:10pm

Sherri Detweiler Purcell: I hope you enjoy...I just had dinner with 2 of your daughters.
July 14, 2009 at 5:29pm

Drenda Lane Howatt: Ooh good! How are they doing? And the third daughter? Hope all is going well at camp~
July 14, 2009 at 6:54pm

Sherri Detweiler Purcell: Rachel and Ellie are part of our weekly staff, and for some reason, the staff tables are labeled this year...SS, TCL, Horse Staff, and weekly

staff...so I don't see Anna at meals. I haven't seen much of her, She was videoing from a kayak today...Well, it is counselor hunt game now...Ellie is hiding.
July 14, 2009 at 7:41pm

Drenda Lane Howatt will have zap #20 today...as in 20/30. Reduced, that means that after 3:10 this afternoon, she will be 2/3 finished with radiation treatment. And she likes that number. Quite a lot. July 15, 2009 at 5:26am

Sharon Mathews: We like that number too, you're in our thoughts & prayers. So good to see you at Caitlin's wedding, wish we could sit & talk & talk! Love you
July 15, 2009 at 8:56am

Drenda Lane Howatt gets to have a visit with her old friend Jerry today...after labs and vitals. THEN she gets to see Jerry. It's been seven long weeks. July 16, 2009

Drenda Lane Howatt has serious chemo brain. Serious. Neglected to read the drug bottle...did wonder why the Research Department sent so many durn bottles of lapatinib...She has had no side effects from the clinical trial drug BECAUSE SHE HAS ONLY BEEN TAKING 1/6 OF THE AMOUNT SHE IS SUPPOSED TO. yikes. Six of those quite large pills every night, not just one. oops. July 16, 2009 at 10:45am

Sally Park: oops X 6
July 16, 2009 at 10:53am

Drenda Lane Howatt: oops x 6 x 7 days = LOTS OF OOPS
July 16, 2009 at 11:01am

Barb Van Dusen Butler: Well, at least you can claim an

excuse like “chemo brain”. I guess my excuse lately has been “hormonal”. Shouldn’t claim that though if the HRT is suppose to help.
July 16, 2009 at 1:20pm

Wendy Ackley: So this is a story from a bright, smart woman. Can you imagine how most people actually take their meds?
July 16, 2009 at 9:55pm

Linda Waggoner: Bummer! Does that mean you have to take the drugs 6 times longer? - or 3 or 4 times longer to make up for the ones you didn’t take?
July 17, 2009 at 1:21pm

Drenda Lane Howatt: I was afraid it would mean I couldn’t be in the clinical study...but I guess lots of people mess up somehow...
July 17, 2009 at 5:04pm

Linda Waggoner: I am sure a lot of people do mess up with the drugs! I am glad they didn’t kick you out of the clinical study! When are we going to Disneyland or???
July 18, 2009 at 4:01pm

Lost: Extra Credit Points

Friday, July 17, 2009 at 6:24pm

I got to see Jerry yesterday.

It had been seven weeks (!) since the last appointment. That means, I think, that it has been 8 weeks since my last chemo treatment.

How time flies.

Even though I was the first appointment of his day (10:30 a.m. -- pretty sweet time to start work), Jerry made me wait 30 minutes. I realize that doctors do other things than see patients. Perhaps he had to go to the hospital? Or just got a late start after relaxing with his cup of coffee and the newspaper?

All is well.

My white blood counts are still low, but not lower than to be expected.

I have lost some of my extra credit points with Jerry. For all of his earlier praise, I really messed up.

I did not live up to my reputation as 'the perfect patient'.

Because I was not so intelligent.

For some strange reason, I did not read the label on the bottles of lapatinib, the clinical trial drug, before I started taking it. I did wonder, when Don brought home the package from the

Post Office, why the research department sent me so darn many pills. Four bottles of 90 pills each.

I dutifully began taking the lapatinib on Thursday, July 9th.

But I didn't read the label.

At all.

I took one 250 mg pill at bedtime every night for a week.

And then I saw Jerry.

Normal dosage of lapatinib is 1500 mg daily. I need to be taking 6 pills every night.

OH MY GOODNESS!

Jerry said "Drenda, what did the label on the bottle say?"

"Well, I can't say that I read the label."

"Really?"

At that moment, I felt incredibly stupid. Careless. Unsafe.

How could I not read the label? (Note to Legacy Research: In the future, please say, over and over if necessary, how many pills a patient should be ingesting...) I AM smart. I AM! Usually. Not this week.

But Jerry, bless his beating heart, did not say anymore.

I love a man that knows when to keep his mouth closed.

Especially when I am really stupid.

Jonna Wilkinson: Perhaps Jerry, in his wisdom and experience, was able to see that you are definitely not stupid, but perhaps a bit overwhelmed, considering all you are going through. And he, too, felt stupid for not making sure that you realized in advance what your dosage would be when indeed you received your postal prescription. Don't be hard on yourself, just be here...
I'm praying for you.
July 17, 2009 at 7:28pm

Sally Park: Well put, Jonna. My goodness Drenda that is just a tiny little woops in the huge overwhelming saga you have been enduring for these many months. Do a little dance in the morning and see the humor ♥
Love you!!
July 17, 2009 at 9:20pm

Andi Pedersen Jordan: Yes, Jonna. You are right on. You are strong and courageous and not a bit stupid. That is a word I refuse to be spoken in our home ... and it should be in yours too! Strong and courageous!!
July 17, 2009 at 10:25pm

Drenda Lane Howatt: Thank you, all, for the kind words. No worries about my self-esteem...I KNOW I am not stupid, but taking medication without reading the label is acting in a less than intelligent manner.

I am getting really really tired of cancer and all that comes with it. Very tired. But I will strive for strong and courageous, and move away from tired and discouraged.
July 18, 2009 at 8:39pm

Sally Park: Don't blame you on that, it is a full time job!
July 19, 2009 at 7:10am

Drenda Lane Howatt is not at all ready to have Monday morning so close.
July 19, 2009 at 4:19pm

Drenda Lane Howatt time to start the bbq...
July 20, 2009 at 4:42pm

Sally Park: Steaks? Chicken? Kabobs?
July 20, 2009 at 5:07pm

Sally Park: btw, we received a package from our man in brown and it had a message from "Donnie". lol
July 20, 2009 at 5:08pm

Drenda Lane Howatt: polish sausage.
July 20, 2009 at 6:16pm

Don Howatt: The "man in brown" you are referring to, is actually "Ma'am in Brown"-her name is Jane.
July 20, 2009 at 7:26pm

Drenda Lane Howatt is up and attempting to cool down the house...open those windows! July 21, 2009 at 4:02am

Sharley Massman: hey...that's what I do...cheers to old school cooling the house down. :)
July 21, 2009 at 8:37am

Drenda Lane Howatt 80%...which means only one more treatment to the entire area, and the last five are targeted to the tumor bed. She may get out of this radiation treatment without blisters...
July 21, 2009 at 4:49pm

Maureen Gatens Thompson: I hope you escape the blisters...I didn't. You go, Girl!
July 21, 2009 at 5:27pm

Lori Buckelew: I didn't either but they say that not everyone gets them, I am praying you are the "not everyone"!
July 22, 2009 at 6:21am

Mom and Dad and the Good Lord Above

Tuesday, July 21, 2009 at 5:46pm

I know that I have posted many things about hair.

One might think I am obsessed with it.

I am not.

But some things that happen along this cancer trail just beg to be documented.

Last week, I was showing an apartment that is for rent. One of the women looking at the apartment said "I LOVE your haircut!"

"Thank you."

"Is your hair naturally curly?"

"Yes."

That was the word that came out of my mouth.

The words knocking around in my head were much more sarcastic.

"With hair this short, how on earth would I curl it?"

But I didn't let those words out.

When I saw Jerry last week, he commented on my hair growth.

(Apparently, I am past the “semblance of fuzz”.)

I relayed to him part of the “is it naturally curly?” conversation.

Jerry’s response?

“It’s the chemo.”

Why thank you, Jerry. It is the chemo. But it is also ME.

Because I have/had curly hair.

So now, if I’m asked if my hair is naturally curly, I will be torn.

Shall I say “yes, it is natural”?

Or “no, it is drug induced”?

I am willing to allow the chemo to take credit for the white hair.

But I am not sure I am willing to let chemo have credit for the curls. I think Mom and Dad and the good Lord above should get credit for that.

So, if asked again about the curls, I will smile and say “yes, it IS natural”.

Thank you.

Barb Van Dusen Butler: I think your BLONDE hair looks great and I don’t think you are obsessing about it at all. I have been loosing tons of hair (still don’t know why yet) and Dan thinks that I am obsessing about it (which I probably am). I am always commenting on how great a head of hair a person has and

yours looks like it's coming back thick. Fortunately for me I can still make what I have left look "fluffy".
July 21, 2009 at 11:05pm

Ginger Clausen: I would have said, "I'm not sure I like the short hair- I may grow it back out again- it's been a drastic change for me..." I'm so glad you haven't lost your sense of humor, Drenda!
July 21, 2009 at 11:14pm

Maureen Gatens Thompson: Of course it's natural. I had friends who lost their curly hair and it grew in straight...it is what it is. Mine was straight as a board and grew in curly. Go figure, Jerry!
July 21, 2009 at 11:36pm

Lori Buckelew: mine was straight too and it grew in curly...although they said it might be a different color too they just didn't tell me it would be GRAY!!!! Here's me praying for red or blond for you!
July 22, 2009 at 7:22am

Caitlin Lopez: Drenda, I LOVE reading your blogs. You are so transparent and open. It's a beautiful thing to see. You are a brave woman. An inspiration to me. Thank you.
August 14, 2009 at 10:56am

Cindy McElmurry: I love the gift of writing out just what you are thinking. I love your hair. I think it might look better with a tan. We are thinking about our discussion and we need to talk!
August 15, 2009 at 8:30pm

Drenda Lane Howatt was excited to learn, at the precise moment she saw the flash, that today was camera day. July 22, 2009 at 2:31pm

> Ginger Clausen: Uh, oh... That doesn't sound like a good surprise. I've had my picture taken like that before. July 22, 2009 at 4:04pm

Drenda Lane Howatt is unhappy that side effects are temporarily halting the clinical trial drug. Perhaps for only two days...
July 23, 2009 at 5:17pm

> Abigale Mary Lane: Yuck...what side effects?
> July 23, 2009 at 5:23pm
>
> Sally Park: Oh, darn. Not serious I hope?
> July 23, 2009 at 6:10pm

The clinical trial drug, lapatinib, had some pretty nasty side effects. Constant diarrhea, uncontrollable itching. The diarrhea was the side effect that caused a break.

Drenda Lane Howatt is at 90%...with only “mild” site reaction (to quote Dr. Wang). Yahoo!
July 25, 2009 at 8:56am

> Drenda Lane Howatt: Monday, Tuesday, Wednesday, DONE!
> July 25, 2009 at 8:57am
>
> Kim Burns: Yeah...Must be about time to celebrate with a girls weekend away! I can hardly wait.
> July 25, 2009 at 10:24am
>
> Becky Annus: When is the “yahoo - I’ve completed another step on my journey” celebration?
> July 25, 2009 at 10:25am
>
> Drenda Lane Howatt: Kim, I am counting the days! And we must decide about the hotel for Saturday night... Becky, how about Wednesday or Thursday dinner?
> July 25, 2009 at 10:47am

Becky Annus: How about Thursday?
July 26, 2009 at 7:51am

Becky Annus: Soooo dinner at Sweet Basils on Thursday?
July 27, 2009 at 6:08pm

Drenda looking at the radiation machine. (July 2009)

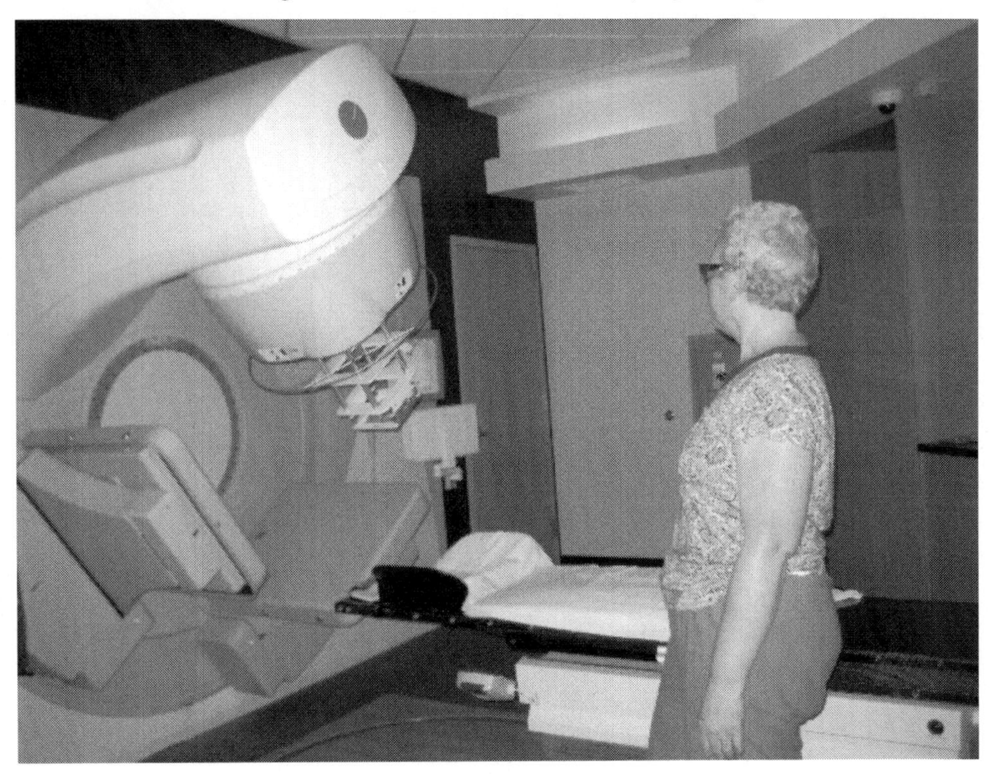

Drenda with her radiation technologist. (July 2009)

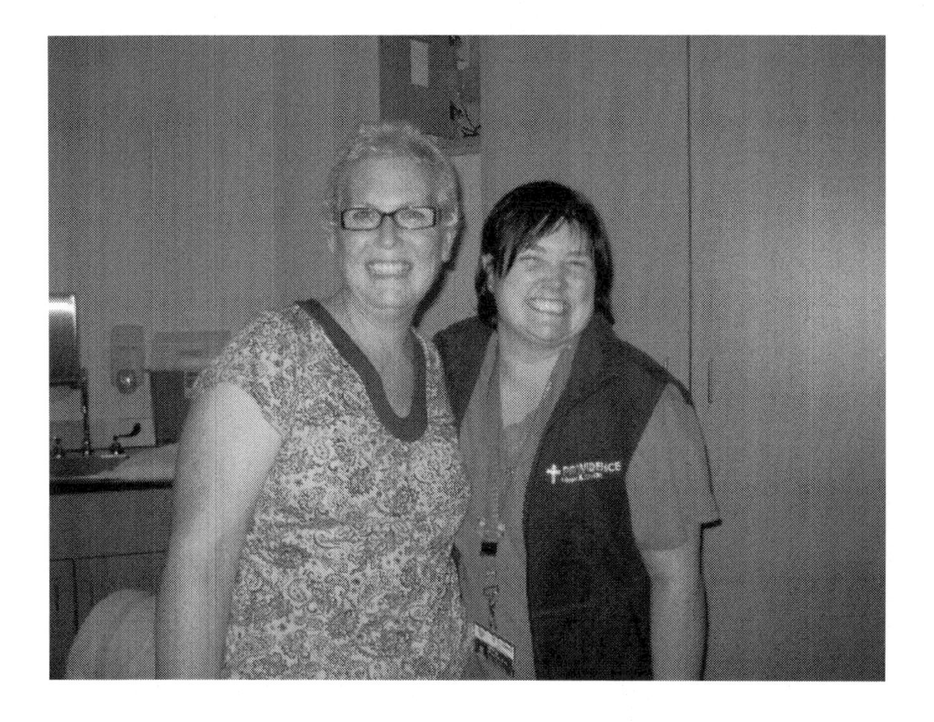

Drenda Lane Howatt Dear Anna It is Ed. No. Wait. It's Kipton. Oh, never mind.
July 27, 2009 at 8:54pm

Drenda Lane Howatt is getting ready, in two days, to reclaim a little bit of her past life. After Wednesday, she will be free from daily or weekly doctor and hospital visits (monthly visits will be the new normal), free from showing her body to strangers every day, free from photo flashes.
July 28, 2009 at 5:46am

> Becky Annus: Looking forward to the declaration "cancer free"! Strong and Courageous AND cancer free.
> July 28, 2009 at 7:08am
>
> Andi Pedersen Jordan: Wooo-HOOOOO!!
> July 28 , 2009at 8:35am
>
> Linda Waggoner: You made it! And with an amazing amount of courage and dignity! I am so proud of you! I love you!
> July 28, 2009 at 9:41am
>
> Nancy Newton: That's awesome!
> July 28, 2009 at 11:44am
>
> Chelsea Lincoln Lane: Drenda, that is WONDERFUL! You are an inspiration to all :)
> July 28, 2009 at 12:20pm

Drenda Lane Howatt can hardly believe that today brings her to 100%. Good thing. Because certain parts of her body cannot take much more exposure. To radiation or to people.
July 29, 2009 at 6:02am

Tina Stinson: Glad to hear that part is done (or close to done).
July 29, 2009 at 7:41am

Nancy Newton: This is the best news. You have been so amazing throughout this ordeal.
July 29, 2009 at 12:10pm

Drenda Lane Howatt did it. 100%. Amazing. So glad to be done with the daily zaps. Has diploma to prove successful(?) finish. Now, she is excited to be able to use deodorant once again. Oh, the sweet joys.
July 29, 2009 at 3:21pm

Amanda Lane: Happy dance!
July 29, 2009 at 4:07pm

Andi Pedersen Jordan: There needs to be something better than a LIKE button!
July 29, 2009 at 4:27pm

Molly Watney Younge: Woo Hoooooo :)
July 29, 2009 at 4:28pm

Sherri Detweiler Purcell: YAY!!!!!
July 29, 2009 at 4:41pm

Laurie Lane: Are you back on the experimental drug?
July 29, 2009 at 6:35pm

Drenda Lane Howatt: Yes, and desperately attempting to mitigate side effects so I can stay on it. I would like to keep cancer out of my brain.
July 29, 2009 at 6:44pm

Maureen Gatens Thompson: One of the positives of

radiation is not having to use deodorant on that armpit...ever again, with no stinky side effects. :-)
July 29, 2009 at 6:57pm

Drenda Lane Howatt: hmmm. I didn't know that. I'll have to test it out...no one complained to me the last 6 weeks, so maybe you ARE right!
July 29, 2009 at 7:17pm

Maureen Gatens Thompson: 24 years later and no one has complained to me. Very little arm pit hair as well. TMI! LOL
July 29, 2009 at 7:18pm

Drenda Lane Howatt: Glad to hear that there are at least some positive side effects.
July 29, 2009 at 7:20pm

Drenda Lane Howatt's husband just encouraged her to write more... "Better get going, Drenda. Your last blog was July 21st". Don't worry, Don, the words are already knocking around in Drenda's head. They will spill out soon.
July 30, 2009 at 6:41am

Don Howatt: I'm not worried, I'm just sayin'...
July 30, 2009 at 6:45am

John Lynch: Yes. This is a good thing for all concerned. John
July 30, 2009 at 6:50am

Janette Wilkinson: You two live together and yet you communicate on Facebook?
July 30, 2009 at 6:56am

Drenda Lane Howatt: Isn't that the way married people are supposed to communicate? On the internet in front

of everyone?
July 30, 2009 at 7:18am

Lori Buckelew: Milt and I do it all the time...he writes me notes on the IM as well...but I can't tell you about those though ;) Congrats on finishing the doctor journey...looking forward to reading your newest blog!
July 30, 2009 at 7:22am

Drenda Lane Howatt thinks 1001 cranes all together is a beautiful sight. Thank you.
July 30, 2009 at 9:56pm.

Drenda Lane Howatt: Is there ANY way possible to have a list of all those involved -- and their connection?
July 30, 2009 at 9:56pm

Denise Lane: Congratulations on your treatment completion Drenda!
July 31, 2009 at 12:59am

Steven Lane: Happy also Drenda that your treatments are over. And thank you to our Lord for standing beside you.
July 31, 2009 at 9:28am

Drenda, with her five sisters and her daughter Rachel, showing their 'strong and courageous' chain links. (July 2009)
Left to right: Sally Park, Laurie Lane, Becky Annus, Drenda, Rachel, Linda Waggoner, Janette Wilkinson

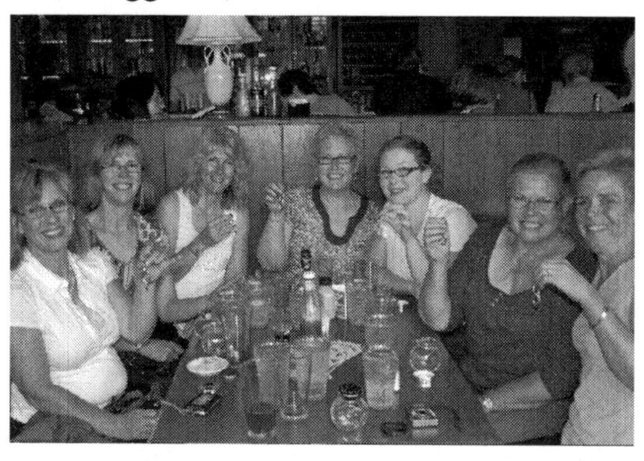

Strong and courageous chain links. We are not strong on our own, but together with God and family/friends, we hold each other up. (July 2009) Photo by Rachel Howatt

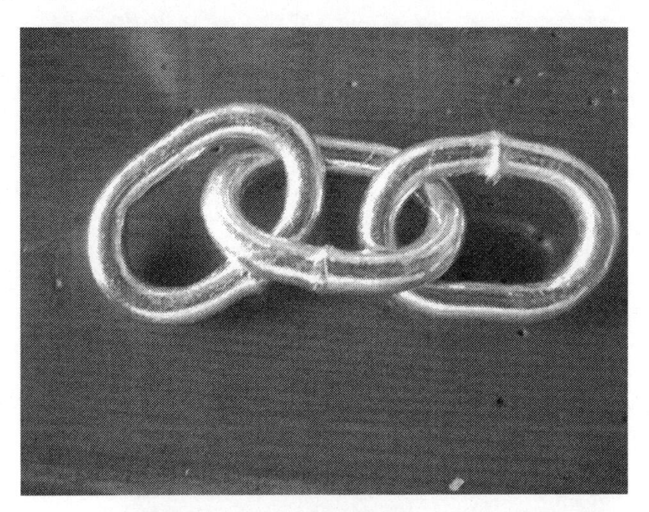

1001 Cranes

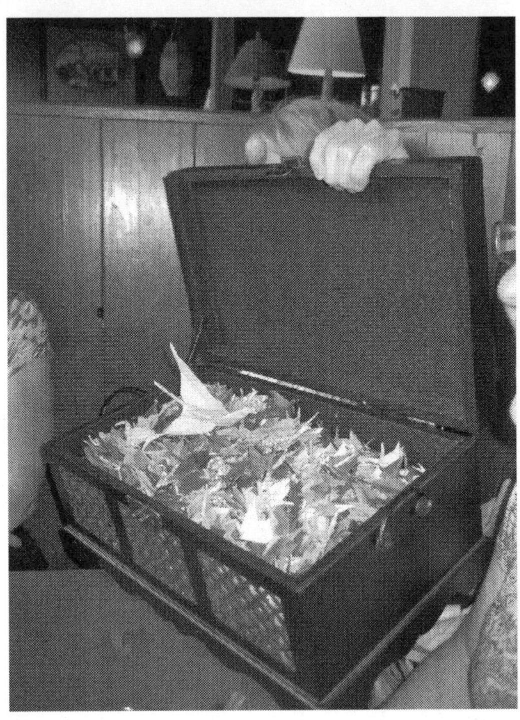

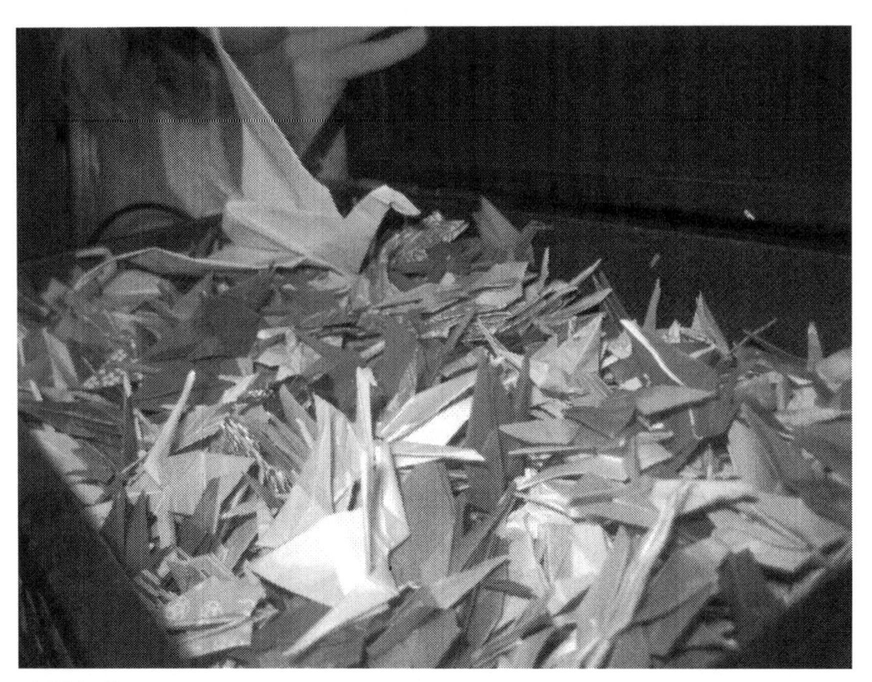

1001 Cranes

An ancient Japanese legend promises that anyone who folds a thousand origami cranes will be granted a wish by a crane, such as long life or recovery from illness or injury. The crane in Japan is one of the mystical or holy beasts (others include the dragon and tortoise), and is said to live for a thousand years. In Asia, it is commonly said that folding 1000 paper origami cranes makes a person's wish come true.

Drenda Lane Howatt had the pleasure of meeting one half of the population of the city of Portland...at Costco east. Came home and had a nap. Three hours.
July 31, 2009 at 5:12pm

> Wendy Ackley: Be nice when you are talking about my social event of the week.
> August 1, 2009 at 1:00pm
>
> Drenda Lane Howatt: Do you mean the trip to Costco or the nap?
> August 1, 2009 at 4:39pm
>
> Ted D.C. Waggoner: Love you Aunt Drenda! Your strength is inspiring and fills me with awe! (sorry for being gushy...) :-)
> July 31, 2009 at 11:05am
>
> Drenda Lane Howatt: I love gushy...
> Thank you
> July 31, 2009 at 11:08am

Drenda Lane Howatt is headed to Eagle Fern Camp to pick up Miss Ellie...with a SBUX stop first, of course.
August 1, 2009 at 7:51am

> Marilla Park: Jealous!! I am on a Starbucks diet =(
> August 1, 2009 at 9:40am
>
> Wendy Ackley: That means all you eat or drink is Starbucks
> August 1, 2009 at 12:55pm

Jerry, My Friend...

Sunday, August 2, 2009 at 8:15am

I am anxious to see Jerry.

Really anxious.

Anxious in a good way.

Because I don't know what to think.

I finished radiation treatment last week.

And all around me, I heard "Drenda is finished with cancer treatment!" "Yay! Drenda is done!"

But I didn't feel so excited. Finishing radiation was good. Great. But I had been viewing it as just one more step taken in a marathon.

I had never considered the end of the totality of chemo and radiation to be the finish line.

I still have the clinical trial drug to ingest until the end of February ish. Of NEXT year.

Brain MRI every year, echo-cardiograms all the time, probably other tests I don't even know about yet.

I still have other drugs to take...for FIVE years.

And then more after that.

But maybe my friends and family are right.

Maybe the "cancer" treatment IS done.

Treatment has been my life for almost 9 months. It has consumed my time, my thoughts, my writings; it has fed my fears and changed everything. Killing cancer. cancer War. Zaps.

Perhaps the next steps in the journey should be considered prevention...like taking vitamins. You know, to STAY healthy.

So I must see Jerry.

And I will ask him.

I will ask him to say the words.

"cancer Free".

If he will not, I will be disappointed. Maybe still scared.

I will ask anyway, knowing I may be reminded that cancer is not done in my body.

But he just might say them. Maybe.

And if he does, if those words come out of his mouth, oh what a day that will be.

August 20th.

Laurie Lane: You've come so far yet the journey continues.
August 2, 2009 at 8:23am

Deborah Davis: It's on my calendar. :-)
August 2, 2009at 9:59pm

Becky Annus: prevention, vitamins and staying healthy...I like that.
August 2, 2009 at 10:04pm

Present is Priceless

Sunday, August 2, 2009 at 7:53pm

I have written much about the support I have received as I have stared cancer in the face.

So many people have been by my side.

Some have gone before me. And then came to take my hand and lead me into the darkness. And they held a light onto my path.

Some have walked beside me the entire time. Their presence makes the darkness less scary.

Some are so frightened by breast cancer that they need to hear my story so they can find the differences between us. For if we ARE different, then they are "safe" from breast cancer. And once they feel safe, some are still there, and others are gone.

Some I do not even know. They read my blog, or hear my story from someone close to me, and then they reach out to let me know I am in their prayers.

But some are absent.

Pretty much completely.

And those that are absent make me wonder.

Are they afraid of me now?

Scared to say anything for fear of saying the "wrong" thing?

Afraid that cancer may be contagious?

Afraid of being a bother?

Or, perhaps, not realizing that reaching out does make a difference?

I don't know the answer.

But their absence does make me realize that I have been "absent" for others before.

And that makes me sad.

Because now I realize, truly, how important it is to be "present".

And what a difference that those "present" can make.

Priceless.

Elizabeth Honeycutt: So true, Drenda. It's better to say something in love than to be quiet for fear of "offending." I'm so glad that you are doing well!
August 2, 2009 at 8:01pm

Chelsea Lincoln Lane: I've said this before, but you are in inspiration. I faced the threat of breast cancer last year. Even though I don't know you well, you give me hope and strength. I know you do the same for many, even if it is unspoken.
August 2, 2009 at 8:05pm

Laurie Lane: Your journey is not unique to cancer. Often loved ones, or others, do not know what to say or how to say it. I have experienced similar things during difficult times in my life and

have treasured the comments and reaching out by others. I know it is sometimes hard, but we need to know someone is listening.
August 2, 2009 at 9:07pm

Deborah Davis: Some who seem absent may really be present but silent supporters. When my daughter was born with life-threatening birth defects, a student nurse was at a loss for what to say, so she sat and cried with me. It was just what I needed. And after the crisis was over, I learned of many, many people I never knew who prayed for us. There are surely many doing the same for you. It would be nice if everyone praying for you would be present for you too. But be assured you have a multitude of silent supporters.
August 2, 2009 at 9:55pm

Sally Park: I love you Drenda Mary Lane Howatt!
August 2, 2009 at 11:59pm

Kim Burns: So true... I think often people are just so busy and so self absorbed they just do not realize the need for connection. They do not realize how much a word of encouragement means to someone going through a tough time (cancer or other trials in life). It is a good reminder to look around you and make that call or write that note. It does make a difference. Thanks for sharing.
August 4, 2009 at 4:03pm

Drenda Lane Howatt has not been too happy to learn that more severe and painful side effects can show up a week AFTER radiation is over. That is just not right.
August 6, 2009 at 6:11am

Cindy McElmurry: Anything that I can help with or do?
August 6, 2009 at 8:05am

Connie Hohensee: Sorry, to hear about that, I hope everything is OK, and can't wait to see you on Saturday
August 6, 2009 at 8:13am

Sally Park: Are you experiencing those side effects now?
August 6 at 8:31am

Evy Marks Tyler: Drenda, I do not remember having side effects from radiation after it was over. I did have the "sunburn" that tended to be painful during the process, but it seemed there was nothing but relief when it was over. Of course, it has been seven years and one's memory tends to forget such unpleasant things. I'll be praying that the doctor is wrong and that none of those side effects hit you.
August 6, 2009 at 9:15am

Kim Burns: Good grief... enough is enough with these side effects.
NO MORE!
August 6, 2009 at 4:12pm

Drenda Lane Howatt: Good grief is right! Blisters and raw burn in places that should be treated carefully and never see things like sun...or radiation...ouch.
August 6, 2009 at 6:17pm

Maureen Gatens Thompson: Remember, this too shall pass...

August 6 at 9:22pm

Sally Park: Oh dear. That sounds painful! I am sorry.
August 6, 2009 at 9:42pm

Drenda Lane Howatt: I am fine...it is just a pain, literally, to deal with. I am getting accustomed to the face/scalp rash (almost), and the other side effects from the trial drug. But when the blisters appeared...oh my! In the whole scheme of things, these are minor inconveniences IF the treatment kills cancer and keeps it away. Even if only for a few years.
August 7, 2009 at 6:31am

Drenda Lane Howatt has a busy busy Friday. Day off? Not really...laundry, shopping, cleaning, paperwork. Plus, Rachel is hosting the Lunch Table Kids tonight at the Howatt House. Party time!
August 7, 2009 at 6:36am

Drenda Lane Howatt has another busy day...full of reunions! First family, then school. And afterwards, more time with great friends.
August 8, 2009 at 7:51am

Tara L Koch: See you tonight!
August 8, 2009 at 8:27am

Becky Annus: Have fun, you've got a great little get away planned with the girlfriends...
August 8, 2009 at 9:37am

Drenda Lane Howatt is home from the beach after a most wonderful time with girlfriends, thankful for friendships that

endure over many years (since 3rd grade). Now back to the real world. Oh my.
August 11, 2009 at 7:43pm

The Clarity of Crystal

Tuesday, August 11, 2009 at 9:14pm

Reunion Day.

August 8, 2009.

First, family.

Odd to see family members that I haven't seen in over a year.

To realize they do not know who I am.

And to see the shock on their faces when they take a look at my name tag.

"Drenda???!!"

Yes, it's me.

It may be a small world, but it is still a world where some news doesn't make it all the way around.

So the afternoon had a lot of "punched in the stomach by cancer" moments.

A lot of surreal moments.

Explanations of the last nine months. Reassurances to others that the worst for me is over. Surface descriptions of the terror.

I heard my voice say words that were unbelievable.

But they were true.

Rush home to prepare for the school reunion.

Again, no recognition.

Blank stares. Perhaps I was a spouse of a graduate, and not a member of the class?

I was in a room with 115 people, most of whom I had not seen in 30 years. Lots of looks at the name tag -- not unusual at a class reunion. The second glances did not bother me. But when some had to take four or five looks at the name tag and then back at my face, that was a bit disconcerting.

I realize that my classmates remembered me as a red headed girl. And now, as a white haired woman, I didn't fit into their memory.

And the problem was mine.

I realized that I did not feel safe in a large crowd where just a few people knew my story. I was thankful for the presence of Kathy and Kim and Kris.

I realized that I have become accustomed to being surrounded by people who know me, people who know my story and struggles. People who work with me. People who care for me. People who have been with me on the journey through breast cancer. I have not had to explain much lately to "my" people. So I have been comfortable. It's easy (as in "easier") to be comfortable with people you know well. And it is easy (again, as in "easier") to be comfortable with complete strangers. Not so much, apparently, with those you know "sort of".

At the reunion, I found myself wanting to explain away my appearance.

Perhaps I am not as comfortable with the way I look as I have led myself to believe.

I don't like to be different.

I don't like to stand out.

I don't like to have breast cancer.

Saturday's reunions made that crystal clear.

Wendy Ackley: You are a gifted writer, I felt I could hear your voice explaining your feelings perfectly, and I understood.
August 11, 2009 at 9:42pm

Laurie Lane: Guess you're human with all the feelings associated with having cancer paired with a 20th year reunion.... What a combination!

I agree with Wendy, you are a gifted and honest writer! Thanks for sharing.
August 11, 2009 at 9:56pm

Becky Annus: ...you are loved by "your" people...
August 11, 2009 at 9:57pm

Deanna Purcell Skirving: Drenda, My eyes are welled with tears as I read what your heart feels. I too love you and am so relieved this is behind you. No one cares what your appearance is when they can see directly into a heart like yours.
August 11, 2009 at 10:26pm

Gail Stempel Hilderbrand: I am stunned right now, as I felt (feel) your every word. You are braver than I. I did not go to my

reunion, nor am I going with Jeff to his this weekend. I can't do it. I am comfortable behind this computer screen, and at home, and with people who know and understand. You my dear are brave. I wish I was.
August 11, 2009 at 10:29pm

Andi Pedersen Jordan: Ah, Drenda, you felt the problem was yours, but, really? I think not! It's in the eyes, not the hair. The eyes show your heart and your soul, not the hair.
August 11, 2009 at 11:02pm

Sally Park: Glad I'm one of "your people" ♥
August 12, 2009 at 12:09am

Pam Smith Axmaker: I am on the other side, a spouse with cancer. His appearance may never be the same (The hair may not grow back), the worst for him is not over, it is yet to come. Being a male he doesn't talk a lot about it, but when he is in the mood we do talk. You have helped me understand what he has not said himself.
August 12, 2009 at 10:06am

Linda Waggoner: And I like your hair! Different from before but so attractive! I am so glad you are my sister! Your willingness to share has helped so many people - people you don't even know. You are amazing! I love you!
August 12, 2009 at 11:34am

Drenda Lane Howatt is preparing to be supported. As in making her first visit to a breast cancer support group. Not too sure she's ready, quite yet, but, um, ok.
August 13, 2009 at 5:28pm

> Mary Olson: Go Drenda! Woo! We're all lovin' and prayin' for ya:)
> August 13, 2009 at 5:57pm
>
> Christina Elford: You go girl...I thought maybe you were looking to be supported as in "bra shopping"...but yours is much better...God Bless...Janet....;)
> August 13, 2009 at 6:45pm
>
> Laurie Lane: My thoughts are with all of you!
> August 13, 2009 at 7:58pm
>
> Drenda Lane Howatt: ok. I had the wrong information...the meeting tonight was a cancer family support group. Baja Fresh for dinner, then family scrapbook activity. Fun, sort of. Apparently, the usual order of business is to separate into age groups - children in one, teens in one, and adults in another. We may try it again next month. Not sure.
> August 13, 2009 at 8:43pm
>
> Drenda Lane Howatt: Not a breast cancer support group.
> August 13, 2009 at 8:43pm

Drenda Lane Howatt wonders why it is so difficult to get some time away with her husband and all three of their daughters. Finally find the dates (not so easy when her husband is still low on UPS's seniority totem pole -- even after 20 years...), and then find out the venue is no longer available. aarrrgghhh.
August 14, 2009 at 7:12am

Cindy McElmurry: What!!!!!! You are not serious!
August 14, 2009 at 4:19pm

Um...Maybe

Friday, August 14, 2009 at 8:05am

Last night was the Family Support Group at Providence. The Howatt Family's first time attending.

For families that are experiencing some type of cancer.

I went by myself; Don and Ellie were stuck in traffic and were late arriving.

So a cancer patient by herself-- even for a short time -- at a Family Support Group. I didn't like that. All alone in a sea of cancer people.

More surreal moments.

A family came and joined me at my table. Until they sat down, I thought the support group was for breast cancer.

No. Any cancer.

The father in that family, I found out later, is battling brain cancer.

And he did not look good. He did not look like he was winning. He came with his wife, daughter and his mother. His daughter couldn't be older than 10.

He asked his wife "where are we?" And then, upon her answer, he asked "why are we here?"

My heart broke.

I thought "this is not a place for me".

But I wasn't there for me.

I was there for Ellie.

I was there because I wanted her to be there. I wanted Anna and Rachel to be there, too.

I was there because I want my babies to know they are not alone.

That it is not just their Mom who is battling, and WINNING, against cancer.

But do I want them there if it is apparent not everyone is winning the war?

I am not sure. Maybe.

As we left, though, I felt better.

I asked Ellie "do you want to come next month?"

And I was surprised by her answer.

Because I expected an absolute "NO".

Instead, I heard her say "um…, maybe".

Maybe being in a room with other families, with children young and children teens, helped. Even if cancer was not discussed.

Um, maybe.

Becky Annus: “um...maybe” is a good start
August 14, 2009 at 9:11am

Ginger Clausen: Was it helpful?
August 14, 2009 at 9:35am

Adrienne Fajen: parenting is such an art! I will pray that God helps you interpret maybe.
August 14, 2009 at 11:24am

Drenda Lane Howatt slept in, had her breve', did a load of laundry, washed the exterior of 13 windows (not counting all the little panes), trained up her jasmine, and is now headed to the grocery store. Oh, and pulled a few weeds, too. What a morning!
August 15, 2009 at 11:51am

> Robin Reilly: You wore me out just reading your post! You go girl. :-)
> August 15, 2009 at 11:52am
>
> Wendy Ackley: You are an inspiration! Now get up Wendy!!!
> August 15, 2009 at 11:56am
>
> Shannon Swope: I slept in later...just woke up...and feel like a total lazy butt compared to your day. See you tonight!
> August 15, 2009 at 2:04pm
>
> Lori Buckelew: After reading your post...I need another nap....
> August 15, 2009 at 8:05pm

Drenda Lane Howatt is paying the price for her industrious day yesterday. Too much, too soon and oh my goodness. But those windows...aside from just a few streaks, they're actually see-through now.
August 16, 2009 at 7:40am

> Evy Marks Tyler: Amazing, how the body complains about overwork, once you have been through surgery, radiation and chemo. Even seven years later painting for two hours, holding a bucket in one hand and a paint brush in the other sent me scurrying for a diagnostic

mammogram to make sure nothing nefarious was going on.
August 16, 2009 at 3:28pm

Drenda Lane Howatt: Time is running out to join team Strong and Courageous at the Komen Walk for the Cure...Walk on Sunday, September 20th...deadline to register on-line is August 31.
August 16, 2009 at 3:42pm

Evy Marks Tyler: Drenda - I'm afraid I'm clueless regarding where I go on line to register for your team. I definitely want to be there.
August 16, 2009 at 3:51pm

Jennifer Stady: Oh I want to do that. What is it? Is it something you are going to do?
August 16, 2009 at 7:09pm

Drenda Lane Howatt: Yes...I'll find the link. It is September 20th...my sister Becky organized Team Strong and Courageous...I'll post the link.
August 16, 2009 at 8:55pm

Evy Marks Tyler: I'm signed up for Strong & Courageous family and friends on the 5k untimed walk. Looking forward to this new adventure.
August 16, 2009 at 10:19pm

Sandy Hagstrand: See you girls there!
August 16, 2009 at 10:26pm

Drenda Lane Howatt was asked today, again, what her prognosis is. She thinks it should be "hope". Yes. That is the prognosis. At least that is what she wants it to be.
August 17, 2009 at 9:15pm

Abbi Howatt: I like it. That is a good prognosis.
August 17, 2009 at 9:17pm

Evy Marks Tyler: For my money I'd say your prognosis is LIFE!! You have fought the fight, you have been strong and courageous. You have chosen LIFE and I say Kudos to you.
August 17, 2009 at 9:41pm

Prognosis HOPE

Monday, August 17, 2009 at 9:38pm

Prognosis.

In the last week, I have been asked a number of times about my prognosis.

I don't like the question.

Because it makes me face my mortality each time I hear it.

I don't know what Jerry will say about my prognosis. I am working on the courage to ask him when I see him on Thursday.

But I know what I hope it is.

I hope that cancer is gone from my body.

Never to return.

I hope that I will never have to be as terrified, ever again, as I have been these last months.

I hope that my dear husband will not have to be so strong for me again for a long long time.

Because, in many ways, cancer has been harder on him than it has been on me.

I hope I can return to being a wife and mother who takes care of her family, instead of her family having to take care of her.

I hope that my precious babies will not have to be concerned with breast cancer again. I hope that they will be able to look back on this time and not be scarred from the trauma.

But all these "hopes" are not my prognosis.

My prognosis HOPE is the assurance I have in Christ.

My prognosis HOPE is the peace that comes amidst the terror.

My prognosis HOPE is the strength and courage that come from the fount of life.

Prognosis HOPE is what I cling to.

Because any other prognosis is not sure.

Marilla Park: Yay for prognosis hope =)
August 17, 2009 at 9:40pm

Sally Park: I agree "Yay for prognosis hope" !!
August 17, 2009 at 10:09pm

Maureen Gatens Thompson: A clinical response: Jerry will probably say the first 3 years is the most important because it is with BC. Then 5 years & on we go. I still struggle with this nagging thought almost 24 years later. ♥
August 17, 2009 at 10:27pm

Chelsea Lincoln Lane: Your prognosis gives us all Hope Drenda...In addition to our Hope for you, you have given us strength and showed us how strong the human spirit can be. We all need Hope and faith. In your battle, you have been a

mentor to more than you know...Yay HOPE!
August 17, 2009 at 11:36pm

Cindy McElmurry: My friend, I will agree with you that our hope is in Christ. He is in control. I love you my friend!
August 18, 2009 at 6:15pm

Drenda Lane Howatt had a busy busy day with work, doctor, volleyball camp, date with Hollace (yeah!), back to volleyball camp, now home. whew. Time to try and cool off.
August 19, 2009 at 6:35pm

Drenda Lane Howatt will visit NW Cancer Specialists today. First, lab work (..."Is that a one inch needle? No? You need to use the one inch needle"), then she will see Jerry. She has missed him. Yes she has.
August 20, 2009 at 7:05am

> Sally Park: Keep us updated tonight, k?
> August 20, 2009 at 8:36am

The Words

Drenda Lane Howatt heard, with her own ears and not just her heart, the wonderful words "cancer free" today. Yep. Jerry said she is cancer free. FREE.
August 20, 2009 at 12:35pm

> Danielle Becker: WHOO HOOOOOO!!!!
> August 20, 2009 at 12:40pm
>
> Tracy Cram: I am so happy to hear that, Drenda! Outstanding news!!!
> August 20, 2009 at 12:44pm
>
> Anna Rose Swope: Awesome!!
> August 20, 2009 at 12:54pm
>
> Kortney Stewart: I more than like this...I Love this!!! :) What an answer to prayer!
> August 20, 2009 at 12:59pm
>
> Bobbi Mapes: Very good news yeppie!!!!!!!!!!!!!
> August 20, 2009 at 1:06pm
>
> Susan Rasmussen Lane: What wonderful news!
> August 20, 2009 at 1:20pm
>
> Amy Hickman: So glad to hear it, Drenda! You have gone thru the valley, but God has been faithful!
> August 20, 2009 at 1:48pm
>
> Amber Lynn Montgomery Lane: HURRAY!
> August 20, 2009 at 2:00pm
>
> Andi Pedersen Jordan: Yipee!!!!!!!!
> August 20, 2009 at 2:29pm

Jennifer Stady: I'm incredibly happy.
August 20, 2009 at 2:53pm

Caitlin Lopez: PRAISE GOD!!!
August 20, 2009 at 2:54pm

Erin Frazier Miller: Beautiful!!
August 20, 2009 at 3:38pm

Adrienne Fajen: Super like! What great news :)
August 20, 2009 at 3:45pm

Jonna Wilkinson: Awesome!
August 20, 2009 at 4:10pm

Linda Waggoner: What great news!!!!! I am so happy for you!!!!!!
August 20, 2009 at 5:33pm

Sherri Detweiler Purcell: YAY Drenda-- Praise the Lord!!
August 20, 2009 at 5:34pm

Craig Glass: Wonderful news, Drenda!!
August 20, 2009 at 7:47pm

Sharley Massman: That is FABULOUS!!!
August 20, 2009 at 8:30pm

Say the Words, Jerry!

Thursday, August 20, 2009 at 6:02pm

August 20th.

Oh what a day this has been!

Jerry, bless him, gave me the words I have been longing for.

"cancer Free".

It wasn't as easy as it may sound.

I asked Jerry if, after all the treatment, I was considered cancer free.

His response?

"Oh yes. Absolutely!"

That wasn't enough for me.

As I choked back tears, I said "can you just say the words? Can you say them for me?"

"You are cancer free."

Giddiness.

Butterflies in my stomach.

Tremendous relief.

OH MY GOODNESS!

Don asked how he knew I was cancer free. Jerry said that the MRI of my brain, the MRI of my breasts, the continual blood tests all confirmed it.

Jerry went on to say that if, indeed, he was wrong and there was still cancer in my body, it would be microscopic and the lapatanib would kill it.

And, if I weren't on the lapatanib, I would be only seeing him every 3 months. But because of the lapatanib, he wants to see me every month. I will have an echo-cardiogram in November and February. Brain MRI annually.

A concern with breast cancer is that, if it spreads, it often shows up in the bones. Jerry told me if I have bone pain that doesn't go away, he wants to know about it. If I have headaches, he wants to know about it.

So I will fight down the terror if/when those aches appear.

But for now, I will work on finding parts of my old normal.

I will work on building back my strength.

I will look for more energy.

And I will spend it.

I can't wait.

Laurie Lane: Cancer FREE--- what beautiful words. These beautiful words, Cancer FREE, free you for moving on with your

life. YEAH!
August 20, 2009 at 6:06pm

Gail Stempel Hilderbrand: I am so happy for you! You won, you are a survivor! Congratulations Drenda, well done!
August 20, 2009 at 7:55pm

Elizabeth Lundquist Calhoun: Amazing!!!!! I can only imagine the emotions you are going through right now. I am praising God with you!!!
August 20, 2009 at 8:23pm

Sandy Hagstrand: How magnifcent those words are! Blessed be the LORD and HIS marvelous grace.
August 20, 2009 at 8:59pm

Sally Park: Wonderful, Glorious news !!!!!!
August 20, 2009 at 8:59pm

Deborah Davis What a happy, happy day. Praise God from whom all blessings flow.
August 20, 2009 at 10:05pm

Drenda Lane Howatt: Thank you all! Your comments are a testament to the fact that I was not, and am not, alone on this journey. I appreciate each one of you so much. Your words are always a great encouragement to me. Thank you for traveling along with me. Words cannot express my emotions.
August 21, 2009 at 7:49am

Becky Annus: strong and courageous AND cancer free! Happy Dance!!!!
August 21, 2009 at 8:42am

Emily Chandler Lawler: Woo hoo!! And dinner at Acapulco to celebrate! :)
August 21, 2009 at 10:00am

Drenda Lane Howatt: I must tell you that the restaurant choice was not a good one...
August 21, 2009 at 11:19am

Ginger Clausen: Praise the Lord! Prayers answered!
August 21, 2009 at 1:28pm

Amber Lynn Montgomery Lane: A WONDERFUL kind of FREEdom!
August 21, 2009 at 9:43pm

Wendy Ackley: I am very happy.
August 22, 2009 at 4:39pm

Susan Rasmussen Lane: YAHOO! Wonderful news!
August 23, 2009 at 6:08pm

Zachary Lane Kovall: Love those words. :D Congrats.
August 25, 2009 at 8:21am

Drenda Lane Howatt is loving the past tense. Present tense is pretty intense. It is no longer "I have breast cancer". It is now "I HAD breast cancer". OH YEAH!
August 21, 2009 at 7:21am

> Becky Annus: We're loving the past tense with you!
> August 21, 2009 at 8:53am
>
> Evy Marks Tyler: I wonder how many people having heard "You are cancer free" after having heard "You have cancer" have a whole new appreciation for life?
> August 21, 2009 at 10:55am

Drenda Lane Howatt is sick. bleh. No day trip to the beach. Drats.
August 22, 2009 at 8:29am

> Ginger Clausen: I'm sorry. I can relate... I'm missing my neice's wedding today for the same reason.
> August 22, 2009 at 8:39am
>
> Cindy McElmurry: What kind of sick???? Do you think it might be dust poisoning?
> You said you were deep cleaning yesterday! I got in the mood to clean as well and had to take allergy meds.
> August 22, 2009 at 9:05am
>
> Drenda Lane Howatt: I have to stay very close to the facilities. I thought it may be the new medication I started yesterday, but then the chills came...
> August 22, 2009 at 9:11am
>
> Ginger Clausen: Wait, no! Not the SAME reason- sick, yes, running to and from bathroom- no. Sneezing loudly and often- sore throat, etc. Either way feel like I've been

run over by a truck. This, too, shall pass.
August 22, 2009 at 9:14am

Hollace Howatt Chandler: Oh, I'm so sorry Drenda. About the beach trip and the sick thing. Not fair!!
August 22, 2009 at 10:45am

Drenda Lane Howatt has a day of vacation. Stay-cation. Paperwork. Reduce and organize the piles. Mission Organization continues.
August 24, 2009 at 6:36am

Kimberly Tibbetts Roberts: Sounds like something I need to do. Way too much clutter. Have a picture I would like to send you I found of your girls and the McGees and Katie. Would love to send to you. Don't know where to send it. You know where to reach me if you would like a copy of it. Hope you are doing well. URLVD Kim
August 24, 2009 at 10:59am

Drenda Lane Howatt made great progress on Mission Organization. The Mission is now on hold for who knows how long...
August 25, 2009 at 6:08am

Drenda Lane Howatt Time is running out to join the team! On-line registration closes next week! Join Team Strong and Courageous on the Komen Walk for the Cure, Sunday September 20th
August 25, 2009 at 11:49am

Drenda Lane Howatt: We're doing the 5K untimed walk....
August 25, 2009 at 11:51am

Amanda Lane: Thanks for the reminder!
August 25, 2009 at 12:18pm

Hollace Howatt Chandler: Can Weak and Wimpy people join Team Strong and Courageous?
August 25, 2009 at 1:35pm

Evy Marks Tyler: Hollace, join me, we can be weak and wimpy together.
August 25, 2009 at 3:21pm

Drenda Lane Howatt: Weak and wimpy welcome!
August 25, 2009 at 4:11pm

Carolyn Kempf: Drenda, you doing well? Not much going on here in Missouri, Work and a little Play! Not much!
August 26, 2009 at 5:14am

Rebecca Groner: Can people just show up the day of the walk and participate?
August 26, 2009 at 7:36pm

Drenda Lane Howatt: not sure...Becky is our captain and she knows everything...are you friends with Becky?
August 26, 2009 at 9:29pm

Rebecca Groner: Yep…I'll ask Becky.
August 27, 2009 at 4:59pm

Drenda Lane Howatt is going to have a bit of summer in the coming days. Lazy days starting next week...8 of 'em. Oh yeah!
August 28, 2009 at 8:24am

Cindy McElmurry: Have a great week at the beach!
August 28, 2009 at 11:59am

Drenda Lane Howatt is smarter than her children may think....
August 29, 2009 at 3:48pm

Adrienne Fajen: On the other hand you may be able to cheat more successfully at cards...
August 29, 2009 at 5:48pm

Drenda Lane Howatt ~only 1 1/2 days left for on-line registration...Join Team Strong and Courageous for the Komen Race for the Cure (we're doing the 5k Untimed Walk)...
August 29, 2009 at 9:33pm

Drenda Lane Howatt had a wonderful evening with family and friends, and now a lazy Sunday morning filled with a breve' and a quiet house. Oh yes.
August 30, 2009 at 8:05am

Don Howatt: "ah ahem" Where'd you get that brevé? It didn't make itself!
August 30, 2009 at 8:50am

Andrea Midge McKeehan Robinson: Gotta love a good hubby and his breve' skills!!
August 30, 2009 at 8:58am

Drenda Lane Howatt: My apologies...my morning was filled with a breve' provided by my wonderful husband...and a quiet time in the library sitting next to him.
August 30, 2009 at 9:13am

Barry Andrews: You have a library in your house?? Oh, yeah. I hadn't seen the house until the other day when we were moving. Is it, like, "old"?
August 30, 2009 at 9:18am

Elizabeth Lundquist Calhoun: That sounds like heaven
August 30, 2009 at 10:07am

Drenda Lane Howatt will, before morning disappears, head out the door and be on her way to the Oregon Coast. Neskowin, here come some of the Howatts!
August 31, 2009 at 6:51am

Marilla Park: I was there this spring!
August 31, 2009 at 10:02am

Gail Stempel Hilderbrand: Hope you have a blast!
August 31, 2009 at 8:51pm

Drenda Lane Howatt is enjoying Neskowin...sun, blue skies, slight breeze, and lots of books!
September 2, 2009 at 12:39pm

Linda Waggoner: I LOVE Neskowin!!!!
September 3, 2009 at 10:42am

Drenda Lane Howatt enjoying Neskowin...what a wonderful week!
September 5, 2009 at 1:04pm

Drenda Lane Howatt is home from a week in Neskowin...a restful and restorative time. Now, back to the real world and AUTUMN!
September 7, 2009 at 2:47pm

Jennifer Stady: Welcome back to the REAL WORLD! Glad you had a good time. I love that house (high school memories).

September 7, 2009 at 6:09pm

Drenda Lane Howatt: The house is wonderful! Yes, the REAL WORLD awaits...but the good news is that it feels as if I have been gone longer than one week.
September 7, 2009 at 8:07pm

Sally Park: You deserved it! The beach makes you relax; the air...
September 7, 2009 at 9:20pm

Sack of Fear

Monday, September 7, 2009 at 8:41pm

It has been 10 months since my life changed drastically.

In the first months after I was told I had breast cancer, I wondered if cancer would ever be out of my consciousness.

Would it ever move out of my eyesight?

Or out of earshot?

Would it ever be anything other than my entire world?

Stop consuming every thought?

Stop feeding and creating terror?

I asked Evy and Maureen, friends who are also breast cancer survivors, those questions. Really.

I remember standing in the reception area at work and asking Maureen "does cancer ever move away from right here?" as I held my hand two inches from my face.

At Applebee's with Evy, I sobbed (literally) that same question, in many different forms.

Their answers were calming and reassuring.

But I didn't believe them.

I just returned from 7 days at the Oregon Coast.

It was Beautiful.

Beautiful weather.

Beautiful time with my family.

Beautiful time with God.

Beautiful in the freedom of nothing. No schedule. No list. Nothing.

I read books -- entire books -- for the first time since last summer. Even non-fiction. That means chemo brain is relenting. Somewhat.

And I did read one novel. It wasn't anything great or remarkable. In fact, almost a waste of time. But there was one quote in the book that hit me over the head.

That quote answered my question about the terror of cancer moving out of my consciousness.

In the book, one character says to another:

"do not pick up a sack of fear and carry it with you everywhere, just waiting until the next test and diagnosis..."

Perhaps cancer terror can move out of my consciousness...but it is up to me.

There are lots of different things in life that I can fear.

Cancer.

Baldness.

Surgery.

Chemotherapy.

Death.

Life itself.

But, perhaps, if I refuse to pick up the sack of fear and carry it with me everywhere, perhaps then I can see past the cancer.

I won't forget the terror.

I won't forget the blessings.

But I will not continue to be terrorized by cancer.

I will not pick up the sack.

I refuse.

Andi Pedersen Jordan: Maybe that is our note to self ... I am going to do some fall cleaning and put all of those horrible things that I can in a bag, maybe even pick it up and I'll throw it out ...
Ever so proud of you, Drenda. Ever so proud.
xoxo
September 7, 2009 at 9:52pm

Wendy Ackley: Thanks Drenda for sharing. I really like the quote. The book was not a waste of time!
September 7, 2009 at 10:29pm

Evy Marks Tyler: Refusing fear is a very good thing. Not picking up the sack of fear is a good visual. JUST SAY NO!!! Yeah! It

may be more complicated than just saying no, but it is a place to start whenever one is attacked by that thief.
September 7, 2009 at 10:57pm

Laurie Lane: Walk away from the sack of fear, you have moved so far in your journey. Thanks for taking us along!
September 8, 2009 at 6:52am

Jennifer Stady: Good for you Drenda. Thank you so much for sharing that...
September 8, 2009 at 7:26am

Kimberly Tibbetts Roberts: That is so beautiful. God carries you through all fears, pain suffering and eventually into his loving arms and the loving arms of our waiting friends and family. It is all his timing. I have had several close calls in my life and he still carries me back to my life to love all, help all and do his good work. You are loved!
September 8, 2009 at 10:16am

Amanda Lane: perhaps if that fear ever starts to creep back in, try answering the question "so what?" as in, if the cancer comes back, so what? Then you answer. and the answer is that you kicked it thoroughly and soundly this time and you can do it all over again if necessary. And as far as the baldness goes, you may just want to keep it in the back of your head how great you look(ed) with no hair. you didn't just survive, you thrived, and you have given so much to all of us just by knowing you through this. I hope that you never again have cause to worry about the cancer, but know that no matter what you will have the same resources you had this time, but even stronger! You will still have god and your family and friends to walk with you, no matter what road...
all my love♥
September 10, 2009 at 12:04pm

Drenda Lane Howatt realizes, anew, that the only problem with going on vacation is that one has to return from vacation and re-enter the real world, and face all the piles of work that await.
September 8, 2009 at 5:55pm

Sherri Detweiler Purcell: Yeah...sometimes you need another vacation after catching up from being on vacation...did that make sense?? I think I must be tired...It was a tiring first day at school!
September 8, 2009 at 7:42pm

Drenda Lane Howatt: Yes, perfect sense! Vacation was wonderful, and restful, but there is still no food in the house, not too many clean clothes, and lots of work from both jobs waiting for me. Some of it is still waiting...
September 8, 2009 at 8:25pm

Pam Girtman: And thank you both for that bit of encouragement . . . I'll be back on Thursday!
September 8, 2009 at 9:14pm

Drenda Lane Howatt: Pam, you make me laugh! Enjoy your time away from the office~
September 9, 2009 at 5:26am

Maureen Gatens Thompson: Hey Drenda--I'll be thinking of you tomorrow while I am in Bend at the state workforce conference. Have a terrific birthday. I treasure every birthday and look forward every year to the next one. Think how different last year's birthday was and how much has happened in 12 months. Tomorrow's birthday will have a new and special meaning. Celebrate and "dance like no body's watchin'." ♥
September 8, 2009 at 11:00pm

Drenda Lane Howatt: Thank you, Maureen~

This has been a difficult and wonderful year. Difficult in the trials of cancer, wonderful in the blessings of friends and family.
September 9, 2009 at 5:42am

Change the Past?

Wednesday, September 9, 2009 at 6:04am

Would I, if I could, change the last year of my life?

Blot out the pain and awfulness of breast cancer?

Take away the surgeries and chemo?

Reclaim the time spent on so many doctor visits?

Call back the millions of tears?

Erase the sudden and terrific fears?

hmmm.

Interesting questions to ponder.

But there would be more questions that would have to be considered before I could answer any of them honestly.

Would I return the courage and strength that God has granted me?

Take back the boldness of sharing my faith in the God who has promised me that He will be with me wherever I go?

Would I go back to being a stranger to my family?

Release the 'reconnections' with so many friends?

Live, again, with no thought of my own mortality?

Give back the renewed understanding of what a solid, strong, and wonderful man I married?

Take away the pain my daughters have experienced?

Take away the joy they felt hearing the words "cancer free"?

There is no question.

Not really.

And it doesn't take me much time to ponder.

Because I know the answers.

I wouldn't change my life.

I am thankful for the difficulties.

Because I am thrilled with the blessings.

Laurie Lane: Your difficulties have brought us all closer. For that I am thankful!
September 9, 2009 at 7:31am

Barb Van Dusen Butler: My "trials" have not been yours, but I too would not want to change them. I learned things that could not be learned otherwise and I pity those who don't have the assurance in God's love, care, and presence that I do. No, I would not change them, but I never want to repeat them either.
September 9, 2009 at 9:16am

Linda Waggoner: Aside from being so proud of you as you have

traveled this journey (and wishing every day that you didn't have to make this particular journey) I am so thankful to have had the chance to meet my sisters as strong, wonderful women - not just part of my childhood. Your willingness to share yourself over this last year has truly been a wonderful gift!! I love you!
September 9, 2009 at 11:48am

Kimberly Tibbetts Roberts: Happy Birthday Drenda. Hope you have a great birthday.
September 9, 2009 at 4:33pm

Jonna Wilkinson: I understand how you feel. I went thru a lot of "crap" of other kinds to bring me where I am today. It gave me so much that I could share with my high school girls bible studies and overnighters, etc. One, as you now understand, of the blessings that God wants so very much to share with us. But it's like the sun - we can't truly appreciate the warmth of the sun shining on our faces if we've never felt the chilled to the bones cold of rain. Likewise, we can't truly understand or appreciate God's blessings if we've never cried out to Him in our pain and grief. Another is that He put me in a unique place to share and teach to my kids that didn't grow up in the church - that didn't understand God's forgiveness because they couldn't find anyone inside the church that had experienced what they had.
And I know that, however long God gives us here on this earth, you will be faithful. So don't forget because it puts you in a special place to share, as you are here.
God bless you, Drenda.
September 9, 2009 at 4:35pm

Drenda Lane Howatt Thank you, everyone, for the wonderful birthday wishes! It was a great day made even better by receiving an "all-clear" from Dr. Wang, radiation oncologist. Next follow-up with Dr. Wang? FEBRUARY! 09-09-09 trivia: September has nine letters Wednesday has nine letters the 252nd day of the year, which adds up to equal nine.
September 9, 2009 at 10:06pm

> Rhonda Cox: Happy Belated Birthday Drenda. WONDERFUL NEWS! We'll keep on sending positive thoughts from Bend.
> September 10, 2009 at 11:04am
>
> Kimberly Tibbetts Roberts: I'm so glad. Keep going and getting stronger!
> September 10, 2009 at 5:34pm

Drenda Lane Howatt is trying not to stress out...lots to do before reporting for surgery at 7:30 a.m. tomorrow. Deep breath. Ok. She is fine now. Still need to survive nothing in the tummy after midnight. She has received stern words that "nothing" means NOTHING. Not even her morning breve'.
September 10, 2009 at 6:12pm

> Laurie Lane: What's the surgery for?
> September 10, 2009 at 6:22pm
>
> Sherri Detweiler Purcell: What??
> September 10, 2009 at 6:23pm
>
> Drenda Lane Howatt: It is a good surgery...to remove the port. Still done under general anesthesia.
> September 10, 2009 at 6:25pm

Sally Park: Get that out of there!!! Woop! Woop!
September 10, 2009 at 6:27pm

Sherri Detweiler Purcell: Yay!! That is a good surgery
September 10, 2009 at 6:30pm

Sandy Hagstrand: I missed something - what surgery???
September 10, 2009 at 9:22pm

Lori Buckelew: I LOVED the surgery where they remove the port...still have the scar but I call it a battle wound! Congratulations!
September 10, 2009 at 9:39pm

Kimberly Tibbetts Roberts: I will pray for you and for your family. God bless you and keep you,
September 10, 2009 at 10:16pm

Drenda Lane Howatt is off to Providence Portland Medical Center for a little nap. And she was very good this morning. No coffee. No NOTHING.
September 11, 2009 at 6:59am

Laurie Lane: Steps toward normalcy.
September 11, 2009 at 7:11am

Linda Waggoner: I am so glad for you!!!!!
September 11, 2009 at 7:59am

Brian Weeks: Hugs
September 11, 2009 at 8:11am

Drenda Lane Howatt This is a pic of the port Dr. Lehti is removing

www.vitamdonline.com
Source: www.vitamdonline.com
September 11, 2009 at 7:56am

Mary Raethke: I will be thinking about you today Drenda - good luck!
September 11, 2009 at 7:58am

Lori Buckelew: Dr Lehti was my doctor...he removed my port too! congrats on this milestone!
September 11, 2009 at 9:32am

Sandy Hagstrand: Ports are wonderful things, and so is Dr L
September 12, 2009 at 10:03am

Drenda Lane Howatt has seen no sign of any medical professional...except for the lab tech who came to draw blood.
September 11, 2009 at 8:51am

Andrea Midge McKeehan Robinson: **Sigh**
September 11, 2009 at 9:09am

Wendy Ackley: I have been working evenings at PPMC this week. Close...but not the right time.
September 11, 2009 at 9:18am

Andrea Midge McKeehan Robinson: Dave is working at Prov Milwaukie right now, can you drive over there real quick? :P
September 11, 2009 at 9:21am

Drenda Lane Howatt five tries...i.v. finally in. hot towels did not help, apparently. two minutes to scheduled surgery time...but

still waiting for the "good" drugs. gotta love free wi-fi at the hospital~
September 11, 2009 at 10:29am

Chelsea Lincoln Lane: Our thoughts and prayers are with you Drenda
September 11, 2009 at 10:45am

Wendy Ackley: I am pondering the idea of free.
September 11, 2009 at 11:58am

Drenda Lane Howatt: I hope Obama makes sure wi-fi is included.
September 11, 2009 at 2:47pm

Don Howatt: I think the free wi-fi is in the constitution
September 11, 2009 at 3:01pm

Drenda Lane Howatt is home...and loving vicodin. Surgery was less than 30 minutes...woke up in recovery room 40ish minutes after being wheeled into the operating room. Now, time to find a little something to eat and then to bed.
September 11, 2009 at 2:49pm

Andi Pedersen Jordan: Thinking of you!
September 11, 2009 at 3:38pm

Drenda Lane Howatt had a great, drug induced, nap at home, and then a fun dinner at McMenamin's on NW 23rd. After dinner, a nice summer evening's stroll with great friends. What a day!
September 11, 2009 at 10:50pm

Drenda Lane Howatt...and, so far, no pain medication needed since leaving the hospital at 2 p.m. A bit of discomfort, but no

pain. yeah!
September 11, 2009 at 10:53pm

Sandy Hagstrand: I suspected that was the surgery you meant. Glad you enjoyed dinner...
September 12, 2009 at 9:59am

Drenda Lane Howatt is feeling great and now off for a coffee date with her baby sister. She cannot, however, drive. No driving for 24 hours after narcotics. Time to get up, Don! You have a delivery to make...
September 12, 2009 at 7:05am

Kim Burns: What a week. I was wondering why I had not heard from you. I guess I have not been on FB all week. Thrilled to hear your surgery went quickly and you are now free of that port. Oh yes it is a celebration indeed. Dinner, coffee, walks with friends. God is good.
September 13, 2009 at 8:31am

Drenda Lane Howatt would say "yes" all over again. Being married 25 years to a great man is a most excellent thing!
September 15, 2009 at 5:38am

Faith Jossi Lichtenberg: Congratulations, Drenda & Don, most excellent for sure
September 15, 2009 at 5:46am

Evy Marks Tyler: Yes, congratulations! Truly it says a lot about both of you, since marriage is HARD WORK!!! but well worth it because after 31 years I'd say yes to my man too.
September 15, 2009 at 5:50am

Susan Rasmussen Lane: Happy anniversary!
September 15, 2009 at 11:48am

Drenda Lane Howatt heard today, from a total stranger, that the Oregonian published her submission about breast cancer...check out Sunday's (9-13-09) special "Race for the Cure" section.
September 15, 2009 at 10:13pm

Andrea Midge McKeehan Robinson: WHOOO HOOO!!! Told you that you are an amazing writer!
September 15, 2009 at 10:22pm

Brian Weeks: Wow that is awesome!
September 15, 2009 at 11:01pm

Tina Stinson: That is Awesome Drenda!!!
September 15, 2009 at 11:27pm

Andi Pedersen Jordan: uhmm... recycled my paper ... please share!
September 16, 2009 at 3:29am

Drenda Lane Howatt: It was one of my writings about cancer from my blog...the "Who Am I" piece. The "O" wanted breast cancer patients/survivors to write about how cancer has affected their lives.

And what in the world are you doing up on fb at 3:29 a.m.?
September 16, 2009 at 5:29am

Drenda Lane Howatt and Don celebrated their silver wedding anniversary by attending "Back to School Night"...welcome to 8th grade. It's going to be a great year!
September 16, 2009 at 5:33am

Ellie Howatt: Maybe it was a sign that I forgot to tell you

about it~
September 16, 2009 at 7:00am

Susan Rasmussen Lane: Ah, yes. Our anniversary is Sept. 8, and over the years we have spent it many times doing just such things. I don't recommend early Sept. weddings if you plan to have kids. By the way, we spent our silver anniversary taking foster children to free day at the zoo! Our "celebrations" of our anniversary have seldom been romantic.
September 16, 2009 at 9:04am

Chelsea Lincoln Lane: Congrats! You teach 8th grade? You're even more of a hero than I imagined! My hopes are to teach middle school history or high school Spanish...a couple more years to go...I'm applying for the GTEP program this year!
September 16, 2009 at 10:47am

Drenda Lane Howatt: No, Chelsea...not that much of a hero! I work in government/politics...staff to the Clackamas County Board of Commissioners...Ellie is in 8th grade this year; we attended "Back to School Night" as parents!
September 16, 2009 at 11:15am

Deborah Davis: If I'd known, I would have baked you a cake! Or sung "Happy Anniversary to You!" Or not... Congratulations to you.
September 16, 2009at 5:04pm

Drenda Lane Howatt: aaahh. Fall. Love it!
September 16, 2009 at 6:17pm

Amy Hickman: Today seems very officially Fall, doesn't it?
September 16, 2009 at 6:19pm

Drenda Lane Howatt: I can't wait for the fall colors. My FAVORITE time of year. Always.
September 16, 2009 at 6:25pm

Carolyn Kempf: We have lots of maple trees here in Missouri so yes my favorite time too.
September 17, 2009 at 9:04pm

Drenda Lane Howatt has a message for Team Strong and Courageous: Meet at 8 a.m. on Race (Walk) Day at the Salmon Street Fountain (Salmon & Naito Pkwy).
September 17, 2009 at 7:52pm

Amanda Lane: Are we supposed to go register at the expo center tomorrow, or do we just do it the day of?
September 18, 2009 at 11:42am

Drenda Lane Howatt: No...your parents have your t-shirt and registration number. Come on Sunday -- meet at 8 a.m. at the Salmon Street fountain.
September 18, 2009 at 11:48am

Amanda Lane: Those sneaky parents! I didn't even know... ☻
September 18, 2009 at 11:49am

Janette Wilkinson: Parents are like that
September 18, 2009 at 4:43pm

Drenda Lane Howatt is home from Race for the Cure. What an amazing morning. "Thank you to Team Strong and Courageous...your strength and courage keep me going. I could not have come through breast cancer without you." 1 Month Survivor...oh yes!
September 20, 2009 at 12:21pm

Marilla Park: Yay! Wish I could have walked!
September 20, 2009 at 12:23pm

Faith Jossi Lichtenberg: So awesome to hear, glad it was an amazing morning!
September 20, 2009 at 12:33pm

Ginger Clausen: Amen! You go girl!
September 20, 2009 at 5:09pm

Evy Marks Tyler: So, it has been awhile since I've walked that much. After the group split up Kathy Damon and I walked across the Steele bridge to the convention center to catch MAX, home. Imagine our surprise when we are asked about our Strong and Courageous shirts, and we explained we are on the team of a friend. "Is that Drenda Lane?" he asks. "Yes," we reply. "She's my sister-in-law."
September 20, 2009 at 7:30pm

Sandy Hagstrand: Yes, it was a WONDERFUL morning. Sharing it with special friends makes it all the more meaningful! Evy and Drenda, you are true examples of HIS Strength and Courage in your lives as you've walked through this. Blessings to both of you!
September 20, 2009 at 7:55pm

Race for the Cure

Sunday, September 20, 2009 at 8:51pm

Today I participated in my first "Race for the Cure".

The entire morning was filled with conflicting emotions.

Team Strong and Courageous. An amazing team of support.

There for me. To support ME.

There because I had breast cancer.

But that very fact punched me in the stomach a million times throughout the morning.

I kept thinking "I shouldn't be here" everywhere I went.

Survivor City? That is a great thing. A great place. But why was I there?

I said to Becky "this is not right. We should not be here."

And she completely and instantly understood.

We should not have been there because I should not have had cancer. Another "how did this happen" moment.

As we walked to meet up with the Team, we heard the live radio broadcast. Celebrating different survivors.

"We have Mrs. ____, a breast cancer survivor who is 93 years old! She is here in her wheelchair! And she has battled breast cancer FOUR times!"

"Another survivor! Her breast cancer has gone to her brain, and she has battled TWENTY brain tumors! She is here!"

I looked at Becky.

She looked at me.

"ooohh. 20 brain tumors."

I had to fight back the tears.

I guess it is good to know that people can and do battle this monster of breast cancer multiple times.

But not me.

I don't want to.

I want to be DONE.

And I found the radio broadcast disturbing in its reminder that cancer may not be done with me.

So, even though I am cancer free, I will still need to be strong and courageous.

Strong enough to refuse to pick up the bag of fear.

Courageous enough to live.

Amanda Lane: Unfortunately, as I am learning all over again

myself, the hardest part of the battle seems to be right after the wolf is no longer at the door... at first I had ecstatic relief, but now I am stuck with being a survivor. I found myself in a place I don't want to belong, and no more battles to fight. At least during the fight I had a purpose and a goal. It was hell, and I'm sure your battle was even worse. And I am so relieved that you have come out the other side, even more beautiful than when you started. Like it or not, I think you will be stuck with the lot of us for the duration. No matter what. You know already that I love you, but I also admire you. I'd say i'm proud of you, but that word seems too small for what you have done and what you have given me through it.♥
September 22, 2009 at 9:07am

Shannon Swope: Nicely put friend-love ya! That WAS fun albeit a little crowded...anything for you of course! :)
September 24, 2009 at 10:09pm

Team Strong and Courageous members Sally Park, Abi Lane, Janette Wilkinson, Thomas Wilkinson, Henry Wilkinson, Patrick Wilkinson, Scott Lane. (September 2009) Photo by Ron Waggoner

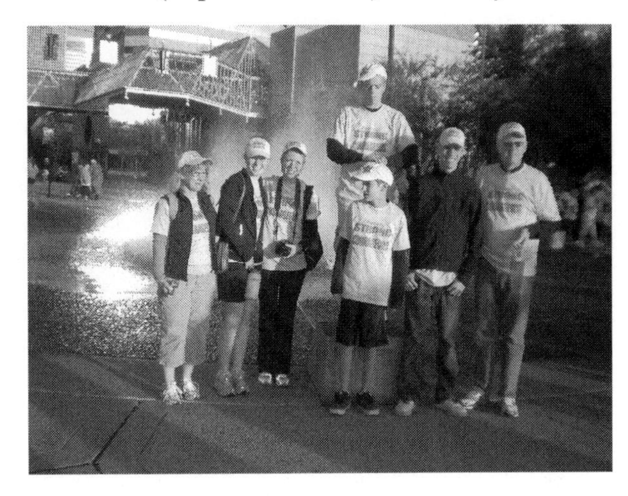

Team Strong and Courageous team members awaiting start of Walk for the Cure. (September 2009) Photo by Ron Waggoner

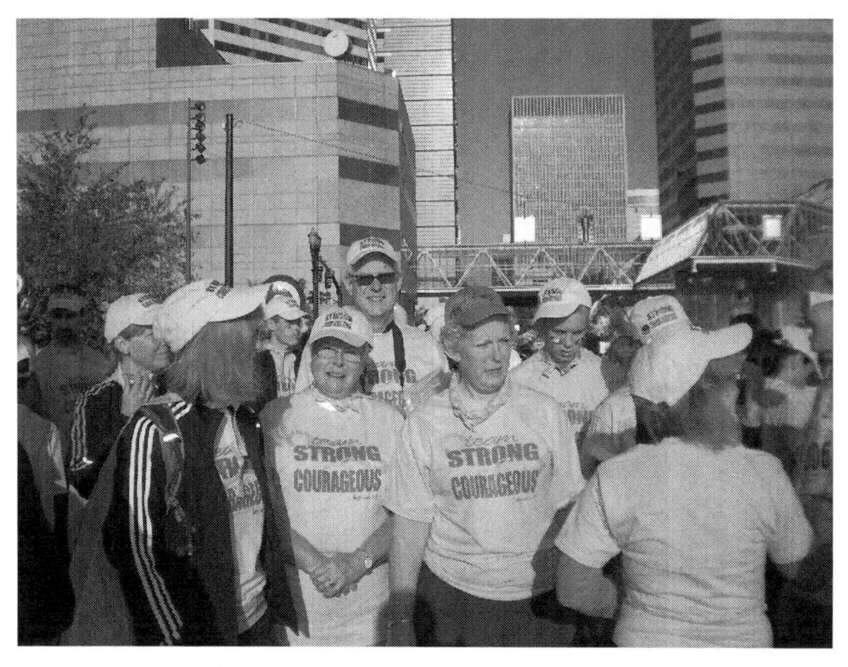

Drenda Lane Howatt will see her surgeon this morning. Just a friendly check-up of the surgical site. Isn't it interesting to have one's own surgeon?
September 23, 2009 at 6:22am

Hollace Howatt Chandler: Better to have an ex-surgeon
September 23, 2009 at 7:27am

Drenda Lane Howatt has her monthly date with Jerry today. He is a good guy.
September 24, 2009 at 6:16am

Annette Mattson: It was great to see you today, even if briefly. I love your curly hairstyle!
September 24, 2009 at 6:53am

Drenda Lane Howatt: Good to see you, too~
My hair is finally starting to look like it could be a real style! Martha made me laugh by saying my hair was "stunning". That is a first!
September 24, 2009 at 7:48am

Drenda Lane Howatt thinks it is unreasonable, and highly irritating, to have a 10 minute lab appointment and a 10 minute doctor appointment take longer than 2 hours. Hello NW Cancer Specialists: Drenda Howatt's time is valuable, too.
September 24, 2009 at 1:22pm

Debbie Bistline: You tell 'em!
September 24, 2009 at 1:23pm

Sally Park: Indeed it is!!
September 24, 2009 at 5:42pm

Elissa Gertler: Why is it like stepping into another time zone when entering a medical office? You would never

keep someone waiting like that at your job-- darn right your time is equally valuable! mmmph!
September 24, 2009 at 5:52pm

Hollace Howatt Chandler: So are you going to tell them?
September 24, 2009 at 6:03pm

Drenda Lane Howatt: I did. Nicely. I said "I've been here long enough to have chemo...except I didn't get a nap." The receptionist even asked me "why have you been here so long?" "Good question", said I.
September 24, 2009 at 7:17pm

Maureen Gatens Thompson: Yep, you're lucky this is the first time. One time I billed my doc....he got the message really fast!
September 24, 2009 at 11:12pm

Wendy Ackley: No it isn't. Of course we know it is valuable but truly they don't.
September 25, 2009 at 7:25pm

Drenda Lane Howatt is not entirely sure what happened to the day...
September 25, 2009 at 6:59pm

Drenda Lane Howatt is off to Beaverton for Ellie's volleyball game.
September 26, 2009 at 11:33am

Drenda Lane Howatt is waiting for Miss Rachel to arrive for her 17 hour visit...
September 29, 2009 at 8:12pm

Andi Pedersen Jordan: oooh, wouldn't want her to

overstay her welcome!
September 29, 2009 at 8:17pm

Drenda Lane Howatt: Yep! A six hour roundtrip on the train...all for 17 hours at home. She is coming for a doctor appointment, and the bonus is that we get to see her for a little while! She won't be back until Thanksgiving. boo hoo.
September 29, 2009 at 8:20pm

Laurie Lane: Whenever we have the opportunity to spend time with our children it is GREAT!
September 29, 2009 at 9:14pm

Laurie Lane: Enjoy your time with Rachel! I won't see Zachary or Nathan until Christmas... :~(
September 29, 2009 at 9:15pm

Hollace Howatt Chandler: Have fun! Loved Rachel's Health video to you.
September 30, 2009at 3:01pm

Drenda Lane Howatt left Rachel at the train station...she is on her way back to Seattle. So good to see her~
September 30, 2009 at 3:06pm

Drenda Lane Howatt is happy for Thursday, which in county land is Friday. Woo Hoo!
October 1, 2009 at 6:11am

Amanda Lane: Maybe I live in the wrong county land... ☻
October 1, 2009 at 9:14am

Ellie Howatt: Yep! If only school was like that.
October 1, 2009 at 12:19pm

Drenda Lane Howatt: Amanda, yes, you do. Clackamas is the only county to work for.
Ellie, interesting comment...especially since you have both Thursday AND Friday off of school this week. Silly girl.
October 1, 2009 at 5:03pm

Ellie Howatt: Well...I wasn't talking about this week I was talking about all the weeks kind of like Zander and Sophie only have a four day week every week
October 1, 2009 at 5:50pm

Drenda Lane Howatt: Oh, yes. Corbett. All schools should have Corbett's schedule. Good idea!
October 1, 2009 at 5:52pm

Becky Annus: I agree - a 4 day school week is AWESOME!! Zander and Sophie love it!
October 1, 2009 at 7:27pm

Drenda Lane Howatt is happy to have a normal day in front of herself...coffee, work, watching a little volleyball practice, home again. And such beautiful weather to experience. Life is good!
October 6, 2009 at 5:22am

Nature

Tuesday, October 6, 2009 at 9:36pm

It happened again.

"Love your hair! Is it naturally curly?"

And, this time, I answered without hesitation.

"Yes. Thank you."

And then exchanged a knowing glance with my husband. One of those glances we call the "we should be married" looks. A look that says everything.

The remarkable thing about this verbal exchange is that it took place at Jerry's office.

The woman doing the asking WORKS there.

So, Jerry, if it IS in fact the chemo that makes my hair curly, apparently not everyone who works with cancer patients understands that.

I am sticking to my answer.

The curls are natural.

Absolutely.

Maureen Gatens Thompson: Yes, they are and so were mine! ♥
October 6, 2009 at 10:01pm

Drenda Lane Howatt has her first day of class today...North Clackamas Chamber's Leadership Clackamas County 2010. Today's assignment? Challenge course. Quite challenging indeed.
October 7, 2009 at 6:06am

> Sally Lane Park: Good luck!
> October 7, 2009 at 6:30am
>
> Wendy Ackley: Tell me more about your class.
> October 7, 2009 at 9:32pm
>
> Shannon Swope: Did you arise to the challenge or pull the ------ card? hmmmm.....fun?
> October 8, 2009 at 10:57am
>
> Drenda Lane Howatt: My understanding, Mrs. Swope, is that I own that card now forever. Forever.
> October 9, 2009 at 6:36am

You Are Going To Die

Wednesday, October 7, 2009 at 9:35pm

Everyone wants to relate.

They want to help.

To reassure.

To encourage.

So many people have told me about someone they know who has battled breast cancer.

But very often, as the conversation progresses, the message that is relayed is not so great.

In the middle of the story, the message can be loud and clear.

“YOU ARE GOING TO DIE.”

That is the message.

I don’t believe it is the message intended.

But it is the message delivered.

For I have heard just as many cancer stories that did not end well as those that did.

It seems that people want to tell me about all their close

relatives and friends who are DYING of cancer.

Not so helpful.

So far, I've managed to get through these conversations graciously (I think) -- saving my terror and tears for the dark of night.

"That won't be me."

"Not me. I am done with cancer."

"NOT ME. I AM DONE."

"Right, God? I AM done, right? Right? Please tell me that I am done. Oh, GOD! TELL ME, PLEASE, THAT I AM DONE!"

Sometimes, the storyteller is oblivious to my discomfort.

Other times, I see the upset on their face as they realize their story is going in the wrong direction but they have no idea how to salvage it and end on a positive note.

I know that death is the end result of life.

I know that I will not live forever.

But I do not like to hear that cancer may be my end.

Don Howatt: Whoah It's 9:39 and you're still up?
October 7, 2009 at 9:40pm

Drenda Lane Howatt: Amazing, I know. But the words had to get out.
October 7, 2009 at 9:43pm

Gail Stempel Hilderbrand: Only God knows the how, when, where, and of what we will die from. You will probably be a 90 year old woman in her bed when you go home. Proverbs 3:5-6 Trust in the Lord with all your heart, and do not lean on your own understanding. In all ways acknowledge him and he will make your path straight Trust him Drenda. The cancer is gone, and you are filled with the Holy Spirit.
October 7, 2009 at 10:47pm

Andrea Midge McKeehan Robinson: I trust God with all my heart. I know that He is in control. But I really wish He would text, email, or snail mail me sometimes and tell me it will be alright. No matter what, it will be alright because He is in control. Thank you Drenda for being willing to share your deepest fears with us, maybe God wants to tell you, through us, that with the Father in heaven running the show, it will be alright.
October 8, 2009 at 6:23am

Linda Waggoner: Oh, Drenda! I am so sorry that you can't put Cancer out of your head but I know that it just continues to batter you! You ARE CANCER FREE - You are DONE WITH CANCER! I love you!!!
October 8, 2009 at 12:56pm

Drenda Lane Howatt is happy to have a Friday that is free...that means time for laundry, grocery shopping, cleaning, and other fun and rewarding activities.
October 9, 2009 at 6:35am

> Laurie Lane: Dislike...there should be a button for dislike! I don't dislike that you have a Friday free, I dislike how you are spending your free day! I know, the laundry, shopping, and cleaning await me too.
> October 9, 2009 at 7:23am
>
> Drenda Lane Howatt: But it is wonderful when it is all done (and wonderful that I can actually do it)! Then we have a clean house, clean clothes, and food...at least for a few hours...
> October 9, 2009 at 8:20am
>
> Pam Girtman: I like it that you work at a place that has Fridays off - me too!!
> October 9 at 3:59pm
>
> Wendy Ackley: Am I the only person that likes cleaning and doing laundry? Maybe I more messed up than I thought!!!:-)
> October 9, 2009 at 9:05pm

Drenda Lane Howatt wonders why it is that the Komen Foundation wants to know her ethnicity, the number of people in her home (including the number of children under age 18), and her annual income in order to accept her feedback on Walk for the Cure? "Survivor" should be sufficient.
October 10, 2009 at 7:13pm

> Maureen Gatens Thompson: Are you joking? They don't need any of that info…especially your income. TMI!
> October 10, 2009 at 8:06pm

Drenda Lane Howatt: Not joking. I didn't answer those questions I deemed unnecessary...But I bet lots of people just answer anything asked! Those questions were for "classification purposes only". Classification? Isn't that the same as profiling?
October 10, 2009 at 8:14pm

Maureen Gatens Thompson: Yes, it is absolutely profiling. Shame on them!
October 10, 2009 at 8:26pm

Drenda Lane Howatt is beginning to make a list of dates that would be good 2010 vacation weeks. UPS does nothing without much advance planning. 2010 vacation to be chosen on October 22. 2009.
October 12, 2009 at 6:34am

Gail Stempel Hilderbrand: UGH, I understand! It sure makes it hard sometimes to plan around kids' functions.
October 12, 2009 at 9:24am

Gail Stempel Hilderbrand: Jeff tells me UPS has you pick so early because that is the way the Teamsters wanted it. In case someone wanted a vacation in January.
October 12, 2009 at 3:14pm

Drenda Lane Howatt: Gail, Thanks! I know there are great reasons to pick early, and we are entirely blessed by the amount of vacation time Don earns, but it is hard to know what is coming in 2010! If Don was able to get any summer vacation, that would be a MIRACLE!
October 12, 2009 at 4:39pm

Drenda Lane Howatt is home for the evening. Time for a hot bath before venturing to the kitchen for dinner prep. Gotta love

leftovers. And freshly baked bread compliments of Miss Anna.
October 12, 2009 at 4:41pm

LOTTO

Monday, October 12, 2009 at 7:12pm

Would you play the lottery if you knew there was a 15% chance you'd lose?

What if there was an 85% chance you'd win?

Perspective.

That fateful day that Don and I first met Jerry, he explained the odds in my cancer lottery. Past performance is not a guarantee of future results.

I don't remember the exact numbers. Or the exact circumstances that produced those exact numbers.

But it went something like this:

If, in addition to surgery, I had the 'adjuvant' treatment of chemotherapy, my odds of surviving cancer free for ten years increased.

If, in addition to surgery AND chemotherapy, I had the 'adjuvant" treatment of radiation, my odds of surviving the 10 years without recurrence increased even more. Somewhere in the neighborhood of 85% chance that I would be alive and cancer free in ten years.

Now, remember, I am pretty good at math. Even without a calculator.

And it did not take me long to figure out that 85% chance of survival meant 15% of non-survival. That is where I camped for many weeks.

Don said to me: "Drenda. You have to fight this. You have to get better. You have to fight."

Me?

I cried.

All I could think of was the 15%.

I never, never ever questioned Jerry's wisdom about treatment. Of course I would do all the 'adjuvants'. Absolutely. This Mama has babies that still need her.

But I was camped, in fear, on the 15%. Terror so severe that medication was necessary. So many evenings Don would only need to take one look at me and know.

He'd say "Drenda, do you need a pill?"

Or "Drenda, did you take your medication?"

Or "Drenda, I'll get your medicine."

Strong and courageous? Me?

Hardly.

Strong and courageous? Don?

Absolutely. A rock. My husband who promised...he PROMISED...to love and care for me. In sickness and in health. And he does.

It was a long time before I could rejoice in the 85%.

I remember the day. At work. Etched in my memory.

In response to a question from Lynn Peterson, I was recounting the statistics. And I heard myself say "85% of women with the same type of cancer, detected at the same stage, are alive and cancer-free in ten years".

It was the opposite of a 'punched in the stomach by cancer' moment.

It was weight lifted off of my shoulders.

Literally, I think.

Because I remember saying to Lynn: "wow! those are pretty good odds!" And smiling. A revelation to myself.

15% had turned over to 85%.

I'd certainly buy that lottery ticket.

Yep.

And I'm gonna win!

Chelsea Lincoln Lane: I have no words other than your wisdom, earned in the most courageous way imaginable, needs to be heard by more than you know. I'm headed to bed now, to snuggle with my Rock...after I grab a box of Kleenex. Thank you Drenda. Thank you for sharing your struggles and your fears...and thank you for sharing your victory.
October 12, 2009 at 11:06pm

Linda Waggoner: Absolutely!
October 13, 2009 at 9:40am

Is It Well?

Monday, October 12, 2009 at 7:24pm

When peace, like a river, attendeth my way,
oh, Lord, please send me your peace...

When sorrows like sea billows roll;
I am drowning~

Whatever my lot, Thou has taught me to say,
I will say it but I don't feel it...

It is well, it is well, with my soul.
Make it well. Make it well, with my soul.

It is well, with my soul,
It is well, it is well, with my soul.

Though Satan should buffet, though trials should come,
he is buffeting...trials are here

Let this blest assurance control,
please be my assurance...please control~

That Christ has regarded my helpless estate,
You know! You know my helplessness, my terror...and You are in control~

And hath shed His own blood for my soul.
And You, Christ, shed your own blood for me. For me.

My sin, oh, the bliss of this glorious thought!
amazing...awesome...glorious~

My sin, not in part but the whole,

Is nailed to the cross, and I bear it no more,
Let it go, let it go~

Praise the Lord, praise the Lord, O my soul!

Deborah Davis: Praying for you, Drenda, that God will answer your prayer and give you His peace, that has no rational explanation- it's just His gift of peace.
October 12, 2009 at 8:22pm

Sally Lane Park: Drenda, I am sorry you are feeling stressed. Love you
October 13, 2009 at 7:30am

Drenda Lane Howatt: Thank you Deb and Sally! I wrote this note a few weeks ago and didn't post until yesterday. This hymn has been in my mind for quite some time, and when I 'hear' it, my own commentary goes along side. Praising God brings peace to my soul. I am fine~
October 13, 2009 at 7:36am

Sally Lane Park: Whew!
October 13, 2009 at 7:52am

Drenda Lane Howatt loves evenings at home...with no commitments. Okay. One commitment. Dancing with the Stars Result show. But no commitments that require venturing out into the blustery night. Home, warm, and cozy.
October 13, 2009 at 6:27pm

> Jonna Wilkinson: I don't care what is on, just add a glass of wine, I'm gooooood.
> October 13, 2009 at 6:53pm
>
> Drenda Lane Howatt: Yes...and a hot bath, too.
> October 13, 2009 at 7:16pm
>
> Shannon Swope: I SHOULD have called you last night! One of my patients told me I was a 'rotten nurse' because I couldn't find Dancing With The Stars. Try as I might, I COULD NOT talk them into a better mood. Seems only dancing would do it...I failed miserably. :(
> October 14, 2009 at 8:25am

Drenda Lane Howatt was the perfect shopper today. Perfect, that is, if you're Fred Meyer. Went to purchase apples and bread...left with two pair of shoes, avocados, wine, light bulbs, wood bolts, ice, apples, bread, and $65 less in her bank account. Pretty expensive apples.
October 18, 2009 at 7:07pm

> Don Howatt: Wood screws! #6 X 3/4, wood bolts would be called lag bolts!
> October 18, 2009 at 7:25pm
>
> Drenda Lane Howatt: oh...so sorry. Wood screws, people. Not bolts. That must be why the total bill was $65.
> October 18, 2009 at 7:31pm

Don Howatt: aaahhh!, I don't think so-the wood screws cost a total of $1.19, perhaps you should fess up about the shoes!
October 18, 2009 at 7:34pm

Chelsea Lincoln Lane: I love you both, but I need to side with Drenda. $65 for two pair of shoes...including groceries...not bad sister!
October 18, 2009 at 8:30pm

Drenda Lane Howatt: Thank you! The shoes were on sale, of course...
October 18, 2009 at 8:37pm

Caitlin Lopez: Nice!
October 18, 2009 at 8:43pm

Another note from Rachel:

Cancer(?) Update
Monday, October 19, 2009 at 1:29am
I want to give a cancer update, even though it's not longer a cancer update as my updates have been in the past. This summer, my mom was declared cancer free by her doctor! Cancer free after months of chemo and radiation - the cancer has gone bye-bye! I am so proud of my mom, who has come out of this a fighter. She has come out victorious and been an amazing example to me and, I'm sure, to everyone around her.

Next month, it'll be a year from the night I got the worst phone call of my life, a year from the night my mom told me she had cancer. This has been a year of tremendous growth. So many blessings have come out of it. One of the big ones is that it has brought my extended family together. I think we all got a wake up call of how important family really is - how important having a support system is.

The race for the cure was in Portland the day after I left for Seattle, so I didn't get to walk with my family. That was hard, because I felt like it was such an honor to be able to be on Team Strong and Courageous (my mom's team), but I didn't get to experience it with everyone. I was glad the leadership conference kept me busy, because, like I said, not being able to be there with all my family and celebrating my mom's accomplishment was... hard.

Tonight we had a worship night in Moyer. It was wonderful. We sang songs talking about how we are broken people, and that we need God to console and complete us. We sang about how great God was. How we would live to love Him. How we need Him. Whenever we sing songs about brokenness or hard times, I think of cancer. Cancer broke me. Cancer gave me hard times. I hate cancer. But, God consoled me. He gave me strength, He gave my mom strength, He gave my family strength.

Ok, but here's the deal. The cancer is gone, right? Wrong. It has infected my family forever. I am cancerous. But it does not control me, I am the one in control. It is going to be a part of my life until the day I die. I am always going to remember the year of my life when I had to fight cancer. I will probably always have a small amount of fear that what happened to Mrs. Dowd will happen to my mom; I will always have the fear that the cancer will come back. I will always avoid soy milk and tofu. Wait, there's a reason. It's because they accelerate estrogen production, and my mom's cancer was a result of some sort of estrogen imbalance. So I will always avoid those foods. Always. Maybe that's unnecessary, but I will also always have the fear of someday getting cancer in the back of my head.

I love this quote:
A woman is like a tea bag: you never know how strong she is, until you put her in hot water.

Drenda Lane Howatt: Rachel, I love you.
October 19, 2009 at 6:13am

Bethann Westfall: Wow, Rachel!! Thanks for sharing your heart. You too are strong and God has carried you and your family through this time. He will do it again whenever hard times come. "For God has not given us a spirit of fear but of power and a sound mind" Be strong and courageous in the Lord!
Love you Friend!
October 19, 2009 at 6:17am

Jory Lane: Rachel, thanks
October 19, 2009 at 6:37am

Laurie Lane: Rachel,
Cancer is horrible, but the cancer experience has given us gifts. One gift you mentioned was bringing the extended family

together. I agree!
This experience has also given you an awareness of how strong you, your sisters, your dad and your mom are. You are a strong family!
I love you all!
October 19, 2009 at 7:08am

Linda Waggoner: Rachel, you are an amazing young woman! I am so proud of you!
October 19, 2009 at 7:43am

Cindy McElmurry: Rachel... God has something so special in store for you...I will be here praying and watching expectantly! You (as well as your mom) are... Strong and Courageous! I Love You Both!
October 19, 2009 at 1:46pm

Sally Lane Park: Thank you Rachel for sharing your thoughts and perspective.
We need to hear it. It helps us stay connected.
We Love you!
Sally
October 19, 2009 at 5:16pm

Hollace Howatt Chandler: Thanks for writing this, Rachel. You were brave to go through it and you were brave to write about it.
October 19, 2009 at 5:54pm

Beauty Comes at a High Price

Monday, October 19, 2009 at 8:06pm

I could hardly believe it.

Did I hear correctly?

Really?

“Drenda, your hair is beautiful!”

“Thank you. “

“Do you color it?”

“No.”

“Is it naturally curly? Was it like that before?”

“Yes, it is naturally curly, but not this curly. No, it wasn’t quite like this before.”

“Wow! It must make it all worth it.”

“Uhhh....no.”

“Really?”

Was he trying to be funny?

“Uhhh....no. ‘It’ doesn’t make it all worth it.”

Another “I’m sure they don’t listen to their words” moment.

My hair is beautiful.

And I do like it.

But having beautiful hair does not make up for the pain -- neither the physical pain nor the heart pain.

It doesn’t ‘make it all worth it’.

This hair came at a high price.

Figuratively and literally.

Each chemotherapy treatment cost thousands of dollars. Thousands. Each one. And there were 16 all together.

This hair cost thousands of tears. Thousands.

This hair cost thousands of questions. Thousands.

This hair cost premature aging on the part of three young women who should not have to consider their mother’s mortality at their tender ages. That is expensive.

This hair cost by becoming a defining life “moment” for my babies. It cost much by being etched in the fabric of their lives.

This hair cost tremendous strain on my husband.
My father. My sisters. My brothers. My entire family. My friends.

This hair cost. And the price is high.

And it is not worth it. Not for the hair.

I thought my hair was kind of nice before.

Nancy Newton: Drenda, you were beautiful before cancer and you're more beautiful now...not because of your great hair but because of the amazing strength, courage and grace you have shown throughout the process. I hope that was just a "dumb vs. mean" moment for the person who made the comment.
October 19, 2009 at 8:32pm

Drenda Lane Howatt: I am sure it was not "mean". Just words without thought. I know I often do the same thing...
October 19, 2009 at 8:45pm

Nancy Newton: I HIGHLY doubt you would say something that boneheaded.
October 19, 2009 at 8:55pm

Hollace Howatt Chandler: People just don't know what to say, and don't know how to be quiet when they should be. I'm glad you could say "no, not really" to him. Sometimes people just need to be taught.
October 19, 2009 at 9:32pm

Andi Pedersen Jordan: ditto to Nancy!!
October 19, 2009 at 9:56pm

Maureen Gatens Thompson: I remember when I lost my straight-as-a-board hair and it grew in curly. I had similar comments made to me. "Wow, you must love your curly hair." "Wow, you have eyebrows now." "Wow, your eyelashes grew back in." "You are so lucky you don't have to shave your legs." Nope, I wasn't thinking about the hair on my head or anywhere else on my body. I was thinking about my husband of less than one year and how he really didn't sign-up for the "sickness and in health" vow, 6 weeks after we were married. I was thinking that although we hadn't talked about having kids yet, all the

Specialists said the strength of the chemo would put me straight in to menopause. I was thinking that he didn't sign up for a bald, infertile wife 8 months after we were married. But that's what he was facing. I was thinking our honeymoon had turned into a cancer journey as quickly as it took for us to get the proofs back from our wedding day. Oh, how happy and carefree we looked and me with lots of hair. I was thinking are we strong enough to turn this bad, horrific start of a marriage into a fairy tale? Turns out we were.
October 19, 2009 at 10:09pm

Drenda Lane Howatt: You inspire me, Maureen.
October 19, 2009 at 10:12pm

Drenda Lane Howatt is still in love with normal. Normal days. Normal energy. Normal life.
October 21, 2009 at 6:37am

> Elizabeth Lundquist Calhoun: Normal is the best
> October 21, 2009 at 8:39am
>
> Luann Sader Hoover: Most of us take normal for granted, but normal is awesome!
> October 21, 2009 at 11:54am
>
> Jennifer Stady: I even like boring sometimes.
> October 21, 2009 at 7:21pm

Drenda Lane Howatt gets to see Jerry today. The time just flies by...another month come and gone cancer free. Not that she is counting...but she is. Two months and three days cancer free! Life keeps getting better and better. Some day, in the future, she will forget about keeping track. That day will truly be cancer FREE.
October 23, 2009 at 8:50am

> Evonne Christensen-Mathews: Yay that is wonderful news!
> October 23, 2009 at 11:59am
>
> Evy Marks Tyler: Yes, as I am now passed seven years, I rarely think about it...just enjoy the fact that I am alive and enjoying all the good things that the Lord continues to give.
> October 23, 2009 at 12:24pm

Transitions

Friday, October 23, 2009 at 9:10am

I remember the days.

"How old is your baby?"

"Four days."

"Two weeks."

"Eight weeks."

"11 weeks."

"Three months."

"18 months."

"Two years."

The progression.

I always, in some ways, mourned the transition from days to weeks. Weeks to months. Months to years.

Mourned because time was moving so fast.

I remember each phase of those transitions.

They were not bad.

Just signals that my babies were growing up.

I am back to the transitions again.

"How long have you been a survivor?"

"Three days."

"Two weeks and four days."

"One month." That transition was particularly amazing.

Because the one month anniversary of being declared cancer free was September 20th.

Team Strong and Courageous.

Walk for the Cure day.

I am now at "two months and three days" cancer free.

These transitions bring no mourning.

I am looking forward to making the transition to answering the questions with " one year", "two years". Looking forward to moving from the answers being months to years.

These transitions bring amazement.

Amazement about how much can happen in a few short months.

One year ago, exactly, I participated in Breast Cancer Awareness activities at work.

I had no idea that three weeks later, I would find a lump in my breast and begin the odyssey of breast cancer treatment.

Those months brought transition from regular, normal, stable to indescribable upset.

These months bring transition from that upset back to normal, stable, and regular.

Survivor.

Cancer Free.

Two months.

Three days.

Deanna Davis: Congrats, Drenda! :]
October 23, 2009 at 9:14am

Shannon Swope: Wow-good expression and way with words. It IS amazing itsn't it? I continue the journey with you my friend!
October 23, 2009 at 9:33am

Sherri Detweiler Purcell: We're thankful for your "transitions" and will continue to pray for you as you continue your journey as a survivor!
October 23, 2009 at 10:58am

Maureen Gatens Thompson: Survivor...Cancer free...transition...the progression...24 years...Your Words. ♥
October 23, 2009 at 12:15pm

Sally Lane Park: The Sun does "always rise"!
October 23, 2009 at 7:49pm

Drenda Lane Howatt had great fun hosting a formal dinner party, pre-homecoming dance. Thanks, Patrick and Thomas!
October 24, 2009 at 8:33pm

Drenda Lane Howatt has enjoyed the gorgeous fall morning -- fog, crisp air, hot coffee, newspaper. Doesn't get much better than that~
October 25, 2009 at 9:24am

Drenda Lane Howatt just had a wonderful dinner...homemade zuppa toscana, fresh bread sticks, salad. Thank you, Miss Ellie! And thank you, home management class project~
October 25, 2009 at 5:20pm

> Erin Frazier Miller: What is zuppa Tuscana? Sounds fabulous!
> October 25, 2009 at 5:25pm
>
> Sally Lane Park: Yummmm!
> October 25, 2009 at 6:04pm
>
> Drenda Lane Howatt: Erin,
> zuppa toscana is one of the signature soups from the Olive Garden. We found the recipe... It IS yummy! And Ellie is a fabulous cook...she made the homemade bread, too.
> October 25, 2009 at 6:07pm
>
> Erin Frazier Miller: Oh, I remember! Love that soup! Can you share the recipe?
> October 25, 2009 at 6:29pm
>
> Drenda Lane Howatt: Sure -- I'll send it to you
> October 25, 2009 at 6:31pm

Gail Stempel Hilderbrand: What?! Ellie made dinner...that is awesome!
October 25, 2009 at 6:34pm

Deborah Davis: Yea for Ellie! I'm proud of her too. :-)
October 25, 2009 at 6:40pm

Hollace Howatt Chandler: Wow! Sounds great, Ellie. I hope our Home Ec student does as well.
October 25, 2009 at 7:28pm

Ellie Howatt: Yep you're welcome. I don't think I will make dinner for a very long time though, it takes up a lot of time.
October 25, 2009 at 9:24pm

Hollace Howatt Chandler: Ha ha. My sentiments exactly.
October 25, 2009 at 9:46pm

Drenda Lane Howatt wonders how she survived before Clackamas County went to a four day work week. Ahhh. Friday.
October 30, 2009 at 6:24am

Sandy Hagstrand: I'm with Drenda ... TGIF!!!
October 30, 2009 at 9:38pm

Drenda Lane Howatt can't think of anything much more exciting than shopping for a new refrigerator...oh, the joys of being old and responsible.
October 31, 2009 at 9:03am

Jennifer Stady: Yeah and Standard Appliace and the like are such great places to spend a Saturday...
October 31, 2009 at 9:07am

Maureen Gatens Thompson: ...and a $1,500 tax credit to

boot!
October 31, 2009 at 2:12pm

Drenda Lane Howatt thought of something more exciting than shopping for a new refrigerator...watching the old, dying, nasty refrigerator being removed and the new, shiny, beautiful refrigerator being put in place.
November 1, 2009 at 3:31pm

Becky Annus: Woo hoo! Enjoy the simple pleasures in life...
November 1, 2009 at 6:16pm

Drenda Lane Howatta: Yes. Simple. But expensive.
November 1, 2009 at 8:57pm

Maureen Gatens Thompson: What kind did you buy?
November 1, 2009 at 9:12pm

Drenda Lane Howatt: Kenmore Elite side by side titanium
November 1, 2009 at 9:14pm

Maureen Gatens Thompson: We are looking for a stove and refrigerator. I'll be interested in how you like it.
November 1, 2009 at 9:17pm

Gail Stempel Hilderbrand: Oh you lucky girl!
November 1, 2009 at 9:31pm

Drenda Lane Howatt is having a crazy day: work, errands, errands, errands, home, more errands. In between, she will fit in date night with Don.
November 5, 2009 at 6:04pm

Janette Wilkinson: Whatcha doing for date night? You

know what...never mind...I don't really want to know...
November 5, 2009 at 6:13pm

Drenda Lane Howatt: ♥
I will tell you anyway...
Happy hour at nb
November 5, 2009 at 6:17pm

Hollace Howatt Chandler: I didn't know new beginnings had happy hour. Wow.
November 6, 2009 at 8:20am

Wendy Ackley: What is nb?
November 8, 2009 at 1:22pm

Drenda Lane Howatt: Newport Bay
November 8, 2009 at 6:51pm

Drenda Lane Howatt is heading to Seattle for the weekend -- Mom's Day at SPU tomorrow! But she wonders how in the world her second daughter can be a sophomore in college...
November 6, 2009 at 6:16am

Don Howat, 2009: Don't worry people, I will manage...
November 6 at 7:13am

Hollace Howatt Chandler: Do you know how to make a tuna fish sandwich?
November 6, 2009 at 8:22am

Pam Girtman: There seems to be a big explosion in that tuna sandwich task lately . . .
November 6, 2009 at 10:06am

Drenda Lane Howatt: Don Howatt is a great cook! And anyone (ahem, Tim) who has trouble figuring out a tuna

sandwich has some serious catching up to do.
November 6 at 8:19pm

Drenda Lane Howatt is having a wonderful day with Miss Rachel in Seattle...despite the blustery weather. Brunch, then shopping at Freddies -- important to stock up that dorm room! Women's volleyball game at 4, then dinner. This weekend is going too fast!
November 7, 2009 at 2:52pm

Maureen Gatens Thompson: What a wonderful weekend--sounds like one for the memory books. Have fun and safe travels home.
November 7, 2009 at 3:03pm

Drenda Lane Howatt is home again. ahh. That is nice.
November 8, 2009 at 6:53pm

Drenda Lane Howatt "Where there are many words, transgression is unavoidable, but he who restrains his lips is wise." Translation: the more talk, the less truth; the wise measure their words.
November 10, 2009 at 6:00am

Andrea Midge McKeehan Robinson OH MY GOODNESS!! I need to memorize this one!
November 10, 2009 at 7:13am

Shannon Swope yes :)
November 10, 2009 at 8:49am

One Year

November 12 at 8:25am

A lifetime
Just yesterday

Almost over
Only begun

A burning, throbbing fire
Doused with tears

Strong belief
Weak faith
Or weak belief and strong faith?

Questions
So many

Answers
So few

Totally alone
Overwhelmed by the crowd

Blazing a trail
Ensnared in the stinging nettles

Terror
Strength

Darkness

Hope

Tears
Courage

Love
Care
Provision

Family

Friends

Savior

Faith?
Weak

Clinical Trial?
Or Character Trial?

Yes. Both

Strength in Weakness

Love
Care
Provision

Savior

Linda Waggoner: I was thinking about you all day yesterday but I didn't know why (except that I love you!). Now I know! Stay strong - you made it!!!
November 12, 2009 at 9:20am

Becky Annus: A year full of tears, love and courage. And faith.
STRONG AND COURAGEOUS
We love you!
November 12, 2009 at 9:46am

Abbi Howatt: ♥
November 12, 2009 at 10:01am

Laurie Lane: Love you!
November 12, 2009 at 12:05pm

Forever Stuck

November 12 at 6:31pm

The phrases below are burned on my brain. These are some of the things that were said to me or overheard over the last year. They are burned on my brain. **Burned.**

"Is *anyone* here with you?"

"You came by yourself?"

"We're *very* concerned."

"I want to do a core biospy right now."

"And, Drenda, bring your husband with you."

"I am sorry."

"It **is** cancer."

"We'll get through this."

"I love you."

"I guess this is the "in sickness" part."

"I love you. I LOVE you."

"You'll have surgery to remove the tumor."

"Let not your heart be troubled."

“Dr. Segal is a doctor’s doctor.”

“This will be a part-time job.”

“Cancer takes a lot of time.”

“You are strong and courageous.”

“Dr. Lehti can’t see you until Wednesday.”

“Dr. Lehti will meet you at his office in between surgeries if you can come now.”

“Surgery will be Tuesday morning.”

“Do not be terrified. Do not be discouraged.”

“Come to the hospital early.”

“Wires will be inserted into your breast to guide the surgeon.”

“Even I could tell it’s cancer.”

“The surgeon and two pathologists are confident that all of the cancer was removed.”

“The Lord your God is with you wherever you go.”

“The pathology report is in -- all of the cancer was removed. Clean margins. Sentinel lymph node clear.”

“Stage 1. Grade 3.”

“Agressive.”

“Hormone fed.”

“Often moves to the brain.”

"I am going to take a picture now."

"Curative. Not pallative."

"Good thing you're wearing earrings."

"You have good bones."

"You are amazing."

"Brain MRI is imperative."

"These doctors don't know a damn thing."

"They'll think we're in collusion."

"Can I bring you dinner?"

"You're not going to die from this."

"Have you decided on the clinical trial?"

"If it were my wife, I'd want her to participate."

"The brain MRI is clear."

"Cancer free."

Becky Annus: Strong and courageous.
I love you.
November 13, 2009 at 8:37am

Sally Lane Park: Strong words, I like the last ones!
November 13, 2009 at 8:35pm

Drenda Lane Howatt was punched in the stomach by cancer yesterday. Oh yes. No longer eligible for increased insurance. How could she forget?
November 13, 2009 at 11:38am

Tammy Busby: Wait, what does that mean?
November 13, 2009 at 11:44am

Drenda Lane Howatt: I am now "marked" -- not, presumably, for life (assuming I live into my golden years), but for a very long time. Can't purchase additional insurances -- disability, life, accident, etc...I am a poor 'risk'. But, hey!, I have good credit.
November 13, 2009 at 11:49am

Andi Pedersen Jordan: Who needs health care reform...HA! Sarcasm.
November 13, 2009 at 11:51am

Drenda Lane Howatt: I don't think reform would change anything on this...just cost more!
November 13, 2009 at 11:55am

Faith Jossi Lichtenberg: Feel your pain on that one ;o(after 10 years they will start talking to you again, unless that changes in the next 10 years! Agghhh!
November 13, 2009 at 1:26pm

Gail Stempel Hilderbrand: Look on the bright side, at least they will rethink it after some years pass. Nobody wants me lol. Oh well, we have the best insurance of all, eternal life in Jesus!
November 13, 2009 at 2:18pm

Drenda Lane Howatt is stymied by appliances. New refrigerator...second repair visit scheduled for Monday. Old dryer. Repair visit. Fixed! Old washer...waiting for parts to

arrive after yesterday's repair visit...parts not available until Wednesday, November 25th. That is a loooong time away. People, appreciate your appliances. Life is difficult without them. As in "very".
November 14, 2009 at 3:38pm

Kimberly Tibbetts Roberts: Isn't it a headache but what would we do without them?
November 14, 2009 at 8:43pm

Caitlin Lopez: I can teach you how to hand wash your clothes african style:) Let me know if you'd like a lesson.
November 15, 2009 at 12:57pm

Drenda Lane Howatt: Thanks, Caitlin. I assume there are rocks involved...I will pass on the lesson. I would rather schlep my clothes next door to the apartment laundry room. And besides, you're supposed to be resting!
November 15, 2009 at 4:55pm

Drenda Lane Howatt is taking the day off of work to work at home. Mission Organization continues.
November 18, 2009 at 7:18am

Cindy McElmurry: When you're done you can come and do mine!
November 18, 2009 at 5:30pm

Drenda Lane Howatt: Sorry...my house is a many-month endeavor. We have too much junk!
November 18, 2009 at 5:31pm

Caitlin Lopez: That sounds FUN! All I want to do is organize stuff. gotta love that nesting instinct!
November 18, 2009 at 5:35pm

Drenda Lane Howatt: Yes...it is fun when it is "nesting"

for a new baby...but not so much fun otherwise! It does feel good to have some things in order, though. Take it easy on the nesting; don't do too much at one time...
November 18, 2009 at 5:37pm

Drenda Lane Howatt had a successful day...coat closet cleaned out (including the dead mouse), buffet cleaned out and organized, two other cabinets cleaned and organized. Huge pile ready to be delivered to Goodwill. Salmon baking in the oven...now it is time for that glass of wine. Oh yes.
November 18, 2009 at 4:40pm

Cindy McElmurry: Where's mine?
November 18, 2009 at 5:32pm

Jennifer Stady: Wow, you GO super-woman!
November 18, 2009 at 8:04pm

Sandy Hagstrand: Do you rent yourself out????
November 18, 2009 at 9:29pm

Drenda Lane Howatt is off to Parent/Teacher conferences and then the weekly dinner date. Such a great evening!
November 19, 2009 at 5:59pm

Wendy Ackley: NB?
November 19, 2009 at 7:24pm

Drenda Lane Howatt: No nb tonight. Ended up coming home and having left-overs...round robin conferences take a LONG time.
November 19, 2009 at 8:18pm

Hollace Howatt Chandler: Now, that's a cheap date.
November 20, 2009 at 9:09am

Drenda Lane Howatt: Yes, indeed. No cash required. Nor credit card.
November 20, 2009 at 9:10am

Pam Girtman: How sustainable of you.
November 20, 2009 at 10:23am

Drenda Lane Howatt is headed to the heart room again...time for yet another echo-cardiogram. Note from Drenda to congestive heart failure --"stay away".
November 20, 2009 at 11:53am

Erin Frazier Miller: Good luck!!
November 20, 2009 at 2:28pm

Andrea Midge McKeehan Robinson: WHAT THE????? What is all this?
November 20, 2009 at 8:19pm

Lori Bradshaw Buckelew: OK...so apparently I'm in the dark....OK, so I'm usually in the dark, but in this instance I don't want to be...what's up?
November 20, 2009 at 10:44pm

Drenda Lane Howatt: It is continued testing for the clinical trial...the hope is that the trial drug keeps the cancer out of my brain...the fear is that the clinical trial drug causes congestive heart failure. So regular echos are the norm. So far, everything with my heart has been A-OK.
November 21, 2009 at 8:34am

Drenda Lane Howatt -- Christmas shopping tomorrow. If I don't have your list, you're either not getting anything, or you'll get something I want!
November 22, 2009 at 12:37pm

Laurie Lane: I am so excited! I'll get my list you by early tomorrow!
November 22, 2009 at 1:14pm

Janette Wilkinson: Here goes...good knife set (so my sister, who shall remain nameless, will stop making fun of my knife set), laptop (not big and cumbersome like Jim's but small and cute), salad tongs, $$$$$ for school (five $'s = five figures), health care for EVERYONE so I can stop telling my nineteen year old students, "I am sorry, there is nothing I can do for you regarding health insurance". a pair of cute black flats that I can wear with skirts, pair of gold hoop earrings, airfare to Romania, someone that will complete all my school assignments on time and in "A" quality, tandem bike so that my sweetie and I may ride together on the STP, a really good and easy to use garlic press, world peace, really cute matching bike outfits that also match the tandem so that we will look so cool/cute on that STP trip, very big framed picture of Silver Falls barn (talk to Isaac)....
That is all for now...I hope this is enough to get you started.
November 22, 2009 at 2:54pm

Laurie Lane: Well, forget my list...I know Janette is your favorite and I can't compete with her. By the time you buy her the presents she requested there will be nothing left for me. I will ask for one present, however, and that is health for all!
November 22, 2009 at 3:07pm

Drenda Lane Howatt: It seems that Janette, despite her wish for world peace and health care for all, is really quite obsessed with looking cute. hmm.
Laurie, feel free to still send your list.
November 22, 2009 at 3:29pm

Amber Lynn Montgomery Lane: I'm going to optimistic about your gift giving abilities and just carbon copy Janette's list and sign my name to it. Thanks in advance! November 22, 2009 at 3:29pm

Janette Wilkinson: Well! I just want to look my best when world peace and health care for everyone becomes reality. I can tell my students, "yes you can go see a doctor, because you see you are now going to be treated equally and you now have health insurance." There is nothing wrong with cuteness! Laurie is just trying to make me look bad and so that is why I need all those "cute" things...
Thanks Drenda! This promises to be the best Christmas ever!
November 22, 2009 at 4:49pm

Drenda Lane Howatt: No one is treated equally on anything, even Christmas...
November 22, 2009 at 4:59pm

Janette Wilkinson: Yes but if there is by chance some semblance of equality, I want to look cute when it happens!
November 22, 2009 at 6:35pm

Gail Stempel Hilderbrand: My list is on the way! LOL
November 22, 2009 at 6:57pm

Becky Annus: No on the tandem bike and cute matching outfit...but yes to the big picture of the barn - awesome. AND I'd love a few jars of the Mexican Style Olives from the Olive Pit....
November 22, 2009 at 7:59pm

Linda Waggoner: Christmas party at the Barn -- the 19th???

November 22, 2009 at 9:26pm

Drenda Lane Howatt: What time?
November 22, 2009 at 9:28pm

Sally Lane Park: We will be in California visiting Lonnie's Sis and Disneyland!
November 23, 2009 at 7:53am

Sally Lane Park: And by the way, go ahead and put me on your list of "you'll get something I want", because I know I will like it too!
November 23, 2009 at 7:55am

Janette Wilkinson: Let's join the Parks at Disneyland instead of the barn....Drenda, that is what I want for Christmas...
November 23, 2009 at 8:03am

Linda Waggoner: Me too!!!
November 23, 2009 at 9:15am

Drenda Lane Howatt has a message for Portlanders: "Go ahead and shop at Costco tomorrow and Wednesday...no worries. It shan't be crowded. No. Because everyone from the region, except you, was there today".
November 23, 2009 at 3:50pm

Shannon V Means: lol!
November 23, 2009 at 3:53pm

Maureen Gatens Thompson: That's how I felt when I went to Freddie's. Geez and I thought by taking the day off I would outsmart Turkey Day shoppers.
November 23, 2009 at 4:20pm

Drenda Lane Howatt: I think the entire city had the same

idea...
November 23, 2009 at 4:29pm

Evy Marks Tyler: Actually, going to Costco or any other store as soon as they open saves you from the crowds. We made it to four stores and home again in less than two hours.
November 23, 2009 at 4:42pm

Drenda Lane Howatt: Wow, Evy...what car was Stretch driving? Any flashing lights?
November 23, 2009 at 6:02pm

Jennifer Stady: Thats funny! I highly recommend shopping on-line!
November 23, 2009 at 6:12pm

Sally Lane Park: Indeed! It was way busier that it should have been on a Monday morning, of all days!
November 23, 2009 at 8:06pm

Emily Klepper: Thanks for the tip. I have to head out tomorrow to finish up my shopping. I am NOT looking forward to it!!
November 23, 2009 at 9:09pm

Drenda Lane Howatt is not sure if has the energy to do more shopping...but the end result of being finished with Christmas shopping is very very enticing. Almost there!
November 24, 2009 at 6:27am

Janette Wilkinson: Thanks for adding a little more stress to my life!
November 24, 2009 at 7:16am

Shannon Swope: Nice...finish up and then ENJOY!!!

Worth a little more...chug a chug...
November 24, 2009 at 8:24am

Drenda Lane Howatt is happy to have hair on her head...even if she does look (and feel) like a chia pet.
November 24, 2009 at 6:55pm

Janette Wilkinson: WHAT???? Chia pet???? What is this about????
November 24, 2009 at 7:05pm

Dan D Davis: I never, ever said that out loud! Are you now also a mind reader?
November 24, 2009 at 7:35pm

Barbara Tyler Kochendorfer: Yay for hair!! That is so exciting!
November 24, 2009 at 8:26pm

Lori Bradshaw Buckelew: I loved the feel of my hair when it grew back...all baby feeling!
November 24, 2009 at 9:12pm

Sally Lane Park: Nope! Not. I would give a bundle for that curly hair!
November 25, 2009 at 8:07am

Drenda Lane Howatt is thankful. Thankful for everything. Everything. The good, the bad, and the bald. And, it is important to know, for these things she is thankful TO the Almighty God who was, who is, and who is to come. Take a moment today to consider what you are thankful for, and to whom. Happy Thanksgiving Day!
November 26, 2009 at 6:29am

Jonna Wilkinson: Amen, Drenda, amen.

November 26, 2009 at 10:40am

Maureen Gatens Thompson: Thankful for you...
November 26, 2009 at 11:33am

Drenda Lane Howatt has the Christmas tree up and ready for the decorations. Yeah!
November 27, 2009 at 11:09am

Hollace Howatt Chandler: Wow! I almost have my Thanksgiving dishes done =)
November 27, 2009 at 11:50am

Diane Carrette Tuttle: I have left over pie...but no tree up yet...good job Drenda...
November 27, 2009 at 1:29pm

Kris Howatt: I have the Christmas wreath in place - and lights around the gazebo.
November 27, 2009 at 9:53pm

Sally Lane Park: Me too! Or should I say Lonnie too? I will put the ornaments on tomorrow...or maybe Sunday.
November 27, 2009 at 10:04pm

Linda Lane Waggoner: Ron and Ted got most of the lights up on the outside of the house yesterday - and I am trying to get the Christmas decorations set out around the house - but no tree. I think we will go out to cut ours on the 12th or 13th - depending on when our kids and their families can make their schedule work.
November 28, 2009 at 11:15am

Drenda Lane Howatt is doing her best to ignore the fact that Monday is so close.
November 28, 2009 at 9:22pm

Drenda Lane Howatt ...vacation is over. Back to the real world in the morning. Drat.
November 29, 2009 at 8:26pm

> Elissa Gertler: What, you're not excited and delighted, like I am?
> November 29, 2009 at 9:13pm
>
> Drenda Lane Howatt: Does that mean, Elissa, that you are excited and delighted that I am back to the real world tomorrow, or have you been on vacation as well?
> November 30, 2009 at 6:02am

Drenda Lane Howatt is off to the train station to drop off a special package. Um...she means a special person. Yes, that's it. Good bye to Miss Rachel. Your Momma is going to miss you tons!
November 30, 2009 at 4:59pm

Drenda Lane Howatt ...December 1st and the Man in Brown is working very late...it must be close to Christmas!
December 1, 2009 at 7:41pm

> Bethann Westfall: My heart goes out to you, Ben worked late on Monday, early Tuesday and today.....it may be a long week, he might even work Saturday. :{ I'm not complaining, overtime is a mixed blessing.
> December 2, 2009 at 6:27am
>
> Drenda Lane Howatt: It will be a long month! But, we are so very thankful to have good jobs, and UPS is a great place to work.
> December 2, 2009 at 6:33am

Drenda Lane Howatt wonders where the last month has gone. It is Jerry Day today...always scary and emotional. Good and bad. She is hopeful the bad will be over quickly with "you're doing great! See you next month."
December 4, 2009 at 7:35am

Drenda Lane Howatt heard from her friend Jerry "You're doing great. Come back in five weeks." Good news. Last month's echo-cardiogram and today's EKG show normal heart function. Guess it still works. Yet another consent form to sign for the clinical trial. Paperwork associated with breast cancer is quite overwhelming.
December 4, 2009 at 7:18pm

Scarring is a Good Thing

Friday, December 4, 2009 at 7:44pm

Jerry is not concerned.

Another lump.

In my breast.

Oh my goodness.

Jerry is not concerned.

At all.

That helps a little bit.

He is not concerned because he thinks it is scar tissue from the surgical site. So "not concerned" that he says it will be checked out at the next mammogram, which will be scheduled for early February.

But can there be scar tissue a bit away from the direct incision line?

Take it out.

That's what I want.

But if Jerry is not concerned, I will try not to be concerned. I'll make conscious effort to leave that bag of fear alone.

I will trust that the trial drug, in conjunction with all of my other treatments over the last 12 months, is killing any microscopic cancer cells that may have been in my body.

I am down to less than 15 weeks left of the clinical trial. Good news there.

That means less than 15 weeks left of uncontrolled itching all over my body. Itching at all times. Itching so severe that it sometimes wakes me up in the middle of the night. How weird is that?

Less than 15 weeks left of acne-like skin rash.

Less than 15 weeks left of severe intestinal duress.

My visit with Jerry today was just a year from my first meeting him. December 3, 2008. A day that sent me reeling. A day where I heard words like "grade 3 cancer", "most aggressive", "this cancer can travel to the brain".

The visit today, December 4, 2009. A day where I heard words like "you're doing well", "I don't need to see you so often", "you're tolerating the treatment so well", "I am not concerned".

I like the words I heard today so much better than those from last year.

So, while all those words I heard are true, the ones today are the most true.

I am certain.

Please.

Laurie Lane: Yes, Please!

December 4, 2009 at 8:06pm

Sally Lane Park: Roller coaster But good news today =) Jerry knows and has not led you wrong yet!
December 5, 2009 at 6:39am

Cindy McElmurry: I will stand with you! I will be certain with you. I will trust!
In God and in the Doctor. I am here.
December 5, 2009 at 8:14am

Linda Lane Waggoner: Scar tissue - I would never have thought that could be a good thing! But it is!!
December 5, 2009 at 9:59am

Shannon Swope: I'm sorry for your fear my friend. A tough way to be kept where we are meant to always be-on our knees in humble trust and faith. A weird thing scar tissue is mmmhmmm...yet another miracle of our bodies! :) See you tomorrow-Keep looking UP!
December 5, 2009at 7:21pm

Drenda Lane Howatt is preparing to have another new refrigerator delivered this morning. Replacement for the new refrigerator delivered one month ago that does not work. This new new refrigerator gets one chance, and if it messes up, it is done and a certain store shall have lost a customer.
December 5, 2009 at 7:19am

> Cindy McElmurry: Did you go with a new model? I hope the streets aren't too icy?
> December 5, 2009 at 8:10am
>
> Shannon Swope: May your milk stay chilled, fresh veggies NOT frozen and freezer NOT too cold...yep, not tooooo cold!
> December 5, 2009 at 7:25pm

Drenda Lane Howatt reminds everyone to be especially nice to the men in brown today -- it's cold out there!
December 7, 2009 at 6:16am

> Faith Jossi Lichtenberg: And the women in brown...love our Valerie here in Gresham!!!!
> December 7, 2009 at 9:31am
>
> Janette Wilkinson: Did Don wear shorts today?
> December 7, 2009 at 10:57am
>
> Drenda Lane Howatt: How politically incorrect of me! Of course, the women in brown too...
> And, no, Don did not wear shorts. Amazing, I know.
> December 7, 2009 at 6:18pm

Drenda Lane Howatt made potato soup with ham and cheese for dinner. Had to have something warming to eat for the UPS man.

December 7, 2009 at 6:19pm

Jennifer Stady: I bet he is one happy guy!
December 7, 2009 at 6:24pm

Cindy McElmurry: I made cream of Broccoli. It must be cold outside.
December 7, 2009 at 6:36pm

Drenda Lane Howatt spent the day learning how to be a leader (?), and is now sitting back and letting Papa Murphy be in charge. An important attribute needed in a leader is the art of delegation. Papa, take it away!
December 9, 2009 at 6:03pm

Knocking Cliches

Wednesday, December 9, 2009 at 7:32pm

So those words? They're knocking.

At my head.

They want to come out.

I am going to let them out now:

There is a cliche' about trash.

"One man's trash is another's treasure."

I have changed that cliche' in my mind.

For me, it is "one person's *routine* can be another's *terror*".

And, I silently bless a few people every time I think of this new cliche'.

I bless them because they saw beyond their routine and stepped out.

I bless the ultrasound technician who left her machine and came around to hold my arm and touch me while the radiologist explained that he was concerned and wanted to do a core biopsy right then. I bless her when I remember her squeeze of my shoulder as the doctor asked "are you here alone?" and the tears rolled down my face.

I bless the pre-op nurse who, seeing my terror while I awaited surgery to insert the port, asked me if I'd like a sedative. She saw the wild look of terror in my eyes. Just my eyes. No words from me. Well, ok, there were a few of those silent-type tears slowly making their way down my pasty white cheeks. But no words.

I bless that same nurse who, when she brought me the sedative, put her hand on my arm and squeezed. And told me I'd be o.k. I bless her.

I bless our friend Gilbert who came to the hospital before my first surgery. I later learned that he came to pray with us, but did not get the chance before they wheeled me away. I bless him for his understanding that both Don and I needed support.

I bless Janis, Don's sister (and a physician), who left her warm home that cold November evening to come to be with me and Don...and brought sedatives with her. I bless her for her calm forthrightness and loving kindness.

I bless Beverly, one of the nurses in the chemo room, er..., the *infusion suite*, who, on my first visit for treatment, told me "your care is curative, not pallative". She will never really understand the impact those words had on me. They were a ray....a bar to hold on to.

I bless Dr. Lehti, my surgeon, who said "we took the cancer out. It is gone." I bless him when I remember his words telling me not to feel guilty for skipping my mammograms the previous four years. "Stop. It wouldn't have made a difference in your case. The cancer was found early, and it is out. It wouldn't have made a difference." Bless him.

And Jerry. I bless him. I bless him for his matter-of-fact way of explaining things. I bless him for the way he makes me feel safe. I bless him for being my oncologist.

My point in all of this? I am not sure, really.

Except, we all have routines.

And our routines may not be comfortable for those around us.

Our routine of driving. We take it for granted. But for the poor young man who just received his permit and now has to learn to drive in our crazy world, that routine of ours may be his terror.

Our routine of whipping up a wonderful dessert. That routine may be something that causes panic in someone asked to bring a dessert to a party.

Our routine of public speaking. Sweaty palms, anyone?

Our routine of expecting fast, accurate service at checkstands. For the new clerk, customer service can be pretty overwhelming...especially service to demanding, impatient customers.

Our routines may not be routine to others.

Let's make a point to notice those around us. And maybe take a minute out of our "routine" to be a person.

Who knows?

We may end up being blessed.

Shannon Swope: Bless you, my friend. Thank you for the very encouraging words. As I caressed a frail 91 year old woman's forehead this a.m., I was praying to be a 'balm' to her worries and tears. We ALL have an impact on others-no matter what. SHE, was a blessing to me and perhaps I, because of God's love,

was a small help to her. Keep dishing it out my friend! :)
December 11, 2009 at 2:33pm

Drenda Lane Howatt is preparing for Multnomah University Exodus' Christmas party. At her home. Tonight. Better get off FB and get that house cleaned up.
December 10, 2009 at 3:52pm

Drenda Lane Howatt wishes her hot flashes came on demand. The home furnace is struggling to survive; the house has now reached the balmy temperature of 60 degrees.
December 11, 2009 at 8:42am

> Linda Lane Waggoner: Oh no! We have room if your furnace dies!!!
> December 11, 2009 at 12:10pm
>
> Drenda Lane Howatt: Thanks, Linda! We had a service man look at it and he fixed whatever the problem was.
> December 11, 2009 at 1:00pm
>
> Shannon Swope: Yikes! We beat you though-it was a whopping 47 degrees when the kids and I got home after school yesterday. It seems although there WERE pellets in the stove, it DID not turn on all day. So, I solved the problem by leaving my family in the cold all night (maybe it got up to 60?) and went to the cozy hospital! :)
> December 11, 2009 at 2:28pm
>
> Ginger Clausen: We're not the only ones with a drafty old house! I made chex mix yesterday because it has to bake for a full hour, but even that didn't heat up my kitchen. Today I put soup in the crockpot. What do I have to do- bake a turkey?
> December 11, 2009 at 3:25pm

Drenda Lane Howatt sees that it was not necessary to rush home from the birthday party last night in anticipation of icy

roads...
December 12, 2009 at 8:01am

Janette Wilkinson: Hmmmmm!
December 12, 2009 at 7:51pm

Wendy Ackley: Syd and I escaped Eugene ice just in time.
December 12, 2009 at 8:32pm

Glenda Turnbull: Hard to predict these things.
December 13, 2009 at 10:09am

Drenda Lane Howatt will do her best to stay up and awake until the Man in Brown gets home from work...may not be possible given her early bed time and his late work time.
December 16, 2009 at 5:42pm

Drenda Lane Howatt is not sure where to start...
December 18, 2009 at 7:30am

Kim Burns: I can relate to that statement. Every time I move in one direction I get sidetracked. I give up.
December 18, 2009 at 5:45pm

Gail Stempel Hilderbrand: It is usually best to start at the beginning:)
December 18, 2009 at 6:12pm

Drenda Lane Howatt: hmm...almost makes me want to break out in song...Julie Andrews anyone?
December 18, 2009 at 8:42pm

Gail Stempel Hilderbrand: That's what I was going for!
December 18, 2009 at 9:10pm

Drenda Lane Howatt, even though she didn't know where to start, had a very productive day. Office work, laundry, store returns, banking, drop-off at Goodwill, and grocery shopping at Winco. Oh, yes, and she had the dogs groomed.
December 18, 2009 at 9:14pm

> Maureen Gatens Thompson: Good Lord, woman! You are amazing!!!!!
> December 18, 2009 at 9:36pm
>
> Andrea Midge McKeehan Robinson: You are a STUD!!
> December 19, 2009 at 7:25am

Drenda Lane Howatt is happy to pass the four month mark. Oh yes. Amazing how times just flies by!
December 20, 2009 at 6:15pm

> Becky Annus: Happy days!
> December 20, 2009 at 7:07pm
>
> Deborah Davis: Every day is a gift. Thank you, God.
> December 20, 2009 at 7:22pm
>
> Chelsea Lincoln Lane: My goodness, four months! Here's to the next sixty years of great health, faith and happiness!
> December 20, 2009 at 8:41pm

Drenda Lane Howatt is very excited for Christmas. She has already received the best present, and that is a renewed appreciation for family, friends, and LIFE! ~Merry Christmas, everyone~
December 21, 2009 at 5:31pm

> Ginger Clausen: Merry Christmas, Drenda! :)

December 21, 2009 at 6:10pm

Mary Raethke: I am right there with you Drenda - I too have a renewed appreciation for family, friends and LIFE - everyday is a gift. Merry Christmas!
December 21, 2009 at 8:11pm

Maureen Gatens Thompson: Ditto to what you and Mary said. Blessings to you and yours. ♥
December 22, 2009 at 8:04am

Drenda Lane Howatt -- It's beginning to look (& feel) a lot like Christmas around here!
December 23, 2009 at 12:01pm

Abbi Howatt: Merry Christmas!
December 24, 2009 at 4:47am

Drenda Lane Howatt: ..."Do not be afraid. I bring you good news of great joy that will be for all the people. Today in the town of David a Savior has been born to you; he is Christ the Lord." "For to us a child is born, to us a son is given, and the government will be on his shoulders. And he will be called Wonderful Counselor, Mighty God, Everlasting Father, Prince of Peace." Merry Christmas!
December 24, 2009 at 11:40am

Drenda Lane Howatt: Merry Christmas~ If you are loved, you are blessed. If you have good health, you are blessed. If you have breath, you are blessed. We love because He first loved us...that means that each and everyone of us is loved by the God of the universe who sent His Son as a babe...we are, all, blessed. Merry Christmas Indeed!
December 25, 2009 at 8:51am

Evy Marks Tyler: Amen, Sister. What a great day to give thanks for all the blessings we have as individuals. What a great day to celebrate the GIFT that God gave in sending Jesus. Even with a daughter in Iraq and another daughter, son-in-law and two grandbabies in Minnesota in a foot of snow I will give thanks for all God's grace poured out on me.
December 25, 2009 at 11:18am

Cindy McElmurry: Merry Christmas and Thank you.
December 25, 2009 at 2:12pm

Drenda Lane Howatt -- old bed out...check. New bed in and assembled...check. 3rd floor maid's quarters into new 'hip' apartment-like quarters...check. Oldest daughter happy...check.
December 27, 2009 at 1:19pm

Maureen Gatens Thompson: Wow...I should hope she is happy. A young woman's dream space. And how wonderful that you have the space to do it.
Happy New Year, Drenda.
December 27, 2009 at 2:03pm

Ellie Howatt: Youngest daughter jealous...Check!
December 27, 2009 at 2:07pm

Drenda Lane Howatt: Thanks, Maureen! Happy New Year to you and yours.
December 27, 2009 at 2:08pm

Drenda Lane Howatt: Ellie, dear, no jealousy allowed. You have a nice room, too, when it is picked up and clean....
December 27, 2009 at 2:09pm

Sandy Hagstrand: Ah, the joys of Motherhood!
December 27, 2009 at 5:19pm

Hollace Howatt Chandler: Done...Priceless
December 27, 2009 at 10:41pm

Drenda Lane Howatt: Oh yes, it IS snowing...beautiful, beautiful. Now to make sure all my babies are home safe and sound before driving gets nasty.
December 29, 2009 at 2:51pm

Drenda Lane Howatt, in her quest to make sure all three daughters were home safe and sound, just spent an hour and one half driving Miss Ellie home. From Lloyd Center. 37 blocks. One half of that time spent on 13. blocks.
December 29, 2009 at 5:55pm

Maureen Gatens Thompson: Oh my...at least you are home safe.
December 29, 2009 at 5:57pm

Shannon V Means: Sheesh, you could have walked in that time...
December 29, 2009 at 7:58pm

Drenda Lane Howatt: Yes, Maureen, I am so thankful to be home. Almost parked at 24 hr fitness at 42nd and Halsey and walked home. Then, almost parked at Providence at 45th and Halsey. I told Ellie "time to pray that God will protect us and get us home safely" as we braved the hill at 47th...after some slip sliding around, we made it up the hill and home. whew.
December 29, 2009 at 8:40pm

Maureen Gatens Thompson: During times like these, I often wonder how in the world the early settlers made it

over the mountains in covered wagons during those cruel winters with absolutely no comforts that we enjoy.
December 29, 2009 at 9:04pm

Drenda Lane Howatt is amazed that the Y2K hysteria was ten years ago. A decade. Oh my goodness.
December 30, 2009 at 4:06pm

Bradley Ruhl: At least we have not run out of things to be hysterical about since then...
December 30, 2009 at 4:19pm

Drenda Lane Howatt brought the all-night party-ers home...nothing like a group of 12 and 13 year olds wanting to get to sleep! Quiet houses today at the Howatt, Annus, and Wilkinson homes~
December 31, 2009 at 9:36am

Amanda Lane: hmm... not wanting to be overly mean, but what were they/you as the parents thinking?!? You are supposed to stay up all night tonight, NOT last night. The new year will be anti-climactic if you just sleep through...
December 31, 2009 at 10:28am

Drenda Lane Howatt: It was an "old-year's party" for the jr. highers...and the trick on New Year's Eve (for all parents out there in fb land), is to turn the clocks ahead a couple of hours. shhh. It's a secret.
December 31, 2009 at 10:30am

Amanda Lane: Won't they catch on when it's time for the countdown?
December 31, 2009 at 10:31am

Drenda Lane Howatt: The idea is that you do your own

count-down!
December 31, 2009 at 10:33am

Amanda Lane: But then you have to count! And backwards…
December 31, 2009 at 10:36am

Ginger Clausen: My house, too! Were they at the overnighter at Spring Mountain? I love your idea, but if they turn on the T.V., the countdown clock will be up and running.
December 31, 2009 at 11:48am

Amber Lynn Montgomery Lane: The big NYE party here will have a New York New Year's. No trying to hide the fact that midnight will happen at 9:00pm.
December 31, 2009 at 12:42pm

Janette Wilkinson: Still sleeping...I have had a gloriously quiet day!
December 31, 2009 at 2:02pm

Amanda Lane: When you sleep, where do your fingers go?
December 31, 2009 at 2:03pm

Janette Wilkinson: I tend to keep them with me...
December 31, 2009 at 2:15pm

Drenda Lane Howatt: Ginger, yes they were at Spring Mountain. Ellie invited 3 of her cousins, and it sounds like they had great fun~
January 1, 2010 at 9:02am

Ginger Clausen: Kai did, too. He assured me he wasn't tired and didn't need to go to bed when he got home. I told him to go anyway, then I woke him up at 4:30 when Ben Sanford arrived to spend the night. They

banged pots and popped pop-its with surprisingly barefoot neighbor boys for about 15 minutes, then bedtime was 12:30. I took pictures and enjoyed their merriment.
January 1, 2010 at 12:51pm

Drenda Lane Howatt is on her way to give a good amount of her money to the auto shop. Good that the Howatts can contribute to keeping the economy in recovery mode. Glad to do it.
December 31, 2009 at 12:27pm

Janette Wilkinson: "Glad"! Really?
December 31, 2009 at 2:01pm

Drenda Lane Howatt: Well...glad to have jobs that allow us to pay to have cars that are working and therefore reliable transportation so that we can get to the jobs to pay for the cars that are working...
December 31, 2009 at 2:03pm

Caitlin Lopez: Way to help out Drenda.
December 31, 2009 at 2:49pm

Maureen Gatens Thompson: That's how we feel: one water heater; one stove and two cars all since August! Yikes!
December 31, 2009 at 3:02pm

Ginger Clausen: Us, too. New tires the week before Christmas. Merry Christmas, Les Schwab!
December 31, 2009 at 5:30pm

Drenda Lane Howatt: We bought two new tires, too, after the car repair.
January 1, 2010 at 9:16am

Drenda Lane Howatt is enjoying the wonderful smell of ham and bean soup simmering on the stove all day...mmm
January 1, 2010 at 3:41pm

> Maureen Gatens Thompson: Sounds great...my goal is to cook ham and scalloped potatoes IF my stove ever gets hooked up.
> January 1, 2010 at 4:41pm
>
> Drenda Lane Howatt: Ham and scalloped potatoes sounds wonderful, too~
> We had that last week; the soup is the last dinner from the bone-in ham.
> January 1, 2010 at 4:54pm
>
> Drenda Lane Howatt loves having three Saturdays in one week. Too perfect~
> January 2, 2010 at 10:02am

Drenda Lane Howatt enjoyed "Sunday" dinner at home with Don, Anna, Rachel, and Ellie. Next, she enjoyed a visit with dear friends. Tomorrow, it is "goodbye" to sweet Rachel as she heads back to Seattle, and "hello, again" to routine. Christmas vacation is, almost, officially over.
January 3, 2010 at 5:38pm

Drenda Lane Howatt received great reassurance and encouragement from her oldest daughter. Drenda said "I look like a chia head". And her daughter's response? "No, you don't. It's not green. Or spiky." Thank you very much. That helped tremendously.
January 4, 2010 at 7:58pm

> Susan Rasmussen Lane: Aren't kids GREAT for the self-esteem? Natalie, looking at a book about saints, "This

says this saint died in 389 AD. Were you born then, Mom?" Me, "(Big sigh.)"
January 4, 2010 at 8:29pm

Chelsea Lincoln Lane: It wasn't too long ago when Laney said, "Mommy, when I grow up, will I be as fat as you?" Gotta love 'em...
January 4, 2010 at 8:52pm

Amber Lynn Montgomery Lane: My kids haven't hit the verbal abuse stage yet. Physical, on the other hand...
January 4, 2010 at 9:01pm

Hiroko Peraza: Aika is still 6 weeks old so I'm safe for a while. :)
January 4, 2010 at 10:40pm

Drenda Lane Howatt: There was no intent of abuse, I am sure...she was just making a 'statement of fact'. Absolutely.
Susan, Ellie once asked me if there were grocery stores when I was little...
January 5, 2010 at 4:42pm

Drenda Lane Howatt talked with her former employer today, the good Senator from Oregon, Mr. Wyden. "Hi, I am Ron Wyden." "Well hello, Ron, I am Drenda Howatt." "DRENDA HOWATT? Drenda Howatt? How are you! So good to see you! How are you? I would have NEVER recognized you. Did you get a new hairstyle?" "Well, umm, yes, I did." Good that it is the hair that makes her unrecognizable, and not the age that came with years gone by.
January 5, 2010 at 4:40pm

Susan Rasmussen Lane: Eeww... You'd think after all these years in politics he'd have better social skills than that....

January 5, 2010 at 4:45pm

Drenda Lane Howatt: I was pleased he remembered me!
January 5, 2010at 4:50pm

Amanda Lane: Oh, I think it might work for him... goofy and not slimey with the compliments. You should have asked him to get you some pork ☻
January 5, 2010 at 4:56pm

Amanda Lane: Strike that last bit there... you should have asked for some pork for your favorite niece. She loOoOves the bacon!
January 5, 2010 at 5:00pm

Wayne Vandekraak: Love that guy
January 5, 2010 at 10:09pm

Drenda Lane Howatt color? Really? I can hardly believe it.
January 7, 2010 at 5:33pm

Don Sawchuk: Green?
January 7, 2010 at 5:51pm

Maureen Gatens Thompson: What's up with all these color posts?
January 7, 2010 at 7:19pm

Drenda Lane Howatt: well, Maureen...only women (mostly) are posting...and most colors posted are black. The men posting don't get it, or they do understand and are just a tad odd to wear one...
January 7, 2010 at 7:53pm

Maureen Gatens Thompson: LOL.....OHHHHHHHHH, now I get it--I think. Wonder who started it?
January 7, 2010 at 7:57pm

Milt Buckelew: I think you underestimate us...as a group:-)
January 8, 2010 at 8:07am

Drenda Lane Howatt: my apologies, Milt~
January 8, 2010 at 8:22am

Caitlin Lopez: I know. Size would be more fun:)
January 8, 2010 at 9:13am

Drenda Lane Howatt is going to see her friend Jerry tomorrow, and must remember to ask him all of the questions on her long list...and to tell him about her upcoming travels. Good to have one's oncologist 'ok' trips that will take one far away!
January 7, 2010 at 8:08pm

Andi Pedersen Jordan: Nice to hear Jerry's name ... but I have to admit, it's even nicer not to have to hear his name as often.
Hope you are feeling the love of color today.
January 7, 2010 at 10:44pm

Linda Lane Waggoner: Where are you travelling to?
January 8, 2010 at 7:17am

Drenda Lane Howatt: Maui in February, and Washington D.C. in March...one for relaxation and one for work~
January 8, 2010 at 7:30am

Robin Reilly: let me guess which is which. ;-)
January 8, 2010 at 9:23am

Drenda Lane Howatt: Robin, you make me laugh! One is for relaxation AND celebration (of cancer survivorship and 25 years of wedded bliss), the other is work (but it

will be fun, too!)
January 8, 2010 at 12:33pm

Drenda Lane Howatt is, instead of posting the color of the bra she is wearing, going to schedule her yearly mammogram. Ladies, please do the same. And for added awareness, she is going to have an MRI of her brain in the morning. There. Aware? Yes, she thinks she is. No question. And no color of the bra.
January 8, 2010 at 12:30pm

Jerry Day

Friday, January 8, 2010 at 3:41pm

Today was "Jerry day".

Labs first. Nothing of note. Use the hot pad to warm up the arm, and then take the blood. And no question about which arm to stick. Of course, I just put out my left arm, so if the wrong arm is not available, all will be well~

Jerry wasn't too late today. Wonderful.

Because of the joint stiffness and pain I have been experiencing (severe -- I hobble around like a really really old person...) Jerry will switch the medication I am taking for estrogen suppression. Hopefully that will help.

I have had a few headaches, so Jerry wants another MRI of my brain. "First available". That is Saturday, tomorrow, 7:30 a.m. Oh my goodness. This time I will take a double dose of sedative in an attempt to have an easier time in the 'machine'.

I have been doing pretty well leaving that sack of fear alone. But not today. "Jerry days" are particularly hard. What will he say? How am I doing? Is the blood work normal? Not to mention the instant panic that arrives upon walking in the door of the Cancer Center. And when that panic rises in the middle of an intense hot flash, I am really in a mess.

As Don and I stood at the counter while Jerry's medical assistant, Sconesha, was making calls to schedule my MRI, echo-cardiogram, mammogram, and EKG, I had another "punched in the stomach by cancer" moment. I had to fight off the tears. As I heard Sconesha say my name, along with the words "history of breast cancer", "headaches", "another echo", I wanted to scream. WHY ARE YOU TALKING ABOUT ME? I AM FINE! STOP SAYING MY NAME AND THOSE AWFUL THINGS. STOP IT. STOP IT. STOP IT!"

Instead of screaming, I stood there and "patiently" waited for her to finish scheduling my next few weeks. And willed myself not to cry.

Another "how did this happen" moment. Another "why me, God" question. I thought I was done with those reactions and questions.

Perhaps I will never be done asking.

That is o.k.

Because I know He will answer -- maybe not on my timeline, but He will answer.

Pam Geddes Girtman: You're a trooper - and aren't Fridays the best invention over the past say year and a half??
January 8, 2010 at 4:14pm

Wendy Ackley: I was looking for you a bit as I was at PPMC, however you may not go there for followup. I saw a guy that looked a little like Don and I think he thought I was stalking him.
January 8, 2010 at 7:37pm

Drenda Lane Howatt: No, I go to NW Cancer Specialists Rose Quarter -- on Broadway right across from the Rose Garden. I

will be PPMC tomorrow for the MRI, though~
January 8, 2010 at 7:39pm

Linda Lane Waggoner: Perhaps you won't ever be done asking those questions Drenda but, hopefully, they will come less and less often. Grief has a funny way of doing that.... showing itself less and less often. I love you!
January 9, 2010 at 8:23am

Andi Pedersen Jordan: Glad Don was with you. You are ever so "Strong and Courageous"!
January 9, 2010 at 9:26am

Drenda Lane Howatt has her earplugs and her sedatives...MRI, here she comes~
January 9, 2010 at 7:16am

> Rebecca Groner: earplugs and sedatives...sounds like a day in the classroom
> January 9, 2010 at 5:03pm

Drenda Lane Howatt MRI? No problem. No problem at all. Just take two xanax, and it will be over and done oh so quickly!
January 9, 2010 at 8:35am

> Becky Annus: I'm thinking of you.
> January 9, 2010 at 9:40am
>
> Drenda Lane Howatt: It was easy this time. I am so glad. I think the difference, besides the extra xanax, was the lack of fear. The first brain MRI I had done last year was at the beginning of this terror-filled journey. Now, not nearly as much terror!
> January 9, 2010 at 10:24am
>
> Faith Lichtenberg: Wow, you are already done with this one? You're my hero ♥
> January 9, 2010 at 10:28am
>
> Drenda Lane Howatt: Who knew Providence Cancer Center did MRI tests at 7:30 on a Saturday morning? It was pretty quiet around there!
> January 9, 2010 at 10:32am
>
> Faith Lichtenberg: Nice to have the express service on something you want to get out of the way that badly!
> January 9, 2010 at 10:34am

Becky Annus: Good! I'm glad for you that it's over and it wasn't nearly as scary as last time.
January 9, 2010 at 12:27pm

Janette Wilkinson: I was sending you anti claustrophobic thoughts all morning! I am glad that it is over!
January 9, 2010 at 3:22pm

Linda Lane Waggoner: I get claustrophobic just hearing about an enclosed space! i would have to be essentially unconscious to have an MRI!!
January 9, 2010 at 4:16pm

Drenda Lane Howatt: I wasn't claustrophobic at all this time...the extra 'pill' helped tremendously, as did the warm blanket, and the cloth I had them put over the little brace over my face. I could still see if I needed to, but it helped me to just keep my eyes closed and relaxed. It was not at all a problem today. God is so good -- answered my prayers that were sent His way all day yesterday and into the evening!
January 9, 2010 at 4:36pm

Linda Lane Waggoner: Yes, God is good - and you are strong!
January 9, 2010 at 6:02pm

Drenda Lane Howatt new medicine to be stored at 77 degrees...brief storage at temps between 59 and 86 degrees is permitted. 77 degrees? How, exactly, does that happen? Heating the Howatt Home to 69 degrees is a very expensive propostion.
January 9, 2010 at 6:42pm

Drenda Lane Howatt Possible symptoms of the new medication,

to name just a few, may include headache, joint pain, hot flashes, hair loss (!), increased (or decreased) appetite, nausea, vomiting, weight gain, constipation, diarrhea, fatigue, confusion, depression, numbness of limbs, severe bone pain, swelling of hands, legs, or feet, dizziness, flu-like symptoms, stomach pain, speech changes, coughing...
seems like some of those listed are opposite of the others-- weight gain/nausea, constipation/diarrhea
January 9, 2010 at 6:44pm

Drenda Lane Howatt: TMI for you all, I am sure. But there are at least one or two of you out there in fb land who are interested, I just know it.
January 9, 2010 at 6:45pm

Faith Lichtenberg: That is some high maintenance medication! Maybe carrying it around in your pocket would make the temp difference it needs.
January 9, 2010 at 6:53pm

Barb Van Dusen Butler: or you could move to a warmer climate. I'd say; "like here" but we've been below freezing for 3 straight days now! Sounds like really scary stuff to be taking, just waiting for all those things to over take you!
January 9, 2010 at 7:17pm

Drenda Lane Howatt: most of the side effects I have already experienced from other treatments!
January 9, 2010 at 7:20pm

Susan Rasmussen Lane: I'm with Faith. That's very high maintenance medication. I hope you don't have any strong reactions to it, except for it working for you for what it's supposed to do.
January 9, 2010 at 7:48pm

Drenda Lane Howatt: Sometimes I think it would just be

easier to remove the organs that produce the estrogen that this medication is supposed to suppress~but the real problem is the fat cells that are producing estrogen. I am finding it difficult to get those cells removed.
January 9, 2010 at 7:54pm

Jonna Wilkinson: I was going to say that it sounds like pseudo-menopause symptoms. as far as the meds, heat 'em up during hot flashes!
January 9, 2010 at 8:11pm

Drenda Lane Howatt: Jonna, I am about as menopausal as possible...thanks to chemo. There is no going back. Intense hot flashes are now a part of my life story! If only the hot flashes could/would occur on demand...
January 9, 2010 at 8:13pm

Jonna Wilkinson: lol... well u know how to keep things warm!
January 9, 2010 at 8:16pm

Barb Van Dusen Butler: So, I hate to ask a dumb question, but can you go on HRT? I understand you need to suppress the estrogen so I guess that kind of negates HRT - as I understand it.
January 11, 2010 at 4:54pm

Drenda Lane Howatt ok, so my parents win!

Drenda's parents get an A+ for originality.
Ranking: 'Drenda' wasn't in the top 2000 baby names for their birth year.
Rarity: 5% of girls had rarer names that year. (Grade: A+)
Peak year: Name too rare. Data unavailable.
Current rank: 'Drenda' isn't currently one of the top 1000 girl's names.

January 9, 2010 at 10:47pm via How original are my parents?

Susan Rasmussen Lane: Ha ha! Yeah, I guess they win, if originality is the only criteria. (Of course, they didn't do so well with Linda in this competition.) But luckily Drenda is a nice name, too, not just original. I've always liked my name, so obviously originality isn't high on my priority list!
January 10, 2010 at 12:15am

Linda Lane Waggoner: I like the name Drenda! It fits you! I wonder why that is?
January 10, 2010 at 10:06am

Drenda Lane Howatt's brain is, perhaps surprisingly, completely normal! MRI results in and everything a-o.k. She praises God for such wonderful, and reassuring, news. Oh yes indeed!
January 11, 2010 at 1:04pm

Susan Rasmussen Lane: Oh, and don't we all? Hooray!
January 11, 2010 at 1:37pm

Caitlin Lopez: woooohoooooooooooo!!!!!
January 11, 2010 at 1:41pm

Hiroko Peraza: Great news!
January 11, 2010 at 4:40pm

Ginger Clausen: Praise the Lord! Glad you didn't have to wait too long to get the results, too.
January 11, 2010 at 4:54pm

Susan Laufman Stevens: No looking back now Sista! Enjoy life!!!
January 11, 2010 at 4:56pm

Janette Wilkinson: So I guess you can't claim chemo brain anymore?!
January 11, 2010 at 7:01pm

Deborah Davis: Oh, I think you have a better than "normal" brain. You're above average for sure.
January 11, 2010 at 8:07pm

Maureen Gatens Thompson: You and your family absolutely postively deserved this news. Blessed Be, Drenda! ♥
January 11, 2010 at 8:31pm

Sandy Hagstrand: Rejoicing with you! Every test is a new milestone to celebraate...
January 11, 2010 at 9:58pm

Maryellen Mann Householder: Wow, that is more than I can say for myself! Praise God.
January 12, 2010 at 6:38am

Drenda Lane Howatt: I had to have the MRI, first available, because I have been having headaches. When Jerry called with the test results, I said "GREAT! Now, when I have headaches I can take tylenol and not worry..." Jerry said "Yes! Well, unless the headaches change...stronger, different, longer, then you call me." Ok, I can do that.
January 12, 2010 at 6:50am

Shannon Swope: Wahoo, that is fantastic news my friend! :) So glad to hear it. I had a very sick pt. last night and she had such great friends laughing and visiting with her. 'Indeed, some of the BEST medicine is shared laughter, stories, encouraging words, etc. with good friends,' I thought as I was caring for her and watching the interaction. It was nice and I was happy for her. I was also thankful for you and what a huge

blessing you are to me! I'm glad you got the 'normal' news-although that's relative and I'm quite glad you're NOT 'normal' for that would be far too boring. :)You have a terrific day and a HUGE hug from me...coffee sooooon! :) I'm going to sleep now...THAT was wordy-sheesh!
January 12, 2010 at 9:32am

Jessica Hernandez: You are a Rock Star!
January 12, 2010 at 11:41am

Drenda Lane Howatt is thankful for leftovers and quiet evenings.
January 12 at 5:14pm

Drenda Lane Howatt: Oh, and hot water in which to soak. Thankful for that, too~
January 12, 2010 at 6:14pm

Sally Lane Park: We need to plan a dinner prep day
January 15, 2010 at 5:55am

Drenda Lane Howatt heard this on the news, and it is a direct quote: "Experienced suicide bombers are few and far between".
January 13, 2010 at 5:39pm

Chelsea Lincoln Lane: Wow, that is REALLY good to know. Now we can rest assured that we have a low-to-moderate chance of encountering an experienced suicide bomber AND that corporate news personnel deliver accurate messages!
January 13, 2010 at 5:51pm

Drenda Lane Howatt: I would think that "experienced suicide bomber" is an oxymoron at its best.
January 13, 2010 at 5:53pm

Michael Schneider: hm...maybe it's ok to say they're experienced (in the events leading up to it) but that the learning curve is 0.00
January 13, 2010 at 7:01pm

Dusti Waggoner: Omg!
January 13, 2010 at 7:21pm

Maureen Gatens Thompson: That's because they are Dead! And they probably took innocent lives with them.
January 13, 2010 at 8:38pm

Drenda Lane Howatt: Yes~ The report was about their behavior giving away their intentions -- suicide bombers are nervous (I assume because they lack experience...)
January 13, 2010 at 8:41pm

Maureen Gatens Thompson: ....nervous about meeting all those virgins in heaven. Good Grief!
January 13, 2010 at 9:33pm

Maryellen Mann Householder: Too funny! Thank goodness they eliminate themselves from the ranks.
January 14, 2010 at 6:04am

Gary Burns: That's something Jay Leno can use on his headlines segment.
January 14, 2010 at 7:08am

Drenda Lane Howatt is getting ready for two dinners at her home tomorrow...first comes lunch with nine wonderful college students, then comes dinner with six great friends. Luckily, there should be almost two hours in between events!
January 16, 2010 at 4:37pm

Drenda Lane Howatt: all of which means that we are going out to dinner tonight!
January 16, 2010 at 4:39pm

Maureen Gatens Thompson: Hmmm....want to test out my new big stove? LOL
January 16, 2010 at 5:17pm

Drenda Lane Howatt: Yes!
January 16, 2010 at 5:25pm

Maureen Gatens Thompson: Probably even better if I do the cooking (following your recipe, of course), serve your guests and do the dishes. After all, what are friends for?! ;-)
January 16, 2010 at 5:28pm

Drenda Lane Howatt: Perfect! Can you be here by noon?
January 16, 2010 at 6:31pm

Drenda Lane Howatt listened to the famous Martin Luther King Jr. speech this morning. He had some great speech writers.
January 18, 2010 at 7:30am

Pam Geddes Girtman: So did we. Good stuff. I like to believe he wrote it himself from the bottom of his heart for the masses.
January 18, 2010 at 8:49pm

Drenda Lane Howatt thinks this short week is actually quite long...
January 20, 2010 at 5:03pm

Drenda Lane Howatt: but it is not a problem that a hot bath can't fix...
January 20, 2010 at 5:07pm

Jennifer Stady: I think it's because the days are, literally, getting longer.
January 20, 2010 at 8:22pm

Drenda Lane Howatt loves Thursdays. Thursdays are the new (not so new, really) Fridays. Oh yes.
January 21, 2010 at 6:55pm

Check-In

Thursday, January 21, 2010 at 8:35pm

Tonight I attended my first breast cancer support group.

There were six other women there. Two of us were new. "First-timers".

What is shared in group stays in group.

Ok.

That is fair. Safe.

But it was good to hear the other women's stories during 'check-in' time.

And to share mine.

Each of the stories brought questions to my mind.

The biggest question?

Will I need to come to a support group five years out?

Ten?

No, I tell myself.

NO.

I won't 'need' to come.

I won't 'need' to come because I will be done with this cancer stuff soon.

Done.

I won't 'need' to come because I will have moved on, away from cancer.

Away from terror.

Away from fear.

Far.

Away.

But maybe I'll 'want' to come.

Perhaps the women who still come years after their diagnosis are not there because they 'need' to be.

Perhaps they were there for me.

Laurie Lane: The women newly dealing with their cancer will need you to be there. They will need your hope and your acknowledging that they are not alone.
January 22, 2010 at 4:30pm

As For Me...

hursday, January 21, 2010 at 9:12pm

I have shared, perhaps too often, the fears that came with cancer.

The terror.

I have never felt anything like it. So scared. So anxious.

Never.

Ever.

I have shared my conflicted heart.

I have shared about what I know to be true about Christ and the salvation He has given me and the conflict that the terror of death has brought. "How can I be a Christian and be so scared of death?"

Surely, my relationship with Christ, if true, would shield me from that terror, right? And if I am not shielded, if I have that terror, what does that mean?

It meant I went back to Him and asked.

Many times.

In the middle of the night.

In the middle of the meeting.

In the middle of the waiting room.

And the answer continues to come.

I am not alone.

The answer came from Sue Walt. When I shared my terror with her, and my upset over the conflict, her words were quick and strong and reassuring. "Drenda, you are not alone."

The answer came from Joyce McElmurry. Same words, again. "You are not alone."

I had never heard anyone admit to that fear. I felt alone. Ever since my Mom died, twenty years ago, I have wondered if she was scared of death. I believe death was a physical relief for her, but was she scared? I don't know. And I've never had the courage to ask my Dad if he knows. I wasn't sure I wanted to know the answer.

But now I know I am not alone.

And today, I was encouraged that there is another who understood. I was reading Psalm 55, a Psalm written by David. Do you know what David says to God?

Psalm 55:4-5
My heart is in anguish within me,
And the terrors of death have fallen upon me.
Fear and trembling come upon me,
And horror has overwhelmed me.

And yet, even in those terrors, David ends the Psalm by writing "as for me, I trust in You."

My heart has been in anguish within me.
And terrors of death have fallen upon me.

As for me, I will trust in Him.

Hiroko Peraza: I wish I could give you a big hug.
January 22, 2010 at 6:39am

Drenda Lane Howatt: Hiroko, I miss you! Let's get together soon -- we have to meet your baby!
January 22, 2010 at 6:41am

Hiroko Peraza: Sure! We can get together for a coffee or something. Aika smiles now. I can't stand how cute she is!!!! :)
January 22, 2010 at 7:03am

Maryellen Mann Householder: Drenda, oh how I know what you mean. There is no shame in being afraid. It is not the measure of your faith. " Even though your heart condemns you, God is greater than your heart". I ask myself "What is it about your love Lord that I am not fully understanding right now?" Doesn't always help but it does help get my mind on the Lord and not on my circumstances. And yes, you are not alone! When you walk through the valley of the SHADOW of death, not the valley of death, you will not fear for God is with you. I'm right there with you sister!!
January 22, 2010 at 10:05am

Irmgard Lam: Drenda, I hope you can come visit us at the Healing Room I volunteer at....we pray for God's healing for any and all illnesses, or situations...we've seen some pretty amazing miracles....it's on Monday evenings at 7:00pm, on NE 103rd & Weidler...right next to McDonalds. It is non-denominational, and we'd love to have you come!

I have not dealt with cancer, but had a very bad scare with another horrible illness a year ago....God healed me of it

completely! In fact it was January 22, 2009 that God told me He was going to heal me of it....we serve an amazing, loving God! He is willing and able to heal us of all our diseases.
January 22, 2010 at 12:56pm

Drenda Lane Howatt: Tomorrow marks 20 years since the world lost an amazing woman. You are missed, beyond measure, Mom.
January 23, 2010 at 8:04am

Cindy McElmurry: I am so glad that I got to meet her.
January 23, 2010 at 9:05am

Drenda Lane Howatt: Cindy, I am, too! Mom really loved knowing our friends~
January 23, 2010 at 9:07am

Rebecca Groner: I have such lovely memories...your family is dear to me
January 23, 2010 at 9:42am

Wendy Ackley: She is still very vivid to me.
January 23, 2010 at 9:50am

Sally Lane Park: I wish my kids could have known her.
January 23, 2010 at 9:52am

Steven Lane: I am so glad that our kids knew what a wonderful grandma she was. I miss Nadine to this day
January 23, 2010 at 10:24am

Gary Burns: I can't believe it's been that long ago. She left behind a great legacy!
January 23, 2010 at 10:39am

Erin Frazier Miller: I remember the beautful tribute to her life. Special indeed!
January 23, 2010 at 10:56am

Drenda Lane Howatt: Karen, I remember Andy's note...Grandma Nadine would use a "whole packet" of hot chocolate...

I believe she would be very proud of all of us. We have a great, strong, and courageous family. Lots of 'ilities"~
January 23, 2010 at 11:33am

Laurie Lane: I miss her so much! I know she would be proud of all of us and would love how large our family has grown. The nice thing is that she has left a little of herself with each of us, we continue her spirit and love through our lives.
January 23, 2010 at 6:12pm

Ron Waggoner: Well said Laurie...I seldom think of my mom without thinking of and missing Nadine. We were all very blessed by her presence.
January 23, 2010 at 9:11pm

Kim Burns: I have so many memories of mom Lane. She was a special woman. Who couldn't help but love her. :)
January 24, 2010 at 8:52am

Drenda Lane Howatt: It is so true, Kim! Our family 'grew' to include so many of our close friends. Mom and Dad had lots of 'adopted' children~
January 24, 2010 at 5:03pm

Drenda Lane Howatt was punched in the stomach again. Those abs must be getting stronger...
January 26, 2010 at 5:36pm

Andi Pedersen Jordan: Uh, oh ... who or what can we punch back?
January 26, 2010 at 5:36pm

Drenda Lane Howatt: Just another "how did this happen/who is he talking about?" moment...and longing for normal that doesn't include chia head hair and creaky stiff bones and and and and.

General whining.
January 26, 2010 at 5:44pm

Linda Lane Waggoner: I am so sorry, Drenda!
January 26, 2010 at 7:26pm

Sally Lane Park: I am sorry. Not so much fun.
January 26, 2010 at 7:29pm ·

Maureen Gatens Thompson: ...we need to talk.
January 26, 2010 at 10:30pm

Luann Sader Hoover: It's okay, someday you'll look back on all this and say...that really sucked!! Seriously, I am sorry Drenda. That must get sooo old. Abs of Steel!!
January 27, 2010 at 8:36am

Irmgard Lam: You're in my prayers!
January 27, 2010 at 12:54pm

Drenda Lane Howatt has *A Thursday* again...medical tests schmedical tests. How can it possibly be time for yet another echo-cardiogram? And a mammogram... Remembering that the cancer is gone, and just hoping her body got the memo.
January 28, 2010 at 7:08am

Ginger Clausen: Trust in the Lord with all your heart and lean not on your own anxiety... Praying for peace for you, Drenda!
January 28, 2010 at 7:15am

Drenda Lane Howatt: Thank you Ginger. Don has taken the day off to accompany me to the appointments today. I don't want a repeat of the "are you here alone?" question.
January 28, 2010 at 8:07am

Ginger Clausen: What a great guy!
January 28, 2010 at 12:11pm

Drenda Lane Howatt: Yes, he is~
January 28, 2010 at 12:57pm

Drenda Lane Howatt is very happy to report that her body did, indeed, get the memo. After another diagnostic mammogram, and a follow-up diagnostic ultrasound (due to her concerns about 'new' lump), Dr. Radiologist gave the all clear. Nothing looks suspicious or of concern. Now, on to the heart test. Congestive heart failure, you're not welcome anywhere near her.
January 28, 2010 at 1:00pm

Drenda Lane Howatt: Diagnostic mammograms for the next five years -- diagnostic means more pictures and greater magnification. All right by me. And a huge thank you to Kathy at PMI for taking extra time to show pictures, comparing to my last mammo (which showed the cancer) and explaining everything. Huge sigh of relief.
January 28, 2010 at 1:03pm

Susan Laufman Stevens: You go girl! Body has many years of healthy memories.
January 28, 2010 at 1:43pm

Irmgard Lam: Praise God! Glad everything came out good - I've been praying!
January 28, 2010 at 2:30pm

Sally Lane Park: Good news!
January 28, 2010 at 4:50pm

Deborah Davis: A huge, collective sigh of relief! Praise

the Lord from whom all blessings flow.
January 28, 2010 at 7:38pm

Maureen Gatens Thompson: Good job, Drenda...we both had "whew" weeks. ♥
January 28, 2010 at 9:17pm

Ginger Clausen: Glad to hear you passed the test with flying colors! :)
January 28, 2010 at 9:39pm

Drenda Lane Howatt is off, soon, to Seattle for the weekend to see Miss Rachel~
January 29, 2010 at 8:15am

Linda Lane Waggoner: Have fun!
January 29, 2010 at 8:21am

Sally Lane Park: Give her a hug for me.
January 29, 2010 at 4:58pm

Cindy McElmurry: Give her a hug for me!
January 30, 2010 at 10:05am

Drenda Lane Howatt: She is happy to see her family!
January 30, 2010 at 10:12am

Drenda Lane Howatt s headed to Pike's...and then shopping to stock a dorm room. Oh, yes, and yarn. Rachel "needs" yarn.
January 30, 2010 at 10:21am

Maureen Gatens Thompson Sounds like a fun weekend...enjoy!
January 30, 2010 at 10:44am

Drenda Lane Howatt had a great day at Pikes, and stocking the dorm room at Fred Meyer's. Capped off the day with dinner at Buca di Beppos. Thanks, Audrey and Wes, for introducing us to Buca!
January 30, 2010 at 6:12pm

Shannon V Means: Oooh, Buca is the best!
January 30, 2010 at 6:15pm

Drenda Lane Howatt: Yes, it is wonderful! Wish there was a Buca di Beppo's in Portland~
January 30, 2010 at 6:31pm

Wendy Ackley: What kind of food is it?
January 30, 2010 at 7:16pm

Drenda Lane Howatt: Italian...family style. Buca's atmosphere is not easy to explain -- but lots of fun! and great food.
January 30, 2010 at 7:37pm

Pam Geddes Girtman: Last time I was at Buca was in Anaheim! Rememba? Fun times - and Bob from Bob's Red Mill!
January 30, 2010 at 8:11pm

Wendy Ackley: Is it one restaurant or a chain...any in Oregon?
Sounds like a girls night out :-)
January 30, 2010 at 8:12pm

Drenda Lane Howatt: Pam - Yes, I was remembering. Tonight, I asked them to turn down the music, and they did!
Wendy, no Buca's in Oregon. We could do a girls' weekend in Seattle, though~
January 30, 2010 at 8:31pm

Drenda Lane Howatt: Wendy, it is a chain...
January 30, 2010 at 8:32pm

Kimberly Tibbetts Roberts: How is Rachel doing?
January 30, 2010 at 8:36pm

Drenda Lane Howatt: Kim, thanks for asking~
Rachel is doing well. Loves Seattle Pacific University.
Studying to teach high school English.
January 31, 2010 at 7:50am

Wayne Vandekraak: Drenda, that place rocks. Enough food to feed a small nation
January 31, 2010 at 11:12am

Teresa Kruger-Brown: I love going to EWU to see my little girl.
January 31, 2010 at 2:07pm

Cindy McElmurry: I think we need to go!
January 31, 2010 at 2:59pm

Shapes?

By Drenda Lane Howatt on Saturday, January 30, 2010 at 11:11am

I am starting to "feel" it.

"Feel" that God is using me.

I take no pride in being used.

At least, I don't want to.

But it does 'feel' good to know that my experiences, my fears, my trembling, are of help to someone else.

To know that God's faithfulness to me, and to my family, is an encouragement to others.

To know that my words that were poured out in pain and terror may help calm that same pain and terror for another.

That was not my purpose.

Perhaps that is His purpose. At least part of His purpose in allowing Drenda Howatt to experience breast cancer.

Platitudes, cliches, and acts are melted away in fires.

The dross is burned. At least some of it.

There is not time to consider what others may think.

To consider how I will look.

To consider if my words ‘sound’ right.

It is what it is.

I am what I am.

That is all ok, because He is who He is. And His promises are true. He is true.

I know cancer will always be a part of me. It will not define me. But it is now a part of who I am.

I know God has allowed it to shape me. Shape my thoughts. Shape my actions. Shape my character.

I will always have the physical reminders that cancer was there.

Scars.

An oddly shaped breast.

The heart reminders will be the helps I can offer others.

And the physical reminders will be the outward sign for me to look for the heart reminders.

Drenda Lane Howatt is having a day off of 'work' to work at home. Wonderful! A bit of time to spend on advancing Mission Organization.
February 1, 2010 at 7:48 a.m.

Drenda Lane Howatt didn't make too much progress on the Mission...but she did do laundry, a bit of work on the taxes, made dinner, AND baked cookies. That's a pretty full day.
February 1, 2010 at 7:38pm

> Pam Geddes Girtman: Missed ya (I took half of it off :))
> February 1, 2010 at 7:39pm

Drenda Lane Howatt was told today that she was brave. It was not the words alone that were so wonderful, but from whence they came. Thank you, Dad!
February 2, 2010 at 7:30pm

> Sally Lane Park: A Man of few words, but when he speaks...
> February 2, 2010 at 7:50pm
>
> Susan Rasmussen Lane: Amen, to that...
> February 2, 2010 at 8:09pm
>
> Drenda Lane Howatt: I know my having cancer has been very hard on him (and on everyone).
> February 3, 2010 at 6:57pm

Hello Mammogram. So Nice to Meet You.

February 3, 2010 at 6:50pm

So, last week I had my 'annual' mammogram.

The first one since my cancer diagnosis. (I did have a mammogram on the morning of the surgery to remove the lump -- but that one doesn't count because its purpose was to guide the insertion of 'guide wires' to assist the surgeon in identifying the outer edges of the tumor.)

The routine is to wait six months after the finish of radiation treatment.

And now I know why.

Because it takes a long long time after radiation is over for the tissue to recover from the inflammation. And mine has not. Recovered. From the inflammation.

OUCH!

This time, I did not go alone.

Don took the day off of work to accompany me for my tests.

Much to the confusion of Kathy, the ultrasound technician, I insisted that Don be allowed to accompany me into the mammogram room. Husband education day! (Surely, others have brought moral support?)

Kathy was wonderful. She explained that, after a diagnosis of breast cancer, diagnostic mammograms are done for the next five years. A diagnostic mammo is different in that more photos are taken, and greater magnification is used.

She asked if I'd like to see the pictures.

So, after each compression, I went back to her computer and compared the picture with the same pose from last year.

And I saw the cancer clearly on last year's picture.

It was not there on this year's picture.

Gone.

Thank God.

I explained to Kathy about the new lump I have felt. She arranged for a diagnostic ultrasound to be done immediately.

The ultrasound technician had me pinpoint the lump. And he went over it again and again with the ultrasound to see if there was anything there.

The radiologist doctor (who is remaining unnamed in this tirade) came in.

He introduced himself to me and said how pleased he was to meet me.

I think, to myself, "um, hello? You met me last year and gave me the worst day of my life. You don't remember me?" Really.

I know, I know. He sees many patients every day. But doesn't my chart tell him that he did the core biopsy? That I would feel so much better if he came in and said "Hello, Drenda. I am happy to see you again. How are you doing?" That I would think I was safe and in good hands if he remembered?

But he did have good news. He said the mammogram results were entirely NORMAL. And then he went over the new lump again and again with the ultrasound. NOTHING IS THERE.

"Drenda, I see nothing suspicious or of concern. Everything is fine. If the lump changes, let us know. Otherwise, I'll see you next year."

Thank God.

Thank God.

I am getting near the end of 'cancer'.

I can feel it.

There is nothing there.

Hollace Howatt Chandler: Wow. What a scary thing, to have felt another lump. You must have been terrified. You didn't tell...Glad it is okay. SO glad!
February 3. 2010 at 9:16 pm

Sally Lane Park: Wow, nice to revisit that room and replace/change the memories . You should write a "nice" note to the radiologist
February 4, 2010 at 7:00 am

Drenda Lane Howatt has a busy busy day. First, Leadership Class. Then off to see radiation oncologist (yes, it has been SIX MONTHS!), and finally, Market Mavens meeting tonight. She loves how routine oncologist visits have become. Right there in the middle of life.
February 10, 2010 at 6:32am

Powerful Nuts

Wednesday, February 10, 2010 at 5:57pm

Today was the day to see my radiation oncologist.

Dr. Alice Wang.

But first, Susie the nurse takes me to the exam room. Susie is a sweet spirit, with a wonderful countenance. She is a smiler.

"List of medications, please."

"Side effects from any of the medications?" Well, yes, actually, there are. And they are not pleasant. "Diarrhea?" Yep. "Taking anything for that?" Nope. "Why?" Because, Nurse Susie, I take too many things already. Too many. And I am tired. And what is a side effect here and there?

"Why did you switch off of arimidex?" Severe joint pain. "Did you take anything for the joint pain? Ibuprofen?" "NO?"

I interpreted the "NO?" to really mean "are you nuts?"

Honestly, I hadn't even thought to take something for the joint pain.

"Do you just power through the stiffness and pain?" Pretty much.

"You need to ask Dr. Wang about taking ibuprofen. You need relief." Well, yes, I do. And I will.

Dr. Wang comes.

She remembers me. Good news.

She is very thorough in her examination. She asks me to show her the range of motion I have in my arms.

I don't have range of motion in my right arm. In fact, I cannot lift it up over my head. Which explains why it is so difficult to undress. So now I am to be referred to physical therapy.

Dr. Wang measures both arms -- around the upper arm, around the lower arm. The length from my elbow to my mid arm. And then she compares the measurements from each arm. If they are not symmetrical, it could be an early sign of lymphedma. That would not be good. The measurements are symmetrical.

Dr. Wang says I should be able to take ibuprofen, but should first ok it through the medical trial gurus. Medical trials complicate everything. So, when I see Jerry on Friday, I will check on the ibuprofen question.

Until then, I will continue to power through.

And I am not nuts.

Sally Lane Park: I hope you are cleared for the ibuprofen. It would be nice to have one less thing to power through. btw, Saturday was a kick! love ya ♥
February 10, 2010 at 8:33pm

Maureen Gatens Thompson: Good news on the lymphedma. I had it pretty bad because they took ALL my lymph nodes on that side and there wasn't anything left to help drain the fluid. I still have bouts of it. Do you do the wall crawl for your arm? So,

Jerry is the next person to check off your “to do” list...Power On!
February 11, 2010 at 10:41pm

Drenda Lane Howatt received another "all clear" -- this time from her radiation oncologist. Oh, the sweetness of simple words.
February 10, 2010 at 5:58pm

> Maureen Gatens Thompson: You go, Girl! ♥
> February 10, 2010 at 6:30pm
>
> Kimberly Tibbetts Roberts: That's great! God is good!
> February 10, 2010 at 7:01pm
>
> Irmgard Lam: Praise God!
> February 10, 2010 at 11:06pm
>
> Linda Lane Waggoner: Hurray!!!!
> February 11, 2010 at 8:13am
>
> Pamela Zarek: That is good news. Thank the LORD, the ONLY ONE who can heal us! I rejoice with you Drenda...HE still does miracles today...
> February 11, 2010 at 9:12am
>
> Kelly Bard: Sooo happy for you! :-) I personally love those "all clear" moments! Did you happen to be in Costco in Clackamas yesterday?
> February 11, 2010 at 11:56am
>
> Drenda Lane Howatt: Thanks, everyone, for all your well wishes!
>
> Kelly, no, I was not at Costco yesterday...
> February 11, 2010 at 11:58am
>
> Kelly Bard: I saw someone that could have been you--looked like your photo on your FB. One day, I'll have to meet you in person. :-)
> February 11 at 12:00pm ·

Drenda Lane Howatt: Kelly, thanks to chemo I do not look much like my fb photo, no more red hair!
I have been unwilling to change the photo because this 'chemo' look will, hopefully, be short-lived~
February 11, 2010 at 12:02pm

Kelly Bard: Speaking of "hair"--mine came in a LOT more grey and super curly/frizzy. I just posted my bald photos on caringbridge the other day...
My hair, a year ago, was about 1 inch long--as you see from my FB, it has grown quite a bit and I've actually had it cut probably 4 times! It is coming back in straight, but still frizzy at the last 5 inches or so.
February 11, 2010 at 12:10pm

Irmgard Lam: My red hair comes from L'Oreal....:)
February 11, 2010 at 4:25pm

Drenda Lane Howatt has, yet again, another Jerry day today. She will remind him of her upcoming adventures and make sure to get any special instructions. And she will ask him about ibuprofen.
February 12 at 6:36am

Drenda Lane Howatt was told by Jerry that all is still well. And ibuprofen is not a problem. And regarding that growing excitement about fewer doctor visits? Well, not so fast. Jerry day every three months for TWO YEARS. And echos at least twice a year for five years. So now the realities of the clinical trial are starting to kick in...
February 12, 2010 at 4:18pm

Susan Rasmussen Lane: Well, at least if you are using a good drug, being part of clinical trials means that you are part of a success story!
February 12, 2010 at 4:37pm

Mary Elizabeth: Yea - all is still well! It's a good thing you see Jerry every three months. It gives you peace of mind!!!
February 12, 2010 at 6:58pm

Maureen Gatens Thompson: Yes, annoying but remember when you were going in almost weekly? They are now further and further apart! I had to have bone scans with contrast once a year and mamograms every 6 months for 3 years...that's alot of squeezing and smashing. ;-) And we both know the alternative is too dreadful to contemplate. You are Recovery!
February 12, 2010 at 7:10pm

Pam Geddes Girtman: Mary and Maureen, you two are also champs! congrats to all for the overcoming :)
February 15, 2010 at 5:34pm

Drenda Lane Howatt is home from a most wonderful weekend at Neskowin. Now it is time for Miss Ellie's 14th birthday dinner out -- restaurant of her choice. Surprise! She chose Robinhood. Again.
February 15, 2010 at 5:22pm

Thom Wilkinson: Does she choose grilled cheese as her food of choice for her birthday?
February 15, 2010 at 5:27pm

Pam Geddes Girtman: What's robinhood?
February 15, 2010 at 5:29pm

Drenda Lane Howatt: Red Robin
February 15, 2010 at 5:30pm

Drenda Lane Howatt: no Thom...buffalo clucks -- hold the bleu cheese~

February 15, 2010 at 5:33pm

Pam Geddes Girtman: ah, we know that one well :)
enjoy!
February 15, 2010 at 5:33pm

Thom Wilkinson: oooo at least thats better then grilled cheese for oh, say, 6 years straight.
February 15, 2010 at 5:34pm

Sally Lane Park: Yum! Love Red Robin!
February 15, 2010 at 6:06pm

Drenda Lane Howatt: Well…I think the clucks record is much longer than 6 years...
February 15, 2010 at 6:46pm

Heaven's Meanderings

Tuesday, February 16, 2010 at 8:34pm

I have been wondering lately.

Quite a lot.

Wondering if people, Christian or not, think about heaven.

And if they do, really, what they think about it.

Do they accept the culture's definition of what heaven will be like?

Or do they go to God's word to learn what He tells us it will be?

Do they get past the cliches?

"It's a better place." It is. But how?

"We'll be together again one day -- in heaven." Maybe. But not everyone will be there.

"Absent from the body is present with the Lord."

"He/she is done suffering."

Do they think about what it will be like?

Do they think what it will be to be in the actual, physical, presence of the Lord?

Do they wonder what they will look like? Act like?

Do they wonder what they will do?

Do they wonder if they will recognize others?

Or do they accept the 'pat' answers?

"She/he is in heaven now."

"She is an angel now, looking over us." (um, people don't become angels when they die, just fyi)

The most precious note was included in our church's prayer note this week.

From a little girl. Savannah.

Who is thinking about heaven.

"I wish I could talk to God, like hear him talk to me. I think you talk about that. It is a very interesting thing. Do you ever wonder what he sounds like or wonder what he looks like? You should talk about that."

Why, yes Savannah, I do wonder.

And one day, I will hear Him talk to me, and I will know what His voice sounds like. I will see Him as He is, and I will know what He looks like.

One day, there will be a new heaven and a new earth, and I will live there forever. With Him.

Only recently have I started past the cliches. The 'pat' answers.

It took staring in the face of the fear of death to get me to consider heaven more seriously. And I've only just begun.

I wonder.

Quite a lot.

Stephanie Fiskum: I am reading the most incredible book next to the Bible called "Heaven" by Randy Alcorn. Have you read it yet? I can't put it down and find I re-read things in it. I love to share it with the family too. Amazing! Really so much I thought I knew and I guess I really did not.
March 23, 2010 at 11:47am

Drenda Lane Howatt: I am in the middle of that book, too! I will need to re-read it, I am sure.
March 23, 2010 at 12:53pm

Stephanie Fiskum: What can I say? Great minds think a like. Isn't it a great book?!
March 23, 2010 at 6:57pm

Linda Lane Waggoner: Drenda, the priest who celebrated the funeral mass for our friend on Monday said that Peggy asked him what heaven is like. He said he told her that he thinks it is just like her life. I don't really understand that completely but I think he was saying that her life gave bits of heaven to all those lucky enough to know her. Maybe a lesson to me about how I live my life and how I can give bits of heaven to those I know?
March 24, 2010 at 8:38am

Just received the news that Jon, my niece's husband was diagnosed with melenoma in his brain. Jon is 37 years old and a Father to five. My family is still in 'recovery' from my cancer experience. Why do we have more?

Drenda Lane Howatt is convinced that there is entirely too much cancer in this world. Entirely. Too much. And, she thinks that her cancer should have filled the quota for the Lane family. Over-filled.
February 16, 2010 at 9:00pm

> Jessica Hernandez: I agree. Truly feels like evil incarnate.
> February 17, 2010 at 7:37am
>
> Amber Lynn Montgomery Lane: Agreed.
> February 17, 2010 at 4:08pm
>
> Erik Lane: Yes, exactly!!
> February 17, 2010 at 8:53pm

Drenda Lane Howatt is attempting to refuse to allow the 'to-do' list to cause undue stress. Preparation for vacation should not be stressful. 23 hours before she has to be at PDX. Pshaw. That's lots of time!
February 18, 2010 at 9:16pm

> Susan Laufman Stevens: Breathe and don't sweat the small stuff! Sounds like an adventure...hope you have a good time.
> February 18, 2010 at 9:22pm
>
> Maureen Gatens Thompson: Where are you off to?
> February 18, 2010 at 9:25pm
>
> Drenda Lane Howatt: Thanks, Sue~
> Maureen, Don and I are off to Maui. I am so looking forward to doing nothing. I have to be careful of the sun (always, but the meds I am taking make me extra sensitive) -- that just means a beach cabana!
> February 18, 2010 at 11:08pm·
>
> Gail Stempel Hilderbrand: Sooo jealous! I wish I was going, don't forget the sunscreen:)
> February 18, 2010 at 11:09pm
>
> Drenda Lane Howatt: spf 70
> Gail, that would be too fun!
> February 18, 2010 at 11:14pm
>
> Maureen Gatens Thompson: Yep, just hangin' out under a Gilligan's Island hut would be so sweet and maybe a pina colada or two. Enjoy, you both have earned this trip...your Olympic Gold Medals. Savor the moments. ♥
> February 19, 2010 at 12:30am
>
> Luann Sader Hoover: Have a great time!!!

February 19, 2010 at 9:45am

Ginger Clausen: I'm praying God blesses your trip! Enjoy!
February 19, 2010 at 12:32pm

Susan Laufman Stevens: Wow! We are leaving in exactly one month from today! Will you Facebook a picture?! Have a great time, you both deserve this awesome trip.
February 19, 2010 at 5:59pm

Drenda Lane Howatt Aloha~
February 19, 2010 at 6:37am

Sherri Detweiler Purcell: woo-hoo...Enjoy
February 19, 2010 at 6:39am

Andrea Midge McKeehan Robinson: You're in HI????????? sniff sniff. Have a wonderful time. You absolutely deserve it!!!!
February 19, 2010 at 8:23am

Elissa Gertler: I want to see some sunset photos! Enjoy!!
February 19, 2010 at 8:34am

Drenda Lane Howatt: Midge,
we're at pdx
flight leaves at 10
Elissa- I will do my best on the photos!
February 19, 2010 at 8:57am

Hollace Howatt Chandler: Have a great time.
February 19, 2010 at 9:25am

Pam Geddes Girtman: I thought you were going in March! I'm not prepared :) (I know, you thought I'd make a scene at PDX . . .)

have a wonderful time and soak up the sun, sand and surf for me!!! wish we could celebrate more birthdays there
February 19, 2010 at 11:42am

Emily Klepper: Enjoy your time together in the lovely sunshine!!!
February 19, 2010 at 2:02pm

Kim Burns: just said a prayer for your safety and for some great R&R.
I can picture it now...lounge chair, good book, sunshine... awwwww trying not to be jealous. :)
February 19, 2010 at 2:34pm

Barbara Tyler Kochendorfer: Slightly jealous:) Have a fabulous time:)
February 19, 2010 at 6:05pm

Lindsay Chandler Mandjek: have a great trip!
February 20, 2010 at 9:27am

Drenda Lane Howatt: Thanks, everyone! We are relaxing...Today's schedule includes...wait, there is NO schedule!
February 20, 2010 at 9:35am

Becky Annus: toes in the sand, beverage in hand, life is good. enjoy!
February 20, 2010 at 4:52pm

Drenda Lane Howatt: indeed!
February 20, 2010 at 4:59pm

Sally Lane Park: Yup
February 20, 2010 at 7:20pm

Drenda Lane Howatt is on the lanai, in her swimsuit, and it is 8:10 a.m. Beach, here she comes. Now, really, this is the way to celebrate the day! Today marks SIX MONTHS CANCER FREE!
February 20, 2010 at 10:11am

Susan Laufman Stevens: I have goosebumps!! Have a wonderful day.
February 20, 2010 at 10:39am

Theodore G. Waggoner: THAT IS AWESOME AUNT DRENDA!!!!!! WOOT WOOT!!!! :)
February 20, 2010 at 11:53am

Maureen Gatens Thompson: Oh, Yeah...have a pina colada for me.
February 20, 2010 at 5:57pm

Pam Geddes Girtman: ahhh - good for you!
February 20, 2010 at 9:39pm

Abigale Mary Lane: Ahhh...warmth!
February 21, 2010 at 8:40am

Amanda Lane: yess!!!!!
February 22, 2010 at 8:58am

Sally Lane Park: 6 months! Congratulations Drenda!
February 21, 2010 at 8:23am ·

Drenda Lane Howatt: Thank you, Sally~
In some ways, it seems like such a long time ago that Jerry said the words...and only yesterday. This past six months have flown by much faster than the 9 months of treatment! And I have to take the clinical trial drug for only 11 more days!
February 21, 2010 at 9:49am

Sally Lane Park: Can you feel Spring? You are

experiencing it!
February 21, 2010 at 9:58am

Drenda Lane Howatt: I can indeed. I am so very thankful for life, and my family and friends.
February 21, 2010 at 10:41am

Linda Lane Waggoner: Drenda, would you tell us again (sorry!) what the name of the trial drug you are taking?
February 21, 2010 at 12:54pm

Drenda Lane Howatt: Tykerb is the "brand" name...it is lapatinib. Goes into the brain. Thus, my "chemo brain" excuse endures...
February 21, 2010 at 3:30pm

Theodore G. Waggoner: At least you have a legitimate excuse! i certainly don't!
February 21, 2010 at 6:35pm

Linda Lane Waggoner: Drenda, the post above was from me not Ted -- I didn't realize he hadn't signed off before I posted the comment. TeeHee.....
February 21, 2010 at 6:43pm

Theodore G. Waggoner: This is Ted speaking now... I was really confused, seeing as I didn't remember writing the above post... I thought I was losing my mind... haha
February 21, 2010 at 7:01pm

Sally Lane Park: lol
February 21, 2010 at 7:30pm

Drenda Lane Howatt: you guys make me laugh. Thanks!
February 21, 2010 at 7:50pm

Drenda Lane Howatt is faced with very difficult decisions....oh,

where to start the day? Beach or pool?
February 22, 2010 at 9:17am

Robin Reilly: such dilemmas...
February 22, 2010 at 9:19am

Andrea Midge McKeehan Robinson: Brat, brat and brat!
February 22, 2010at 9:30am

Nancy Schifferdecker: My question was clean the toilets or mop the floors? Hmmmm. What a rip. I shall taunt you from the Mexican Riveria in a few weeks!
February 22, 2010 at 9:50am

Drenda Lane Howatt: Nancy, the toilets and floors are waiting for me...but that is ok. They can wait. Mexico for spring break? Kids too? Have a great time!

Midge, sorry~ If you were still needing those pearls for your name badge, I'd get them for you.

Robin, yes, hard choice. But we've decided to put off the decision and go to Whalers Village first.
February 22, 2010 at 10:19am

Robin Reilly: Even better! :-)

robin
February 22, 2010 at 10:24am

Irmgard Lam: Walk on the beach...then dip in the pool...ahhhh..I'm living vicariously through you!
February 22, 2010 at 1:48pm

Amanda Lane: hmm... i'd say no matter where you are, a good caffeinated beverage is always a safe bet to start the day ☻ enjoy!
February 22, 2010 at 3:26pm

Drenda Lane Howatt: Amanda, of course! French press coffee every a.m.
absolutely
February 22, 2010 at 4:17pm

Maryellen Mann Householder: The best thing about a vacation is after you come home you can still go back there. Mental snapshots! I am in Kaui at this very moment in my mind. Next trip Maui! You will have to fill me in. Can we have you guys over when you return?
February 23, 2010 at 6:12am

Drenda Lane Howatt: Maryellen, that is so true about the mental snapshots~
We'd love to come over when we get back! I will only be home a few days before I am off to D.C. for work, but after March 10th, life slows down.
February 23, 2010 at 9:36am

Drenda Lane Howatt is happy to be home...but the rain. Oh the rain. And the cold. Yikes.
February 26, 2010 at 12:01am

Irmgard Lam: Yes, but did you see all the trees blooming? Whoohooo, it is spring!
February 26, 2010 at 2:32pm

Pam Geddes Girtman: welcome home - sorry :)
February 26, 2010 at 4:38pm

Drenda Lane Howatt had a most excellent day! The house is cleaned, laundry in progress, the windows were opened, fresh air circulated throughout at least three levels, dogs at the groomers, and grocery shopping done. Spring is trying to spring.

February 27, 2010 at 6:04pm

Maureen Gatens Thompson: OMG, you must have gotten the energy bug in Hawaii. What a productive day!
February 27, 2010 at 6:21pm

Drenda Lane Howatt: Oh, and dinner is in the oven! No energy bug in Maui --energy comes from knowledge that there is little time before I leave again for a week, this time to D.C.
February 27, 2010 at 6:24pm

Drenda Lane Howatt: and I didn't do the cleaning...so I really didn't do much, but am enjoying the fresh house!
February 27, 2010 at 6:24pm

Maureen Gatens Thompson: LOL...are you going to NACO?
February 27, 2010 at 7:48pm

Drenda Lane Howatt: yes
February 27, 2010 at 8:08pm

Irmgard Lam: What is NACO?
February 27, 2010 at 9:11pm

Maureen Gatens Thompson: Lucky you...hope the weather in DC is better. Too bad it's too early for the Cherry Blossoms.
Irmgard: National Association of Counties. :-)
February 27, 2010 at 10:24pm

Drenda Lane Howatt: Just checked the weather report -- snow next week. ugh. But it will be a good trip.
February 27, 2010 at 10:26pm

Maureen Gatens Thompson: DC is ALWAYS a wonderful

trip. If you have a free evening do the bus tour of the monuments. They are even more breathtaking at night plus you won't get cold.
February 27, 2010 at 11:02pm

Drenda Lane Howatt oooh...vacation officially over. Back to work today! Good thing I like my job.
March 1, 2010 at 6:27am

Andrea Midge McKeehan Robinson: I have come to the decision that you should lead a womans study group. (because you have so much free time!)
March 1, 2010 at 7:07am

Linda Lane Waggoner: You are very lucky to have such a great job! Have a great day!
March 1, 2010 at 11:02am

Irmgard Lam: Yes, how wonderful to love your job!
March 1, 2010 at 2:03pm

Drenda Lane Howatt: Yes, it is so nice to have a job that is interesting!
Midge, you come to interesting decisions! And what, exactly, have you decided the study is that I lead? Have you decided the where and when and who as well? These things would be good to know...
March 1, 2010 at 4:52pm

Drenda Lane Howatt is alarmed to find out that regular, moderate consumption of alcohol increases the risk of breast cancer for all women. For women who have had early stage breast cancer, consumption of an average of 3 drinks a week increases the chance of recurrence by 30%. One drink = one 5 ounce glass of wine, or one shot of liquor, or one 12 ounce beer. Ladies, be careful out there!
March 1, 2010 at 5:33pm

Barry Andrews: Wow. Thanks for the info.
March 1, 2010 at 6:21pm

Danielle Becker: Isn't it interesting that Mike's Hard Lemonade merchandises its Pink Hard Lemonade with a Brest Cancer Ribbon on it? "Drink Mikes... we will donate money towards breast cancer research... because we are the ones giving it to you!"
March 1, 2010 at 11:02pm

Kelly Bard: Interesting. I also just read that the consumption of wakame and mekabu seaweed suppresses breast cancer growth by causing cell death. Mainly due to idodine content.
March 2, 2010 at 9:19am

Drenda Lane Howatt is waiting, wondering, and praying. Waiting to hear an update. Wondering what the neurosurgeon had to say. Praying for a good report. Nephew-in-law Jon Krohn is battling recently diagnosed brain cancer. Jon is strong and courageous.
March 1, 2010 at 7:16pm

Jonna Wilkinson: Praying with you
March 1, 2010 at 7:34pm

Amber Lynn Montgomery Lane: Ditto...
March 1, 2010 at 7:37pm

Maryellen Mann Householder: Drenda, wow, feels like an epidemic!! We will be praying. Let us know what kind and grade. Hearts to you and your family.
March 2, 2010 at 6:44am

Drenda Lane Howatt is thankful she was gone from the Pentagon and the Pentagon Metro station just before the shooting yesterday. Whew!
March 5, 2010 at 6:00am

Laurie Lane: Me too!
March 5, 2010 at 7:05am

Linda Lane Waggoner: Scary!
March 5, 2010 at 8:06am

Drenda Lane Howatt had quite the great day. Coffee at Starbucks, tour of the White House, staff-led tour of the Capitol (thank you Congressman Schrader's staff!), including a stop in the House Gallery, and then walking around the exterior of the Capitol. Across the street from the Supreme Court, and the Library of Congress. Ah, Government is invigorating!
March 5, 2010 at 7:22pm

Jonna Wilkinson: Sweet!
March 5, 2010 at 7:49pm

Wendy Ackley Scott: wants to know when it is his turn to go.
March 5, 2010 at 8:09pm

Linda Lane Waggoner: Me too!
March 5, 2010 at 8:15pm

Laurie Lane: I've never been to DC. I think it's my turn!
March 5, 2010 at 8:16pm

Amy Hickman: Sounds great!
March 5, 2010 at 8:30pm

Amber Lynn Montgomery Lane: Will you be going to the Mall on this trip as well?
March 5, 2010 at 8:50pm

Irmgard Lam: Lovely photos! Are the cherry trees in bloom yet?
I got to go to DC back in '84 when I was on a road trip, while getting ready to go on my mission trip to Austria…I really enjoyed seeing all the beautiful monuments…we were there in April, and the cherry trees had finished blooming.
They're all blooming now here in Portland though…fluffy, pink visions of loveliness!
March 5, 2010 at 11:12pm

Scott Lane: How come we didn't get advance notice about this trip. You'd think I was out of the loop or something. Did you like the Pentagon?
March 6, 2010 at 6:10am

Drenda Lane Howatt: Well...family, all you had to do was invite yourself along...
Amber, I am working today, but Becky is on the Smithsonian trek today. We're going on an evening tour of the Mall/monuments tonight. Irmgard, no blossoms on anything here yet!
March 6, 2010 at 9:37am

Erik Lane: Kind of hard to invite yourself along if you never knew it was happening in the first place...
Not that I would have had the time/money to do it right now in any case! :)
March 6, 2010 at 10:02am

Drenda Lane Howatt: only have to read fb status to know what's coming up...first it was Maui, then D.C. You would not have been welcome to tag along to Maui, though~

March 6, 2010 at 10:03am

Amber Lynn Montgomery Lane: I'm SO glad you're there. I absolutely LOVE Washington D.C.
March 6, 2010 at 10:04am

Drenda Lane Howatt: It is amazing!
March 6, 2010 at 10:06am

Drenda Lane Howatt: Scott, the Pentagon tour was disappointing. The tour guides, military men in full dress uniform, were not the best representatives of their branch of the military or of the United States. We did stand in the spot where the plane impacted the building on 9/11, and went to the small memorial chapel right next to the affected area. That was really very sobering.
March 6, 2010 at 10:08am

Erik Lane: Funny - it feels like I check Facebook too often - usually a couple times a day.
As good as DC is, I think I might have preferred Maui... Some day I'll get to go to Hawaii! Looks like you had a blast!
March 6, 2010 at 10:34am

Irmgard Lam: DC is a very cool place...I super enjoyed it, especially The Smithsonian and the Museum of Air & Space! Loved walking the Mall too, and riding the mass transit train (kinda like MAX)...I forget what they called it over there....
We got to visit a bunch of other places too on our Missionary Road trips...a really amazing time...traveling and seeing different places is so interesting and fun...I highly recommend it.....I'm glad you are able to do this, Drenda!
I wish I had had a digital camera when I did it...because I don't have very many good pictures of my travels...
March 6, 2010 at 1:34pm

Drenda Lane Howatt is attending the National Association of Counties Legislative Conference...anyone interested in the Environment, Energy, and Land Use Steering Committee? Because the issues before the Steering Committee will fill today and tomorrow. Full.
March 6, 2010 at 9:50am

> Maureen Gatens Thompson: Yep, Weatherization for low -income folks---probably through the Department of Energy.
> March 6, 2010 at 9:57am
>
> Drenda Lane Howatt: And Monday and Tuesday will bring visits to Oregon's Congresional Delegation (Representative Blumenauer, Senators Wyden and Merkley), the Department of Energy, and Housing and Urban Development.
> March 6, 2010 at 10:37am
>
> Sally Lane Park: Give 'em your two cents!!
> March 6, 2010 at 5:27pm

Drenda Lane Howatt is off to Capitol Hill for meetings with Congressman Blumenauer's staff and then to the Department of Energy.
March 8, 2010 at 8:35am

> Elissa Gertler: how'd that work out for ya?
> March 8, 2010 at 2:28pm
>
> Drenda Lane Howatt: Elissa, it worked out GREAT! The Department of Energy meeting was amazing, and we managed to expedite federal dollars coming to the county. Tomorrow will be even better.
> March 8, 2010 at 6:45pm

Kris Howatt: A member of our board will be there next week as part of a team accepting an energy efficiency award for our district. Whoot!
March 8, 2010 at 9:37pm

Kim Burns: How exciting Drenda. What a great experience. Keep up the good work. When do you return home?
March 9, 2010 at 7:41am

Hate

Saturday, May 1, 2010 at 8:30am

I hate cancer.

Hate it.

Even though I am thankful for the things I've learned and the ways I've grown because of cancer, I hate it.

I hate that it silently creeps in and rips normal routine out of families' lives.

I hate that it tears into the hearts of our children. I hate that it causes life-defining moments for them. I hate that it makes little ones consider the mortality of their parents.

I hate that it has the power to create panic that knows no bounds.

I hate that it is everywhere.

I hate that it still has the power to punch me in the stomach. Hard.

I hate that it causes questions over EVERY little ache or pain. Every one.

I hate that I have the knowledge now of what it feels like to hear unimaginable words.

I (unlike the rest of the world, apparently) hate the pink ribbon.

I know what it means. I know it is good. I often wear one. I still hate it.

It is good that I can be of help to others who are battling cancer. It is good that I can accompany my dear niece and her strong and courageous husband on their appointment with the oncologist. And I am so glad they asked me to come.

But I hate the reason I am there.

Even being at the 'cancer center' with them punches me in the stomach. Inside, my head is screaming *"why are you here? OH! YOU'RE HERE BECAUSE YOU HAVE CANCER!"* And then, my rational side takes over. *"NO! I **HAD** cancer. '**HAD**' is PAST TENSE."*

All this screaming and discourse going on in my brain while I am listening to the oncologist explain next steps to Jon and Dustine. I want to protect them from the terrible words they are hearing. I hate cancer.

In a post I wrote on my birthday last September, I said that I am thankful for the difficulties of cancer because I am thrilled with the blessings. I wrote that I would not change the past.

I wouldn't.

Really.

I ***am*** thrilled with the blessings. I stand amazed at what God has done in me and through me because of the trials of cancer.

But I still hate it.

Sally Lane Park: Your journey has had many blessings, that I

reap every day. I am aware of all the warm moments in my day and also very aware of the inconsequential small stuff. I don't take for granted quite as much as I used to.
Have I thanked you lately? For sharing your experiences? For being strong enough to be vulnerable? Thank you!
May 1, 2010 at 8:55am

Evy Marks Tyler: I'm with you, Drenda. I'm thankful for what I learned through the process as well, but a list of the pros and cons of cancer, I'm thinking the cons would win.
May 1, 2010 at 11:14am

Joanie Shew: I hate it too. Cancer sucks!
May 1, 2010 at 12:11pm

Dusti Waggoner: Hate, yup, that's the word…
May 1, 2010 at 12:48pm

Amber Lynn Montgomery Lane: Hate Hate Hate Hate Hate. One of the only uses I know where hate is not too strong, and totally appropriate. I, too, hate cancer.
May 1, 2010 at 2:28pm

Maryellen Mann Householder: Yep, me too!!!! Are you hating it right now for any specific reason? Praying all is well in Drenda's body.
May 2, 2010 at 7:02am

One Year. One Lifetime.

Sunday, May 9, 2010 at 4:28pm

"...a year ago on mother's day my strong, beautiful, and faithful momma was bald, going through chemo, and just trying to get through each day. Now my mom is healthy, cancer free, and living life to the fullest. I am so proud to be her daughter and so thankful for her! I love you, mom!"

My daughter, Rachel, posted this on her Facebook today. As I read it, my heart was thrilled. I was happy. My daughter is proud of me. My daughter thinks I am strong. She thinks that I am beautiful. She thinks I am faithful. She loves me. She has no idea the import of those words. They make me cry. Even now as I sit typing this note, I am teary-eyed.

And then her words made me think about the last 18 months. It has been quite the journey.

One year ago. I was going through chemo. "Going through" doesn't give the true picture. I think the word "enduring" is better.

One year ago, I was bald. I was bloated. I was oh, so tired. All the time. And getting through the day was a struggle.

But now?

Now I am healthy.

Now I am cancer-free.

Now I am living life to the fullest.

Thank you, dear Rachel, for the reminder.

And I am proud to be your Momma. Oh so very proud.

Maureen Gatens Thompson: Our Rachels are indeed strong and courageous young women. ♥
May 9, 2010 at 5:05pm

Heidi Witte: I'm teary-eyed reading this! You always amazed me, Drenda! Thank you for being a great example. And Happy Mother's Day! ;)
May 9, 2010 at 6:09pm

Erin Frazier Miller: Sweet. And very touching. Nice work Mama Drenda!
May 9, 2010 at 6:14pm

Debie Owen Willis: Tears =-)
May 9, 2010 at 9:43pm

You're Invited...

Wednesday, May 19, 2010 at 7:14pm
I had a wonderful conversation with one of my sisters today. About many things. So good to really talk.

I asked her if she thought that our family was different now after going through cancer with me. I asked her if she thought that we know how to reach out better to others in our midst who are battling cancer.

She said "yes". She said that she thought that because I had "invited people in" to go through cancer with me that reactions were different. She said that because I was so "open and willing to answer questions" that our family knew what I needed.

Her words made me stop in my tracks.

Invited?

No.

Not really.

I hadn't thought of what I shared as an 'invitation'.

It was more the throwing out of a lifeline, asking, begging, for people to grab the rope and pull me in.

I was drowning and needed to be lifted out of the quicksand that was engulfing me.

I shared my pain and terror and the details of the photographs and the overwhelming tide of chemo and surgeries and radiation and the nausea and the hair loss and the draining of any energy and the sadness not because I wanted 'my people' to know what I was enduring. Or because I wanted people to feel sorry for me.

No.

I shared those things because I knew not what else to do.

I shared those things because, when I lay in bed, the choice was often between more tears or more typing.

I shared those things in writing because to speak the words was more than I could bear. And to keep them inside would kill me.

So, there really was no 'invitation'.

But how thankful I am that you RSVP'd.

Andrea Midge McKeehan Robinson: How funny that you didn't see the invite. I felt so honored to attend. So proud to learn, pray and hope along side your family. Maybe it was a suprise party, held by God?
May 19, 2010 at 7:39pm

Sally Lane Park: Check your FB message
May 19, 2010 at 8:18pm

Drenda Lane Howatt: Midge,
Yes, indeed, a surprise party~
And thank you for saying you felt honored and proud. Thank you for attending so faithfully~
May 19, 2010 at 8:30pm

Kim Burns: Wow

May 19, 2010at 9:31pm

Linda Lane Waggoner: Thank you, Drenda! I love you!
May 19, 2010 at 10:08pm

Gail Stempel Hilderbrand: Thank you for throwing out the rope, because in a way we were holding the rope together. Your words saved me a little each day. Thank you Drenda.
May 19, 2010 at 10:33pm

Sally Lane Park May 19, 2010 at 8:57pm
I read your post and sort of sat back and exhaled. I feel remorse; sorry that I didn't rsvp earlier in your cancer.
To be honest, I just didn't know if I could say the right things, felt very awkward. It kills me that you experienced such pain & terror.
Kills me that I didn't reach out sooner.
Your cancer has changed me. Really changed me.
It has changed our family. All good.
And even though I take that good and cherish it, I would never be thankful that you endured so much. I'm only thankful that I have my sister back and that you are part of my life again.
I love you Drenda and I am proud of you!

Sally

Drenda Lane Howatt May 19, 2010 at 9:19pm
Sally~
Thank you. Thank you for telling me these things.

And let me just say that you rsvp'd immediately. Immediately. In fact, I have an email that you sent the night I got the diagnosis. You offered to bring Rachel home. So you rsvp'd within hours. The email was sent at 8:20 p.m. I'd say that was pretty quick. So no remorse, dear sister, because you WERE there. You ARE there.

Breast cancer was certainly a learning experience for all of us. And I really wouldn't change the past 18 months. I wouldn't want to go through it all again, but the blessings and the good that have come from it I would not trade.

Tomorrow marks the one year anniversary of my LAST chemo treatment. Can you believe it? One year already? Time marches on, and quickly.

Thank you thank you thank you for telling me these things. And for your comments on my earlier writings. I would read your comments, and others, and think "do they really think that? Do they really think I am strong and courageous? Are they really thanking me for sharing?" Your encouragements along the way were such a tremendous help.

I love you~
Drenda

Drenda Lane Howatt is so thankful for the last year. Today marks 365 days since her last chemotherapy treatment. And a few of those 365 days held no thought, and therefore no fear, of cancer. Wow! It just keeps getting better and better.
May 21, 2010 at 7:27am

Jonna Wilkinson: I'm so happy for you, Drenda. That's awesome! Go, God!
May 21, 2010 at 8:44am

Evy Marks Tyler: Each day is a gift! The fire you went through has given you insights and appreciations that others can only imagine. Praise the Lord for CANCER FREE!!
May 21, 2010 at 8:49am

Debie Owen Willis: yes, so happy for you.
May 21, 2010 at 9:19am

Hollace Howatt Chandler: Praise the Lord for answered prayers!
May 21, 2010 at 4:05pm

Cindy McElmurry: I am so thankful for His saving grace and mercy. I love you my friend!
May 21, 2010 at 4:49pm

Sally Lane Park: Ya Baby!!
May 21, 2010 at 5:59pm

Lynn Peterson: Has it really been a year? Wow. Congratulations on such a big celebratory day. I might have to bring something more this evening!
May 21, 2010 at 6:09pm

Joanie Shew: How wonderful and what an encouragement to others who are going through it!

Praise God (from whom all blessings flow!)
May 21, 2010 at 7:27pm

Jessica Hernandez: We love you! ...and I am always thankful for my aunties. :)
May 21, 2010 at 9:24pm

Debie Owen Willis: Yaaaaaaaaay!
May 21, 2010 at 11:16pm

Caitlin Lopez: I'm so very proud of you Drenda! Way to kick cancer's butt!
May 22, 2010 at 8:22am

Darlene Frazier: YEA!!! I am so happy for you!
May 23, 2010 at 7:26pm

Drenda Lane Howatt has "Jerry Day" today...has it really been two months since the last time? Deep breaths and focusing on the fun weekend to come shall assist in getting through walking into the cancer clinic...there is no cancer in her body. None. So she shall (try to) not be stressed about seeing Jerry. Well, maybe a little stressed~
May 28, 2010 at 7:52am

Maureen Gatens Thompson: This too, shall pass. And when you are done today, you will breathe another sigh of relief and start thinkiing about your fun weekend and "to do" list. You will be free of that knot in the pit of your stomach for 59 more days. Trust me, the knot does get smaller as time goes on but never goes entirely away and that's ok. Considering what we've been through, it wouldn't be normal if we didn't have those sporadic "what if..." moments. We are in the Here and Now of life and it is grand. You are blessed, we are blessed.
May 28, 2010 at 8:31am

Drenda Lane Howatt: Maureen, you are so good for me! Thank you. And, if all goes well, after today's appointment, I get to push back to seeing Jerry every 90 days~
May 28, 2010 at 8:52am

Kelly Bard: Praying for you, Drenda. I get to see my onc. June 15 and dreading it!
May 28, 2010 at 10:02am

Drenda Lane Howatt: Thanks, Kelly. I don't think it is seeing Jerry that I dread, it is the clinic. It is quite awful. But Jerry? He's a great guy!
May 28, 2010 at 11:52am

Lisa Spears: All good?

May 28, 2010 at 7:42pm

Maryellen Mann Householder: Boy do I know that feeling. I want predictability, security, and I want things my way! Not much of a faith walk I guess! Working on that one.
May 29, 2010 at 6:49am

Drenda Lane Howatt ...well, Jerry, you were on time today! And you had such great news, you're almost forgiven for all the previous wait times. "Blood work looks excellent, nothing suspicious or of concern..." Those are good words, indeed. Next appointment? September 3! And after that? February 2011. Guess we're moving to the six month schedule after September. Now, exhale.
May 28, 2010 at 11:50am

Drenda Lane Howatt: Don and I were back home exactly one hour from leaving to go see Jerry. That is pretty fast for lab work AND a doctor appointment. Good work, NWCS!
May 28, 2010 at 11:53am

Lisa Weeks Bliss: I'm so glad to hear that, that's great news...Enjoy your holiday weekend!! :-)
May 28, 2010 at 11:53am

Drenda Lane Howatt: Thanks, Lisa. We're off to the coast to spend the weekend with Dad and Verta as a surprise. They went with Linda and Ron today, and the rest of us and our spouses are heading down at different times this afternoon/evening. So, a weekend with my brothers and sisters and in-laws and Pops and Verta. It will be fun!
May 28, 2010 at 11:56am

Elizabeth Lundquist Calhoun: GREAT news!
May 28, 2010 at 12:04pm

Maureen Gatens Thompson: ...and as it should be.
May 28, 2010 at 12:18pm

Andrea Midge McKeehan Robinson: Yeah God!
May 28, 2010 at 12:40pm

Debie Owen Willis: Good for you Drenda
May 28, 2010 at 1:26pm

Jonna Wilkinson: Yay God!!!!
May 28, 2010 at 2:14pm

Jennifer Stady: That's fantastic to hear Drenda!
May 28, 2010 at 6:07pm

Lisa Spears: Great report.
May 28, 2010 at 7:48pm

Beth Sanford Ruhl: That's great news Drenda!
May 28, 2010 at 8:12pm

Cindy McElmurry: I am sooo glad! Have a great time at the beach! Call me when you get back.
May 29, 2010 at 7:55am

Drenda Lane Howatt is having great fun at the beach with her 8 siblings, their spouses, Pops, and Verta. Oh! And Don, too. Beautiful afternoon~ All to celebrate Pops' 90th birthday (July) and Verta's birthday. Not too often one gets to have a get-away with all nine kiddos and their spouses.
May 29, 2010 at 5:09pm

Abigale Mary Lane: I hope everyone is enjoying everyone!!! That's a lot of people!
May 29, 2010 at 5:42pm

Maureen Gatens Thompson: Take tons of pictures!
May 29, 2010 at 6:24pm

Drenda Lane Howatt: Abi, we are! Maureen, my nephew Isaac is a professional photographer and he drove down to Lincoln City today to document the day~
May 29, 2010 at 7:21pm

Abigale Mary Lane: Can't wait to see 'em!
May 29, 2010 at 7:55pm

Debbie Williams: Hey Drenda, hope everything is going well down there - we haven't heard a peep from your crew, not a very roudy bunch, eh?
May 30, 2010 at 12:00am

Susan Laufman Stevens: There are 8 of us in my family, never a dull moment! Hope you take lots of pictures for your memories. It's been many years since we have all been able to get together, your right it's not easy. ENJOY!
May 30, 2010 at 9:54am

Drenda Lane Howatt is sure that all of her brothers and sisters (and the in-laws) are missing each other about now...
May 31, 2010 at 7:24pm

Laurie Lane: I've too much paperwork to complete to miss anyone. My bills, Lenore's bills, and Flora's bills....
May 31, 2010 at 7:52pm

Drenda Lane Howatt: ew. I guess it is that time...end/beginning of the month.
May 31, 2010 at 8:09pm

Drenda Lane Howatt is home...after three days, five sisters, three brothers, one Pops, one Verta, five brothers-in-law, three

sisters-in-law, one husband, one movie featuring a number of Pops' grandchildren, three walks on the beach, one nap, two shopping trips, one photo shoot, one hot tub dip, eight meals...
May 31, 2010 at 4:59pm

> Lisa Weeks Bliss: LOL...OK wow you just made me tired I have to go lay down now…LOL :)
> May 31, 2010 at 5:49pm
>
> Karen Lane: Drenda this was the best weekend. It will be hard to top. I enjoyed it. Hope to do it again. Love to all.
> Steve
> June 1, 2010 at 7:48am
>
> Hollace Howatt Chandler: Nice to be all together, I bet.
> June 1, 2010 at 9:15am
>
> Stacee Carpenter-Jossi: Sounds great! But, I think I would have preferred only one shopping trip and two naps!
> June 1, 2010 at 11:34am
>
> Drenda Lane Howatt: Hollace, it was wonderful to be all together. First time that the siblings/spouses and Pops have been together without grandchildren in many many years.
> Stacee, the second shopping trip was necessitated after finding such great deals on the first trip...
> June 1, 2001 at 6:19pm

Drenda Lane Howatt is wondering how she can possibly be so exhausted at 6:20 p.m. As soon as that dinner is done (re-heated), she is going to bed!
June 1, 2010 at 6:21pm

> Drenda Lane Howatt: And, yes, Ellie, Anna, and Rachel, it is because I am old. And because I work hard.

June 1, 2010 at 6:22pm

Lisa Weeks Bliss: You're so funny that sounds like something my Mom would say too!! :)
June 1, 2010 at 7:05pm

Wendy Ackley: Old?
June 1, 2010 at 8:20pm

Drenda Lane Howatt: Yes, but not old....er
June 2, 2010 at 3:34am

Maryellen Mann Householder: I fell asleep at 7:15 on Monday and slept clear through. I think I am now officially old!
June 2, 2010 at 6:39am

Evy Marks Tyler: Drenda, after hearing about your weekend, I'm surprised you didn't spend all day in bed, yesterday. I don't think it has anything to do with being old!!! Because YOU AREN'T!! However, there is residual from the battle you went through last year. Don't beat yourself up, just go to bed when you need to.
June 2, 2010 at 9:18am

Drenda Lane Howatt: Thanks, Evy~
I realized after this weekend that I am still not 100%. Slow progress, but not back to normal. Doesn't seem right that the residual can last so long...
June 2, 2010 at 5:22pm

Drenda Lane Howatt 's baby graduates from 8th grade today. Tomorrow? A high schooler. The next day? College. Wow. Time moves fast. Congratulations, Miss Eleanor Claire Howatt! You are amazing.
June 8, 2010 at 6:19am

Drenda Lane Howatt Seattle! Bringing Miss Rachel home today. Second daughter's sophomore year of college? Check.
June 10, 2010 at 6:31am

Drenda Lane Howatt perfectly normal
July 9, 2010 at 5:05pm via Text Message

Cavalier. Who? Me?

By Drenda Lane Howatt on Friday, July 9, 2010 at 10:56pm

adjective
a cavalier disregard for danger offhand, indifferent, casual, dismissive, insouciant, unconcerned; supercilious, patronizing, condescending, disdainful, scornful, contemptuous; informal couldn't-care-less, devil-may-care.

"It is what it is."

"What if it comes back? Well, it comes back. And I'll deal with it then."

Dismissive.

Unconcerned. (not really. ALWAYS concerned.)

Casual.

Have I mentioned that every ache and pain causes heart aches and pain?

Have I mentioned that the every day type of headache or leg cramp raises my blood pressure? That every one makes me inhale sharply and talk myself calm? Every one? Every damn one?

Jerry's words to me were that if I had bad headaches, or bone pain, he wanted to know about it. Other than that, he basically told me to go and have a good life.

I have had intermittent and recurring leg/ankle pain in my right leg for a few weeks.

But, I told myself, it was intermittent. Cancer pain would be always there, right?

Yesterday I google searched "bone pain from cancer".

Intermittent and recurring.

Today I called.

oohhh, that was a hard call to make. Hard to quell the quiver in my voice. Strong and courageous? Who? Me? You've got to be kidding.

Jerry doesn't have "advice nurses". He has "triage". I am thinking that 'triage' isn't the best word to use. I shall add that to my list of suggestions for NW Cancer Specialists.

I talked to nurse Kathryn. She was one of my favorite chemo nurses. Don's favorite, too. She is a Mac girl.

So I describe to nurse Kathryn about the ankle and leg pain. She said "so, do you have a question about it, or do you just want the doctor to know?"

Um, yes. My question is if the pain is caused by cancer. That is my question. But instead of asking nurse Kathryn my question, I respond "Jerry said he wanted to know if I had bone pain..."

Nurse Kathryn asks for the best phone number to call me back. I ask when the call would be and she said "probably Monday, possibly late this afternoon".

Imagine my surprise when my phone rings within 40 minutes. Dr. Segal wants me to have an xray today. And don't wait too long to go so that he can get the results this afternoon...in case they have to do an "intervention".

Breathe, Drenda. Breathe. It is probably nothing. Quell the panic. I tell myself that I will feel silly about my upset and fear when I get the news that all is well.

I go to Providence for the xray. No record of the order. Finally found. Sent to xray.

Darrell, the xray tech, asks me why I am having an xray. "Injury?"

"No."

That is all I say. I am laying on the table, and thinking "'no' is enough. He doesn't need to know more." I cannot bear to hear myself say the words that are in my head. I cannot bear to say the words "just ruling out cancer"... or "want to make sure breast cancer has not spread". Can't say them.

Darrell goes to develop the xrays. And he comes back. And spends quite a bit of time at his monitor, looking at the xrays.

Then he comes over to me and asks me to pinpoint for him where, exactly, I am having the pain. I do. He says, "ok. You can go. The doctor will interpret the xrays and then call your doctor, and your doctor will call you."

Cavalier?
Strong and Courageous?

My facade may be all three.

But my heart?

My heart is quivering.

My heart is often fear-filled.

My heart is waiting. For the other shoe to drop.

So I am home now.

Waiting for Jerry to call.

And when that phone rings?

That's when I'll need the strength and courage.

Just to answer.

Drenda Lane Howatt: Nurse Kathryn called with the news that all is, indeed, well. "Perfectly normal." Thank God.
July 9, 2010 at 11:07pm

Sally Lane Park: aaaaak! Why didn't you say something last night, girl? I didn't read this until this morning.
So happy that it turned out to be normal aches and pains.
Love you sister ♥
July 10, 2010 at 8:23am

Linda Lane Waggoner: Oh, Drenda - my heart aches for you! I am so glad that the pain was normal and NOT cancer! I love you!!!
July 10, 2010 at 9:49am

Amber Lynn Montgomery Lane: My heart was racing for you while reading this. I can only imagine how you felt! SO happy for the" perfectly normal!" Let's up that to just plain "PERFECT" shall we?
Laurie Lane: YEAH to NORMAL!
July 10, 2010 at 3:40pm

Abigale Lane: Good, good!
July 10, 2010 at at 6:20pm

Drenda Lane Howatt: Who would have thought that pain could be normal? Actually, the word was that my bones were perfecty normal. I'll see Jerry on September 3rd, so I'll ask then about the pain. Perhaps it is yet another lovely side-effect of my meds? Thank you all for your loving encouragement. This would be a lonely and even more difficult journey without you.
July 10, 2010 at 6:49pm

Rachel Howatt: Mom - I want to know about these things as they are happening - please. I had no idea this was going on and that is not okay with me!
July 11, 2010 at 1:21pm

Drenda Lane Howatt: Rachel, dear,
Sorry...but even your Daddy didn't know until a few days before. No need to alarm you~
July 11, 2010 at 3:01pm

Joanie Shew: Relieved to hear it was normal, and I pray you remain cancer free! It is so very scary!!! Blessings and peace to you!
July 12, 2010 at 12:39am

Drenda Lane Howatt All is, indeed, well. And I do feel a bit silly. But the truth of the matter is that this is my life. Struggles with fear seem to be my on-going battle.
July 10, 2010 at 8:13am

Maureen Gatens Thompson: Ok---first and most important, all is well. That is good. No, not good, that is fabulous! Not silly. Survivors are not silly, paranoid or hypochondriacs. We have survived the ultmate battle and have the scars and post -traumatic stress disorder to prove it. It is what it is. We worry, some days more than others. Some days we tell someone, other days we don't...mostly we don't. Instead, we have that "brain conversation" back and forth with our scared side and logical side. It is exhausting and confusing. Then we come out of the fear and fog, take a deep cleansing breath and move on--sometimes chatising ourselves for being so "silly." No, not silly. We know what it is like--"been there, done that and hated the t-shirt." No speculation, we lived the reality of the diagnosis. Now you can put this experience into the closet and shut the door...it's over. Yep, it will happen again...survivors don't lie to each other or sugar coat it. But we will deal with it, in our own way and it isn't silly. ♥
July 10, 2010 at 8:43am

Drenda Lane Howatt: Maureen,
Thank you. You understand. If I told anyone everything, no one would talk to or listen to me anymore. Thank you. Some days I can hardly breathe. cancer has more power over me than I like to admit. I am working on gaining the upper hand, but it is an on-going battle.
July 10, 2010 at 6:45pm

Evy Marks Tyler: Being strong and courageous is a moment by moment process!! Yes, even after 8 years, there are challenges to not giving in to fear. CHECKING

IT OUT!!! Never has my doctor done anything but affirm that checking it out is the way to go!! I think it is significant that The Lord always puts in Scripture, "Be Strong and Courageous" next to "Do not be afraid or dismayed, for the Lord Your God is WITH YOU." Blessings on you, Drenda!
July 10, 2010at 8:18pm

Elizabeth Lundquist Calhoun: I just read your post, and am so glad to hear that all is well. You did the right thing -- two right things, actually! Getting it checked out, and writing about it. Have a great afternoon, and keep us posted.
July 15, 2010 at 3:21pm

Drenda Lane Howatt has a busy day today. Getting things ready to send Miss Ellie to, ahem, HIGH SCHOOL camp at Eagle Fern. Yikes. Seems like it was just last summer that Ellie was going to her first week at Eagle Fern as a kindergartner.
July 24, 2010 at 9:02am

> Mary Brennan Lopez: Careful-that was the year I met and started dating the boy I married:)
> July 24, 2010 at 3:04pm
>
> Caitlin Lopez: oooooo, Ellie's gonna get married!!!!
> July 24, 2010 at 3:18pm
>
> Mary Brennan Lopez: Ha! Its eaglefern bridal camp:)watch out!
> July 24, 2010 at 3:45pm
>
> Drenda Lane Howatt: Mary and Caitlin,
> You're not helping me. Don't make me panic.
>
> Mary, you were only 14 when you met Luke? Yikes!
> July 24, 2010 at 3:51pm
>
> Mary Brennan Lopez: I was 15-and yikes is right! Ha! Don't you worry tho! Good kids go to that camp!
> July 24, 2010 at 7:38pm

Drenda Lane Howatt is happy...wearing her wedding ring again after 18 months.
July 26, 2010 at 5:20pm

> Rachel Howatt: You should clarify that it is because your fingers were swollen.
> July 26, 2010 at 5:30pm

Drenda Lane Howatt: Well, to clarify, it was because of chemo. But a little time at a jeweler, and a little more $$$, and viola! The wedding ring fits once again.
July 26, 2010 at 5:33pm

Maureen Gatens Thompson: Wonderful…I'd like to do the same with mine!
July 26, 2010 at 7:16pm

Linda Lane Waggoner: Good, Drenda!
July 26, 2010 at 7:31pm

Sally Lane Park: That's wonderful ♥
July 27, 2010 at 1:32am

Coming Back

By Drenda Lane Howatt on Thursday, August 12, 2010 at 12:19pm

There are hours, finally, where I live life. I live life -- real life.

Not life lived through the lens of cancer.

And how glorious those hours are!

We were on vacation for a few days this past week. And half way through, I realized that I had not been punched for a few days. No cancer punches to my stomach. Almost able to really relax.

I even forgot the reason for my 'creakiness'. The same medication that inhibits estrogen (and hopefully, cancer) also causes bone pain and joint stiffness. But this week, in my thoughts, I was just 'creaky'... not 'creaky' because I take medication to keep cancer away.

I had thought it would be terribly scary to increase the time between my visits to see my friend Jerry. But, the reality is that that time allows me to be normal. It allows me a break from the journey. A few times, it has even allowed me to think "did cancer really happen? Did I really go through all of that?"

And those questions, those breaks, let me be me.

Just plain old me.

Not Drenda who is strong and courageous. Or Drenda who is

'looking so good'. Not Drenda who is overwhelmed with the terror of cancer.

Just Drenda.

I kinda like her.

And am so very happy she is coming back.

Beth Sanford Ruhl: Awesome.
August 12, 2010 at 9:24am

Linda Lane Waggoner: Drenda, YOU never left - you just pulled from that vast well of strength that we all hope we have but don't know for sure until we are called to face a semmingly insurmountable obstacle. I know that "just plain normal" sounds wonderful to you! Now, let's go play some more "best ball" golf!
August 12, 2010 at 11:24am

Drenda Lane Howatt is CANCER FREE! One year today, and counting...
August 20, 2010 at 2:24pm

Drenda Lane Howatt ...so tomorrow brings yet another heart test. Is it still there? Is it too large? This is a time when being 'big-hearted' would not be so great. Here's hoping the echo-cardiogram shows normal, and that the cancer killing drugs have done no damage to her heart. Congestive heart failure, stay away~
August 24, 2010 at 5:47pm

> Laurie Lane: Yes, STAY AWAY!
> August 24, 2010 at 5:51pm
>
> Linda Lane Waggoner: No congestive heart failure! Not allowed!
> August 24, 2010 at 5:51pm
>
> Sally Lane Park: What time is your appt?
> August 24, 2010 at 5:51pm
>
> Drenda Lane Howatt: 12:45 I think
> August 24, 2010 at 5:52pm
>
> Leah McMahon: Praying.
> August 24, 2010 at 5:56pm
>
> Debbie Mewing: You are in my thoughts and prayers. Keep us updated. We all love and support you!!!
> August 24, 2010 at 6:19pm
>
> Sally Lane Park: You pull a golf cart around on a very hot evening
> August 24, 2010 at 6:21

Sally Lane Park: And...out golf us...best shot all the time; you have a big heart just not one the echo will pick up ♥
August 24, 2010 at 6:26pm

Cindy McElmurry: I will be praying.
August 25, 2010 at 9:46am

Hollace Howatt Chandler: How did it go?
August 25, 2010 at 10:51pm

Drenda Lane Howatt: Hollace,
Everything went fine, but I won't know the results until late next week. Glad to have it over, though. It is not a hard test to have done, but it is stressful~
August 26, 2010 at 6:37am

Glenda Turnbull: I will be thinking about you. It was so nice to see you this summer.
August 31, 2010 at 12:50pm

Drenda Lane Howatt gets to have a visit with Jerry today. She's missed that guy!
Friday, September 3, 2010 at 7:38am

Andrea Midge McKeehan Robinson: Have a wonderful day Ms. Drenda. I really do miss your lovely smile!
September 3, 2010 at 7:42am

Linda Lane Waggoner: Good luck Drenda!
September 3, 2010at 8:43am

Sally Lane Park: Keep us posted on his good news ♥
September 3, 2010at 9:18am

Drenda Lane Howatt: I will, Sally ~ I saw 'my' radiation oncologist yesterday. Everything ok there. How odd to have two of my very own oncologists~
September 3, 2010at 9:28am

Drenda Lane Howatt ...all is well...and NORMAL. Next date with Jerry on December 3rd. Now off to enjoy a long weekend~
September 3, 2010 at 12:18pm

Linda Lane Waggoner: I'm so glad!
September 3, 2010 at 12:20pm

Debbie Mewing: That is great to hear Drenda. Have a fun weekend.
September 3, 2010at 12:23pm

Sally Lane Park Yipee
September 3, 2010 at 1:23pm

Dennis G. Lane great news
September 3, 2010 at 4:41pm

Susan Rasmussen Lane: Hooray!
September 3, 2010 at 10:05pm

Deborah Davis: Wonderful, wonderful!
September 3, 2010 at 10:28pm

Is it Over?

By Drenda Lane Howatt on Monday, September 6, 2010 at 7:54 p.m.

No.

No.

It is not 'over'.

But it is no longer in the driver's seat.

No longer even in the front seat.

I will always have reminders that I have battled cancer.

I have scars.

I have tattoos.

I have memories. Oh, the memories.

Good, bad, and bald.

So I close out this chronicle of my enduring of cancer.

It is not over.

But it is done.

For now.

I have been strong and courageous.

I have been terrified and discouraged.

I have been open with my fears and struggles (perhaps too much/too often?).

I have called out to God, and been answered with great and mighty things which I did not know.

And now, I stop.

I stop because it is time to refocus my life.

I stop because it is time to live my life.

I stop because I want to be normal.

I make no promises. This 'stopping' may be just a momentary break. Or it may be all. I don't know.

But I do know this:

I was not strong and courageous on my own.

I was not going through breast cancer alone.

It was by God's grace that I made it.

And, God used my family, friends, and even complete strangers to surround me, prop me up, and carry me through when I could not take another step.

Not my strength.

Not my courage.

His.

He supplied it.

He promised.

“Have I not commanded you? Be strong and courageous. Do not be terrified. Do not be discouraged. For the Lord your God is with you wherever you go.” Joshua 1:9

2010 Walk for the Cure. I AM a survivor! (September 2010)
Photo by Rachel Howatt

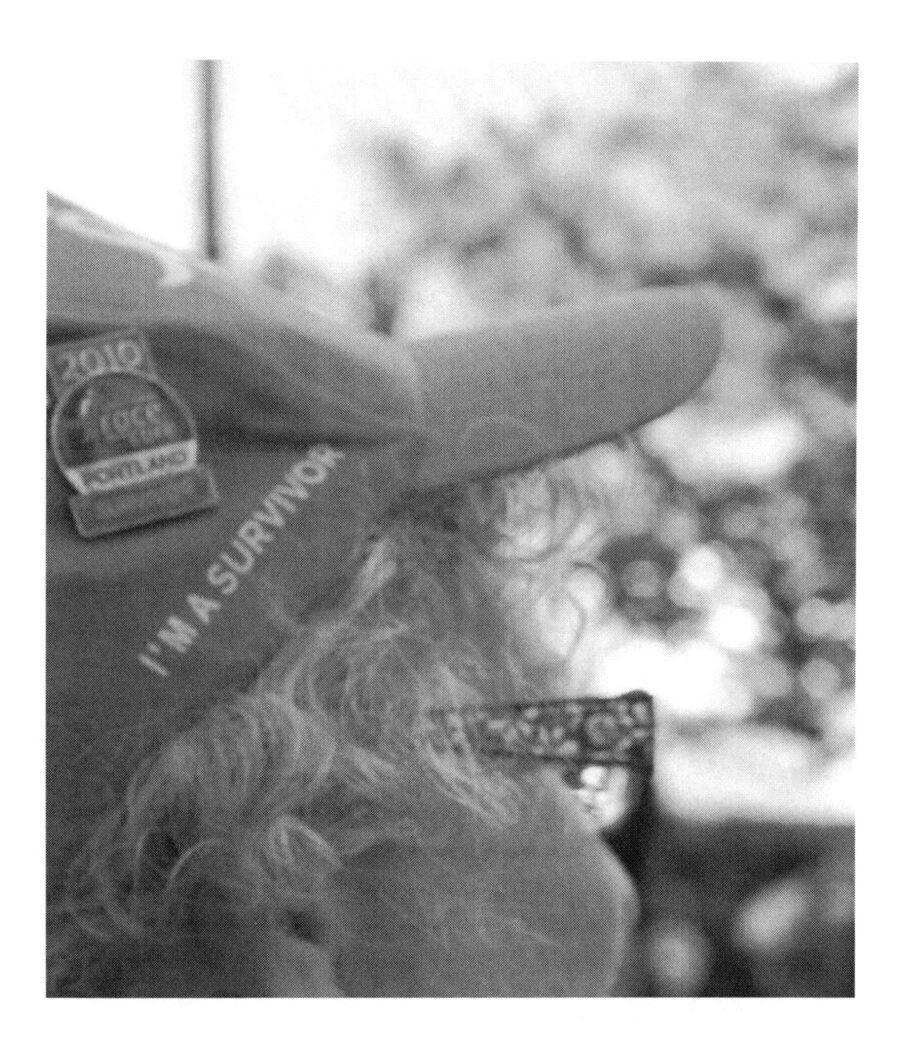

Don and Drenda Howatt with their daughters Rachel, Anna, and Ellie. (September 2010)

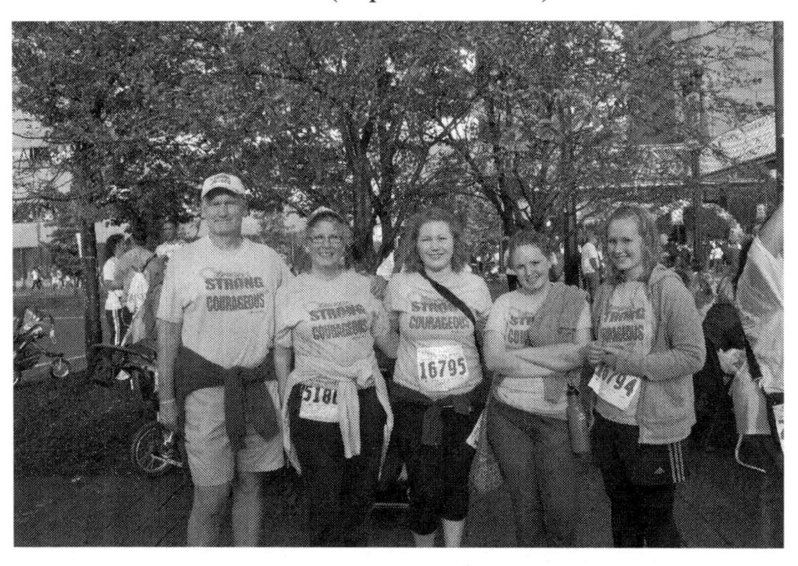

Finishing the Walk for the Cure through the Survivors' Finish Line. (September 2010) Photo by Rachel Howatt

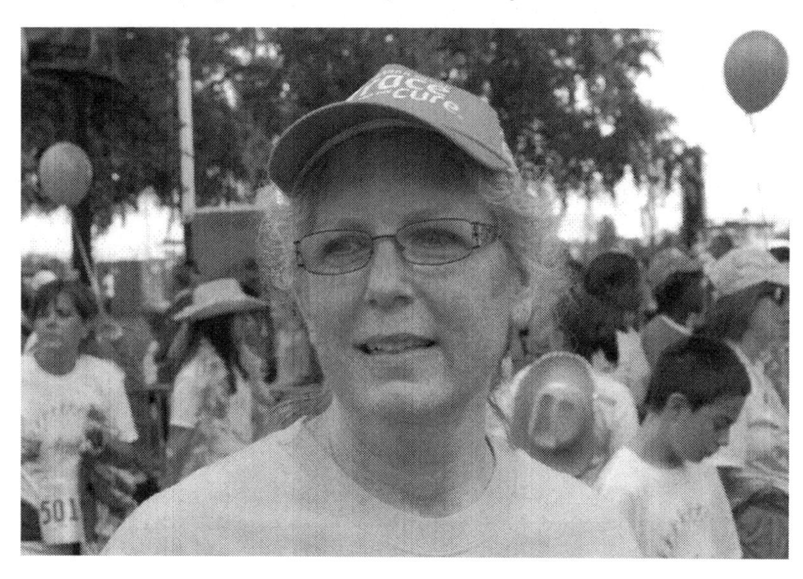

Team Strong and Courageous.
2010 Walk for the Cure
(September 2010)

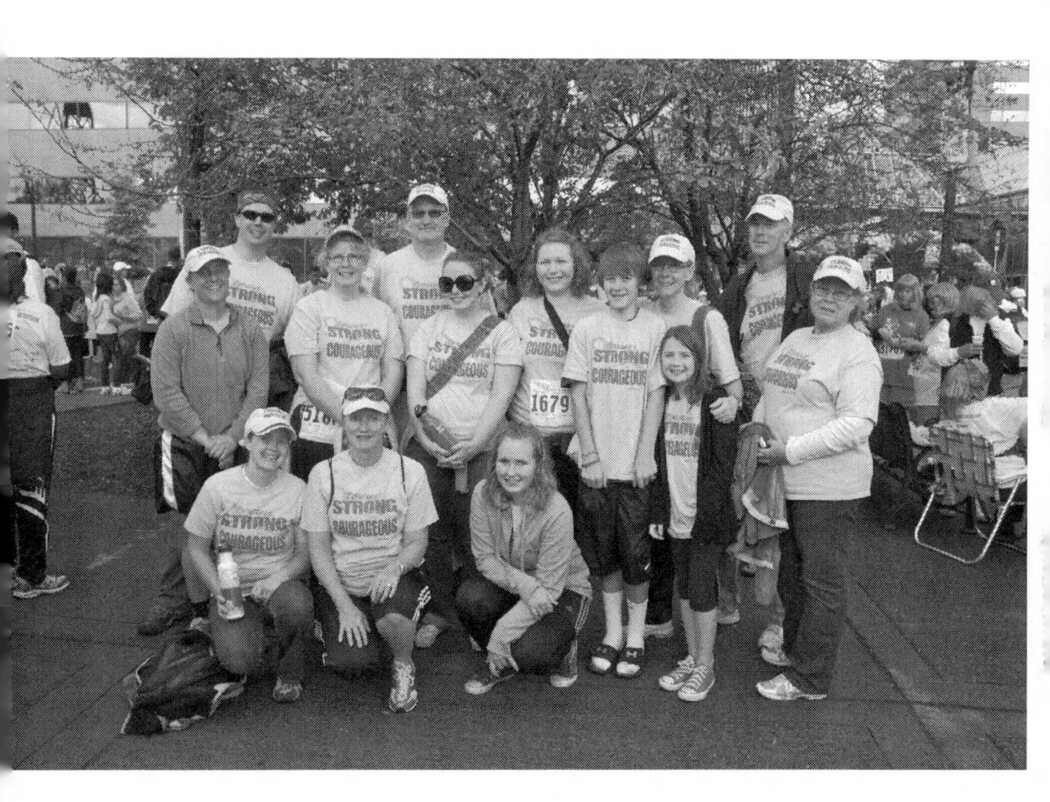

About the Author

Diagnosed with breast cancer in 2008 at age 47, **Drenda Lane Howatt** was declared "cancer-free" in August 2009. She has been married to her husband, Don Howatt, since 1984. Drenda and Don have three daughters, Anna, Rachel, and Ellie. Drenda works as a Policy Coordinator for the Board of Commissioners of Clackamas County, Oregon. Prior to working for Clackamas County, Drenda worked for Congressman Ron Wyden.

Drenda can be contacted by email at
iamstrongandcourageous@gmail.com

Resources

Cancer*Care* National Office
275 Seventh Avenue, Floor 22
New York, NY 10001
Phone
Services: 1-800-813-HOPE (4673)
Administrative: 212-712-8400
Email info@cancercare.org
www.cancercare.org
www.cancercarecopay.org

Cancer*Care* is a national nonprofit organization that provides free, professional support services to anyone affected by a cancer diagnosis: people with cancer, caregivers, children, loved ones, and the bereaved. All of Cancer*Care*'s programs are provided by professional oncology social workers, and are completely free of charge.

Our professional oncology social workers provide counseling to help people with cancer find ways to cope with the emotional and practical challenges of the diagnosis. Counseling is offered in person at our offices in New York, Connecticut, and New Jersey, and over the phone to anyone in the United States, Puerto Rico, and the U.S. Virgin Islands. Our social workers lead numerous support groups that connect people who are faced with a similar situation. Support groups are held over the telephone, face to face, or online, where they can be accessed 24 hours a day, seven days a week.

Our staff also helps people manage financial concerns and provides referrals. Limited aid is available to eligible families for cancer-related costs like transportation, pain medication, and child care. The **Cancer*Care* Co-Payment Assistance Foundation** was established in 2007 to help people who cannot afford their insurance co-payments to cover the cost of medications for treating cancer. The foundation provides up to $10,000 per year in co-payment assistance to qualified individuals who meet the foundation's medical, financial, and insurance criteria.

Education is provided through our Connect® Education Workshops, in which leading experts in oncology provide up-to-date information in free, one-hour workshops over the telephone. Anyone in the world can listen in live to learn about cancer-related issues have their questions answered by workshop presenters. Cancer*Care* additionally offers dozens of free booklets and fact sheets that provide up-to-date, easy-to-read information about the latest treatments, managing side effects, and coping with cancer.

Cancer*Care* provides numerous other services throughout the year including community workshops, therapeutic activities, and special events. Founded in 1944, Cancer*Care* provided individual help to more than 100,000 people last year, in addition to the more than 1 million unique visitors to our websites.

Breast Friends
14050 SW Pacific Hwy #201
Tigard, OR 97224
Phone 503-598-8048
Email mail@breastfriends.com
www.breastfriends.com

Breast Friends is a nonprofit organization dedicated to improving the quality of life for female cancer patients. Our organization teaches friends and family specific ways to offer support, helps them understand what their loved one is going through, and suggests resources for the woman and for those who care about her. A number of programs developed by Breast Friends have proven valuable in assisting and reassuring the patient, her friends and family.

Breast Friends believes that no woman should go through the cancer experience alone; unfortunately, it happens. We find that even women with friends and family nearby often fail to receive the kind of emotional, spiritual or physical support they really need. Our programs are designed to aid in making sure proper support is given *and* received. Every woman in America will be touched by breast or other women's cancers in her lifetime. One in eight women will be diagnosed, and the other seven will know her. Our goal is to reach the seven in order to help the one.

"Until there's a cure...helping women survive the trauma of cancer, one friend at a time."

Made in the USA
Charleston, SC
20 November 2010